Medical Radiology

Diagnostic Imaging

Series Editors

A. L. Baert, Leuven
M. F. Reiser, München
H. Hricak, New York
M. Knauth, Göttingen

For further volumes:
http:/www.springer.com/series/4354

Medical Radiology

Diagnostic Imaging

Andrea Laghi (Ed.)

New Concepts in Diagnosis and Therapy of Pancreatic Adenocarcinoma

Foreword by

Albert L. Baert

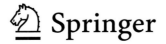 Springer

Editor
Prof. Andrea Laghi
Università di Roma, La Sapienza
Dipto. Scienze Radiologiche
Polo Pontino, I.C.O.T.
Via Franco Faggiana 34
04100 Latina
Italy
andrea.laghi@uniroma.1.it

ISSN: 0942-5373

ISBN: 978-3-540-85380-0   e-ISBN: 978-3-540-85381-7

DOI: 10.1007/978-3-540-85381-7

Springer Heidelberg Dordrecht London New York

Library of Congress Control Number: 2010937237

Cover design: eStudio Calamar, Figueres/Berlin

Printed on acid-free paper

Springer is part of Springer Science+Business Media (www.springer.com)

Foreword

The prognosis of patients with adenocarcinoma of the pancreas remains poor not-withstanding the enormous progress achieved in the imaging of this disease during the past two decades by the introduction of the cross-sectional new imaging modalities including Pet-CT

Because this disease remains an important cause of death, due to oncological cause in men and women, big efforts have been made to clarify its epidemiology and pathology genetics as well as to develop new strategic concepts for therapy. Moreover the large spectrum of available modern imaging methods requires critical scrutiny of their cost-effectiveness.

The editor has adopted a new and original view on the problem of pancreatic adenocarcinoma. On the base of new discoveries in the area of molecular biology the book develops a multidisciplinary approach on the best strategies for diagnosis and therapy of this disease.

Andrea Laghi is an internationally leading academic radiologist, well-known and recognized for his original research and his numerous publications mainly related to abdominal CT and MRI. For this volume he is surrounded by an impressive group of Italian and International experts in the field. The text is concise, well written, and easy to read. The volume is completed by the judiciously selected and numerous up-to-date superb illustrations

I would like to thank Andrea Laghi for his outstanding performance as the editor of this work. I would like to congratulate him as well as all contributing authors for their outstanding contributions offering the latest in our knowledge on the topic.

This book offers an excellent update of our actual insights on the diagnosis and multidisciplinary management of pancreatic carcinoma and can be warmly recommended to certified radiologists and radiologists in training as well as to all other medical and surgical specialists involved in the care of patients with this disease.

Together with the two previous volumes on the pancreas, published earlier in this series, this "trilogy" offers one of the best comprehensive overviews on modern imaging of the pancreas.

I am convinced that this work will encounter the same success as previous volumes published in this series.

Leuven   Albert L. Baert

Preface

Pancreatic adenocarcinoma is the fourth leading cause of cancer-related death in the USA and the fifth in Europe. It is an insidious disease, with the vast majority of patients presenting at an incurable stage at the time of diagnosis. In practice, despite the enormous progress in imaging and therapy, patient prognosis is still very poor; with a 5-year survival rate, which does not exceed 20% even in those suitable for radical surgery.

Patient management is usually complex and typically involves multiple clinical specialists during the course of the disease, namely gastroenterologists, radiologists, pathologists, surgeons, and oncologists. Only a multidisciplinary approach can guarantee the best diagnosis, treatment, and ultimately, care for patients.

For this reason, when Prof. A. Baert asked me to edit this book, I strived to involve leading experts from these different fields in order to provide the readers with a comprehensive and multidisciplinary overview of pancreatic adenocarcinoma. I would like to express my sincere appreciation and gratitude to all the authors, who in their respective discipline made the effort to summarize the immense amount of knowledge in order to provide immediate, concise, and extremely up to date information for the benefit of a larger audience.

The book as we intended it, is recommended for different specialists as well as general practitioners who are eager to keep up to date on new diagnostic techniques as well as treatment options for Patients presenting with pancreatic adenocarcinoma.

The book is divided into three sections. The first is devoted to analyze epidemiology, clinical aspects, and risk factors. In particular, the perspective of potential primary and secondary (in patients at high risk) prevention strategies will be discussed. While pathological aspects, (with the description of the recognized precursors of disease), and genetics, will be presented in a synthetic but exhaustive chapter. The second section focuses on critically exploring the new advances of different imaging techniques: from contrast-enhanced ultrasound to multidetector-row CT, MR Imaging (including the additional value of new sequences), PET-CT and Endoscopic Ultrasound. Cost-effective considerations are also included as a way to propose to readers the most cost-effective and efficient diagnostic pathway to undertake according to the clinical conditions of the Patients. Finally, in the third section, different modern treatments are presented according to Patient status: surgery in those presenting with resectable disease; chemotherapy, chemoradiation therapy, or percutaneous ablative techniques in those with a locally advanced nonmetastatic disease; and systemic chemotherapy for those with metastatic disease. The role of interventional endoscopy in the management of biliary obstruction and pancreatic pain will be discussed as well as the new frontiers represented by drug-eluting stents and brachytherapy.

It is my personal hope that readers will appreciate the efforts made by the authors and find this book useful for their clinical practice.

Rome, Italy   Andrea Laghi
September 2010

Contents

Part III Therapy

Epidemiology, Risk Factors and Clinical Presentation

Gabriele Capurso, Cesare Hassan, Gianfranco Delle Fave, and Emilio Di Giulio

Contents

Abstract

> Pancreatic cancer (PDAC) is a deadly disease. It has an incidence ranging 8–12 per 100,000 per year, with a similar mortality, as more than 95% of patients diagnosed with PDAC will ultimately die.

> Prevention policies are therefore particularly important and they should be distinguished in: (1) Primary prevention, aimed at reducing risk factors for PDAC and possibly favouring protective habits. (2) Secondary prevention, aimed at the early diagnosis through appropriate screening tests in subjects with a particularly high risk.

> The most important risk factors for pancreatic cancer are family history of pancreatic cancer, smoking, obesity, diabetes, alcohol and chronic pancreatitis. Diabetes of recent onset should be considered a possible alarm symptom. In patients with defined genetic syndromes such as "familiar pancreatic cancer", and Peutz–Jeghers syndrome screening for pancreatic cancer as a part of research protocols are performed in selected Centres. There are no sufficient data to suggest that vitamins or aspirin may have a role for PDAC chemoprevention.

G. Capurso (✉), G.D. Fave, and E. Di Giulio
Digestive and Liver Disease Unit, II Medical School,
University "La Sapienza", Rome, Italy
e-mail: gabriele.capurso@gmail.com

C. Hassan
Department of Gastroenterology, "Nuovo Regina Margherita"
Hospital, Rome, Italy

1 Epidemiology and Disease Presentation

Pancreatic ductal adenocarcinoma (PDAC) is not one of the commonest cancer types, with an incidence ranging

A. Laghi (ed.), *New Concepts in Diagnosis and Therapy of Pancreatic Adenocarcinoma*,
Medical Radiology, DOI: 10.1007/174_2010_7, © Springer-Verlag Berlin Heidelberg 2011

8–12 per 100,000 per year, but it is now the fourth lead-ing cause of cancer-related death in the United States, with an estimate of some 35,000 deaths per year, and the fifth in Europe. Up to 80–85% of patients have incurable disease at the time of diagnosis (Jemal et al. 2007; Ferlay et al. 2007). The peak incidence is in the seventh and eighth decades with the average age at diagnosis being 60–65 years of age, with some 10% of cases, indicated as "early onset" occurring in people aged <50 years. The incidence of PDAC is slightly higher in males than females (relative risk 1.35), although this difference is decreasing, and the risk seems higher in black males.

The disease presents in a subtle way, with symp-toms including weight loss, fatigue, abdominal pain, newly diagnosed diabetes mellitus, jaundice and nau-sea, which are non-specific and typically occur late in the course of the disease.

As a result, at the time of diagnosis some 50% of patients have metastatic disease, and only some 20% are considered for potentially radical surgery. The median survival of unresectable pancreatic cancer is 4–6 months, and not surprisingly more than 95% of patients diagnosed with PDAC will ultimately die from the disease (Berrino et al. 2007), and even in these receiving potentially radical surgery the 5-year sur-vival rate is well below 20%. Unfortunately, there have been few progresses in the treatment of the disease either with chemotherapy, and radiotherapy. Prevention policies are therefore particularly important and they should be distinguished in:

1. Primary prevention, aimed at reducing risk factors for PDAC and possibly favouring protective habits.
2. Secondary prevention, aimed at the early diagnosis through appropriate screening tests in subjects with a particularly high risk.

As PDAC is a relatively rare disease, and tests are inva-sive and expensive, screening of the general popula-tion cannot be recommended and a better understanding of the role of genetic and environmental risk factors is particularly important.

2 Risk Factors

Several risk factors have been identified that increase an individual's risk of developing PDAC. They can be distinguished in "genetic (familial)" and "non-genetic (environmental)" factors.

2.1 Genetic Risk Factors

2.1.1 Family History of Pancreatic Cancer

A percentage of PDAC patients ranging from 5 to 10% reports family history of PDAC. A family history of PDAC in a first-degree relative is associated with an increased risk of developing PDAC between 2.5 and 5.3 times. The risk increases if more relatives are affected (see familial pancreatic cancer (FPC)), with a risk of 6.4 in subjects with two affected relatives, increasing to more than 30 if three relatives are affected (Brand et al. 2007). Accordingly, the risk of dying of PDAC is around 4% in relatives of PDAC patients, increasing to 7% if the relative with PDAC was aged under 60 at diagnosis (Del Chiaro et al. 2007).

These data highlight the importance of the genetic component of the disease. However, unfortunately, a specific "familial pancreatic cancer" gene has not been identified, but apart from other genetic syndrome, cri-teria for this condition have been defined in the last few years. These conditions and the related risk of developing PDAC are summarized in Table 1.

2.1.2 Familial Pancreatic Cancer

FPC is defined as a clinical syndrome in which a fam-ily has at least two first-degree relatives affected with pancreatic cancer without accumulation of other can-cers or familial diseases (Klein et al. 2004). It accounts for 1–3% of all PDAC cases (Brand et al 2007), and apart from single reports (Pogue-Geile et al. 2006) not confirmed in other families, a definite gene has not been identified, although the transmission is known to be autosomal dominant. These families are character-ized by an early onset of disease and by the high life-time risk of developing PDAC, therefore are now considered for screening as a part of research protocols in highly specialized Centres in the US (Brentnall et al. 1999; Canto et al. 2006) and Europe (Langer et al. 2009).

2.1.3 Other Genetic Syndromes Associated with PDAC

Familial atypical multiple mole melanoma (FAMMM) syndrome, is an autosomal dominant condition charac-terized by multiple atypical naevi, familial clustering

Table 1 Major genetic syndromes associated with the risk of developing pancreatic ductal adenocarcinoma (PDAC)

Syndrome	Gene	Cumulative PDAC risk at age 70 (%)	Other cancers

Familial pancreatic cancer
    Two first degree relatives
    >3 first degree relatives
	?	
		3
		16	

Familial atypical multiple mole melanoma	CDKN2A/p16	17	Melanoma Breast
Peutz–Jeghers syndrome	LKB1/STK11	60	GI tract Breast
Familial adenomatous polyposis	APC	2	Colon Ampulla
Hereditary non-polyposis colorectal cancer	MSH2, MLH1, MSH6...	2–4	GI tract, biliary Ovary, urinary endometrium...
Breast and ovarian cancer syndromes	BRCA2 BRCA1	5 1	Breast, ovary, prostate...
Cystic fibrosis	CFTR	2–3	GI tract
Hereditary pancreatitis	PRSS1	40	–

of cutaneous malignant melanoma and an increased incidence of other malignancies, particularly of PDAC . The mutated gene is the tumour suppressor gene (TSG) p16, and the estimated cumulative risk of developing PDAC in carriers of the p16-Leiden mutation by 75 years of age is above 15% (Vasen et al. 2000; Borg et al. 2000).

Peutz–Jeghers syndrome (PJS) is a rare, autosomal dominant disease with characteristics features of hamartomatous GI polyps and labial mucocutaneous pigmentation which is associated to a high lifetime risk of developing cancers, including PDAC. The risk of PDAC in PJS has been reported to be as high as some 130 times, with a lifetime risk reported to range from 30 to 60% (Giardiello et al. 2000). Most cases are associated with mutation of the TSG LKB1/STK11. Screening for PDAC in patients with PJS is performed in different Centres, with a relatively high incidence of significant findings.

Familial adenomatous polyposis (FAP) is an autosomal dominant inherited disease caused by germline mutations of the adenomatous polyposis coli (APC) gene, and characterized by thousands of adenomatous polyps in the GI tract. There are few reported cases of PDAC in FAP.

Hereditary non-polyposis colorectal cancer (HNPCC) is an autosomal dominant condition characterized by the development of colon cancers, which are usually of the proximal colon, at an early age. HNPCC is caused by mutations in one of the DNA mismatch repair genes.

PDAC cases have been described, but are not common in HNPCC patients (Lynch et al. 1985).

Familial ovarian and breast cancer (FOBC) is an important syndrome mainly caused by germline mutations in the BRCA1 or BRCA2 genes. The BRCA2 gene is mutated in sporadic PDAC cases, and, at higher rates, in subjects with important family history (Couch et al. 2007). On the other hand, the risk of PDAC is increased significantly in FOBC families, especially when BRCA2 is mutated (Lal et al. 2000; van Asperen et al. 2005).

Hereditary pancreatitis is a rare disorder characterized by recurrent idiopathic acute pancreatitis episodes which usually start at a paediatric age. The disease is autonomic dominant, and most cases are associated with mutations of the cationic trypsinogen gene, PRSS1. The lifetime risk of developing PDAC is pretty high, with reported percentages around 40% (Lowenfels et al. 1997). Smoking further increases the risk (Lowenfels et al. 2001).

Cystic fibrosis (CF) is one of the most common life-threatening autosomal recessive disorders in the Western World, affecting about 1/2,000–3,000 Caucasian newborns. It is caused by mutations in the cystic fibrosis transmembrane conductance regulator (CFTR) gene. The main consequence for the pancreas is pancreatic insufficiency, but heterozygous mutations in the CFTR gene may result in CP. As a result, a slightly increased risk of PDAC has been reported

(Maisonneuve et al. 2003). Interestingly, the CFTR carrier status has also been linked with early onset of PDAC (McWilliams et al. 2005).

2.2 Non-genetic Risk Factors for Pancreatic Cancer

Most cases of PDAC are caused by non-genetic (environmental) risk factors, as summarized in Table 2. Many of them, such as smoking and overweight, may be controlled by definite health politics, with the potential of saving lifes, and eventually reducing the costs due to PDAC cure.

2.2.1 Smoking

Smoking is by far the major environmental risk factor for PDAC. Its role is biologically plausible, clear, and consistently reported in numerous case–control and cohort studies conducted worldwide, and related meta-analyses (Iodice et al. 2008). Smoking causes a 75% increase in the risk of developing PDAC, and explains at least 25% of all PDAC cases. The risk is dose and time related, with former smokers still at risk for at least 10 years after quitting smoking. It has been calculated that if all smokers would quit, the number of new cases of pancreatic cancer in the EU could be reduced by at least 15% (Mulder et al. 2002).

Table 2 Non-genetic factors consistently associated with an increased risk of PDAC

Risk factor for PDAC	Estimated OR compared to non-exposed[a]
Smoking	1.75
Overweight/obesity	1.12 per increased 5 kg/m^2
Heavy alcohol drinking	1.2
Type I diabetes	2
Long standing type II diabetes	1.5
New onset type II diabetes	2
Chronic pancreatitis	14
Occupational exposure to nickel	1.9

[a]The reported odds ratio are estimates of data obtained from the literature, taking in account the highest quality evidence when available (i.e. meta-analyses or large cohort studies)

Smoking is also associated with an higher risk of cancer and a younger age of onset, in sporadic cases (McWilliams et al. 2006; Brand et al. 2009) in subjects with family history of pancreatic cancer (Rulyak et al. 2003), and those with hereditary or chronic pancreatitis (Howes et al. 2004; Talamini et al 1999). Smoking has also been reported to act synergistically with diabetes and family history of pancreatic cancer in a wide, well-designed recent case–control study (Hassan et al. 2007a). There is no evidence for passive smoking as a risk factor (Hassan et al. 2007b), while the risk for pipe or cigars smokers seems much lower, yet significant.

2.2.2 Overweight and Obesity

Overweight and obesity are also biologically plausible risk factors for pancreatic cancer (reviewed in Giovannucci and Michaud 2007). A recent meta-analysis of prospective studies reported a risk of some 12% per increase of 5 kg/m^2, and a risk exceeding 30% in obese subjects (Larsson et al. 2007). The risk has previously been reported to be slightly lower, and close to 20% for obese subjects in a meta-analysis of both retrospective and prospective studies (Berrington de Gonzalez et al. 2003). A case–control study conducted in Italy reported no significant relationship (Pezzilli et al. 2005). However, of course the risk may be underestimated in case–control studies due to recall bias, and to weight loss frequently occurring before diagnosis. Some data suggest that this risk is far more relevant in the US than in Europe, possibly due to the higher prevalence of obesity (Renehan et al. 2008). Moreover, it has recently been reported that the risk of PDAC is related with overweight and obesity throughout lifetime, particularly during early adulthood, with an earlier age of PDAC onset in subjects who have been overweight since adolescence (Li et al. 2009a). This is a very relevant issue, as public health politics deemed at reducing overweight and obesity in children and young adults may tackle this deadly disease.

2.2.3 Alcohol

The evidence for a causal association between alcohol intake and PDAC is much weaker than these reported for smoking and overweight. A minority of the published cohort studies, and some case–control study suggest a moderate risk. However, as alcohol is a risk factor for chronic pancreatitis and diabetes, a "confounding" effect is likely. Moreover, heavy drinkers tend to be heavy smokers and to have a "unhealthy" diet, and most case–control studies are not corrected for these interferences. Accordingly, the risk of pancreatic cancer is not different in alcoholic and non-alcoholic chronic pancreatitis. Some recent well-conducted cohort studies, however, reported a moderately increased risk with heavy alcohol use, particularly for liquor (RR 1.62) (Jiao et al. 2009a), or a risk of 1.22, comparing subjects drinking more than 30 g of alcohol compared to non-drinkers, which is only significant among women, possibly suggesting that this topic deserves further attention. (Genkinger et al. 2009).

2.2.4 Other Dietary Factors and Lifestyle

A high consumption of red meat has inconsistently been reported as a risk factor. Cooking method may be a factor determining the different results (Anderson et al. 2002). Similarly fat intake cannot be considered a significant risk factor (Michaud et al. 2003). Most of these studies were performed in the US or Northern Europe, where consumption of fat and red meat is highly prevalent, possibly masking a small risk difference. However, it is more likely that the entire diet style, and its interaction with other habits, such as smoking and drinking may influence the risk of developing PDAC. Interestingly, a very recent study investigated the role of a "healthy lifestyle score", combining smoking, drinking, weight, diet and physical activity, and found that compared with the lowest combined score, the highest score was associated with a 58% reduction in risk of developing PDAC (Jiao et al. 2009b).

2.2.5 Diabetes

Diabetes is a significant risk factor for pancreatic cancer. Type I diabetes is associated with a significantly increased risk, with a RR=2 in a recent meta-analysis of both case–control and cohort studies (Stevens et al. 2007). Type II diabetes is also a significant risk factor, but in the last few years it has become clear that the risk

is different for long standing diabetes (some 50% increase in risk compared to non-diabetic subjects) and patients with recent onset diabetes in whom the risk is as high as 100% of that of healthy individuals, as reported in a meta-analysis of 36 studies (Huxley et al. 2005). More recent data have confirmed this association highlighting the diabetogenic nature of the neoplasm. Indeed, new onset diabetes, recognized by alterations found up to 3 years before PDAC diagnosis has a higher prevalence in PDAC patients than in controls, and is resolved by surgery in some 60% of patients (Pannala et al. 2008). For this reason a sudden onset of diabetes, especially in people aged > 60 requires particular medical attention (Pannala et al. 2009).

Moreover, amongst diabetic patients, a protective role has been recently reported for metformin, while diabetic patients treated with insulin or insulin secretagogues have an higher risk of PDAC (Li et al. 2009b).

2.2.6 Chronic Pancreatitis

Chronic pancreatitis is a risk factor for pancreatic cancer, while data about acute pancreatitis are scanty and inconsistent. The risk for chronic pancreatitis has been variably reported to range from some twofold to a figure as high as 19-fold (McKay et al. 2008). Initial misdiagnosis of chronic pancreatitis in patients with early cancer may be a confounder, but the risk is still elevated when cases of cancer diagnosed in the first years after chronic pancreatitis diagnosis are excluded (Talamini et al. 1999).

2.2.7 Occupational Exposure

As far as regards occupational exposure, a meta-analysis examining data from 92 studies suggests that exposure to chlorinated hydrocarbon solvents (OR 1.3) and nickel compounds (OR 1.9) is associated with an increase risk of PDAC (Ojajärvi et al. 2000).

2.2.8 Peptic Ulcer and *H. pylori*

Data regarding *H. pylori* infection as a risk factors for PDAC are conflicting, with some older studies reporting an excess risk (Stolzenberg-Solomon et al. 2001), not confirmed subsequently (de Martel et al. 2008). The putative mechanism is also still unknown and speculative, as diseases associated either with acid hypersecretion (peptic ulcer) and hyposecretion (pernicious anaemia) have also been associated with PDAC. Interestingly, the risk after peptic ulcer is only elevated many years after surgery and not increased in unoperated (Luo et al. 2007) subjects, suggesting that an unbalance in the oxidative stress due to achlorhydria, may be the factor associated with an increased risk (Capurso et al. 2004).

2.3 Factors Associated with Decreased Risk and Potential Chemoprevention

Unfortunately, there are few protective factors for PDAC, and no chemoprevention policies are advisable. One of the few protective factors is atopy which amongst other allergic conditions, has been associated with the lowest risk (RR 0.7), in a well-conducted meta-analysis. (Gandini et al. 2005). As far as regards diet, a meta-analysis of pooled data from clinical trials employing vitamin supplement vs. placebo, reported no evidence for a benefit of either beta-caroten, vitamins A, C, E or their combinations (Bjelakovic et al. 2004). On the other hand, there is some evidence for a protective role of folates (Larsson et al. 2006).

Some in vitro data, and observational data also suggested a protective role for statins, which although biologically plausible, should be considered unproven, at least at the clinically employed doses, as suggested by a recent meta-analysis (Bonovas et al. 2008).

Finally, as for other cancers, reduction of inflammation through aspirin and NSAIDS has been considered as a possible therapeutic strategy for PDAC (Garcea et al. 2005). This is supported by findings of increased expression of COX-2 in PDAC and in pre-invasive ductal lesions (PanIn) compared with normal pancreatic ducts, and by in vitro data (Maitra et al. 2002). However, while the use of aspirin and NSAIDs is associated with a reduced risk of most gastrointestinal cancers (oesophagus, stomach, colorectal), this is not true for PDAC in a meta-analysis of case–control and cohort studies adjusted for different doses (Capurso et al. 2007), and some studies even reported an increased risk (Schernhammer et al. 2004).

References

Anderson KE, Sinha R, Kulldorff M, Gross M, Lang NP, Barber C, Harnack L, DiMagno E, Bliss R, Kadlubar FF (2002) Meat intake and cooking techniques: associations with pancreatic cancer. Mutat Res 506–507:225–231

Berrington de Gonzalez A, Sweetland S, Spencer E (2003) A meta-analysis of obesity and the risk of pancreatic caner. Br J Cancer 89:519–523

Berrino F, De Angelis R, Sant M et al (2007) Survival for eight major cancers and all cancers combined for European adults diagnosed in 1995–99: results of the EUROCARE-4 study. Lancet Oncol 8:773–783

Bjelakovic G, Nikolova D, Simonetti RG, Gluud C (2004) Antioxidant supplements for prevention of gastrointestinal cancers: a systematic review and meta-analysis. Lancet 364(9441):1219–1228

Bonovas S, Filioussi K, Sitaras NM (2008) Statins are not associated with a reduced risk of pancreatic cancer at the population level, when taken at low doses for managing hypercholesterolemia: evidence from a meta-analysis of 12 studies. Am J Gastroenterol 103(10):2646–2651

Borg A, Sandberg T, Nilsson K et al (2000) High frequency of multiple melanomas and breast and pancreas carcinomas in CDKN2A mutation-positive melanomafamilies. J Natl Cancer Inst 92:1260–1266

Brand RE, Lerch MM, Rubinstein WS, Neoptolemos JP, Whitcomb DC, Hruban RH, Brentnall TA, Lynch HT, Canto MI, Participants of the Fourth International Symposium of Inherited Diseases of the Pancreas (2007) Advances in counselling and surveillance of patients at risk for pancreatic cancer. Gut 56(10):1460–1469

Brand RE, Greer JB, Zolotarevsky E, Brand R, Du H, Simeone D, Zisman A, Gorchow A, Lee SY, Roy HK, Anderson MA (2009) Pancreatic cancer patients who smoke and drink are diagnosed at younger ages. Clin Gastroenterol Hepatol 7:1007–1012

Brentnall TA, Bronner MP, Byrd DR, Haggitt RC, Kimmey MB (1999) Early diagnosis and treatment of pancreatic dysplasia in patients with a family history of pancreatic cancer. Ann Intern Med 131(4):247–255

Canto MI, Goggins M, Hruban RH, Petersen GM, Giardiello FM, Yeo C, Fishman EK, Brune K, Axilbund J, Griffin C, Ali S, Richman J, Jagannath S, Kantsevoy SV, Kalloo AN (2006) Screening for early pancreatic neoplasia in high-risk individuals: a prospective controlled study. Clin Gastroenterol Hepatol 4(6):684–687

Capurso G, Delle Fave G, Lemoine N (2004) Re: etiology of pancreatic cancer, with a hypothesis concerning the role of N-nitroso compounds and excess gastric acidity. J Natl Cancer Inst 96:75

Capurso G, Schünemann HJ, Terrenato I, Moretti A, Koch M, Muti P, Capurso L, Delle Fave G (2007) Meta-analysis: the use of non-steroidal anti-inflammatory drugs and pancreatic cancer risk for different exposure categories. Aliment Pharmacol Ther 26(8):1089–1099

Couch FJ, Johnson MR, Rabe KG et al (2007) The prevalence of BRCA2 mutations in familial pancreatic cancer. Cancer Epidemiol Biomarkers Prev 16:342–346

Del Chiaro M, Zerbi A, Falconi M, Bertacca L, Polese M, Sartori N, Boggi U, Casari G, Longoni BM, Salvia R, Caligo MA, Di Carlo V, Pederzoli P, Presciuttini S, Mosca F (2007) Cancer risk among the relatives of patients with pancreatic ductal adenocarcinoma. Pancreatology 7(5–6):459–469

de Martel C, Llosa AE, Friedmana GD, Vogelman JH, Orentreich N, Stolzenberg-Solomon RZ et al (2008) *Helicobacter pylori* infection and development of pancreatic cancer. Cancer Epidemiol Biomarkers Prev 17:1188–1194

Ferlay J, Autier P, Boniol M, Heanue M, Colombet M, Boyle P (2007) Estimates of the cancer incidence and mortality in Europe in 2006. Ann Oncol 18:581–592

Gandini S, Lowenfels AB, Jaffee EM, Armstrong TD, Maisonneuve P (2005) Allergies and the risk of pancreatic cancer: a meta-analysis with review of epidemiology and biological mechanisms. Cancer Epidemiol Biomarkers Prev 14(8): 1908–1916

Garcea G, Dennison AR, Steward WP et al (2005) Role of inflammation in pancreatic carcinogenesis and the implications for future therapy. Pancreatology 5:514–529

Genkinger JM, Spiegelman D, Anderson KE, Bergkvist L, Bernstein L, van den Brandt PA, English DR, Freudenheim JL, Fuchs CS, Giles GG, Giovannucci E, Hankinson SE, Horn-Ross PL, Leitzmann M, Männistö S, Marshall JR, McCullough ML, Miller AB, Reding DJ, Robien K, Rohan TE, Schatzkin A, Stevens VL, Stolzenberg-Solomon RZ, Verhage BA, Wolk A, Ziegler RG, Smith-Warner SA (2009) Alcohol intake and pancreatic cancer risk: a pooled analysis of fourteen cohort studies. Cancer Epidemiol Biomarkers Prev 18(3):765–776

Giardiello FM, Brensinger JD, Tersmette AC et al (2000) Very high risk of cancer in familial Peutz-Jeghers syndrome. Gastroenterology 119:1447–1453

Giovannucci E, Michaud D (2007) The role of obesity and related metabolic disturbances in cancers of the colon, prostate, and pancreas. Gastroenterology 132:2208–2225

Hassan MM, Bondy ML, Wolff RA, Abruzzese JL, Vauthey JN, Pisters PW et al (2007a) Risk factors for pancreatic cancer: case-control study. Am J Gastroenterol 102:1–12

Hassan MM, Abbruzzese JL, Bondy ML, Wolff RA, Vauthey JN, Pisters PW et al (2007b) Passive smoking and the use of noncigarette tobacco products in association with risk for pancreatic caner: a case-control study. Cancer 109: 2547–2556

Howes N, Lerch MM, Greenhalf W, Stocken DD, Ellis I, Simon P et al (2004) Clinical and genetic characteristics of hereditary pancreatitis in Europe. Clin Gastroenterol Hepatol 2: 252–261

Huxley R, Ansare-Moghaddam A, Berrington de Gonzalez A, Barzi F, Woodward M (2005) Type-II diabetes and pancreatic cancer: a meta-analysis of 36 studies. Brit J Cancer 92:2076–2083

Iodice S, Gandini S, Maisonneuve P, Lowenfels AB (2008) Tobacco and the risk of pancreatic caner: a review and meta-analysis. Langebecks Arch Surg 393:535–545

Klein AP, Brune KA, Petersen GM, Goggins M, Tersmette AC, Offerhaus GJ, Griffin C, Cameron JL, Yeo CJ, Kern S, Hruban RH (2004) Prospective risk of pancreatic cancer in familial pancreatic cancer kindreds. Cancer Res. 64(7):2634–2638

Lal G, Liu G, Schmocker B et al (2000) Inherited predisposition to pancreatic adenocarcinoma: role of family history and germ-line p16, BRCA1 and BRCA2 mutations. Cancer Res 60:409–416

Langer P, Kann PH, Fendrich V, Habbe N, Schneider M, Sina M, Slater EP, Heverhagen JT, Gress TM, Rothmund M, Bartsch DK (2009) 5 Years of prospective screening of high risk individuals from familial pancreatic cancer – families. Gut 58:1410–1418

Larsson SC, Giovannucci E, Wolk A (2006) Folate intake, MTHFR polymorphisms, and risk of esophageal, gastric, and pancreatic cancer: a meta-analysis. Gastroenterology 131(4): 271–1283

Larsson SC, Orsini N, Wolk A (2007) Body mass index and pancreatic cancer risk: a meta-analysis of prospective studies. Int J Cancer 120:1993–1998

Li D, Morris JS, Liu J, Hassan MM, Day RS, Bondy ML, Abbruzzese JL (2009a) Body mass index and risk, age of onset, and survival in patients with pancreatic cancer. JAMA 301(24):2553–2562

Li D, Yeung SC, Hassan MM, Konopleva M, Abbruzzese JL (2009b) Antidiabetic therapies affect risk of pancreatic cancer. Gastroenterology 137:482–488

Jiao L, Silverman DT, Schairer C, Thie'baut A, Hollenbeck AR, Leitzmann MF, Schatzkin A, Stolzenberg-Solomon RZ (2009a) Alcohol use and risk of pancreatic cancer. The NIH-AARP Diet and Health Study. Am J Epidemiol 169: 1043–1051

Lowenfels AB, Maisonneuve P, DiMagno EP et al (1997) Hereditary pancreatitis and the risk of pancreatic cancer. International Hereditary Pancreatitis Study Group. J Natl Cancer Inst 89:442–6

Lowenfels AB, Maisonneuve P, Whitcomb DC et al (2001) Cigarette smoking as a risk factor for pancreatic cancer in patients with hereditary pancreatitis. JAMA 286: 169–70

Lynch HT, Voorhees GJ, Lanspa SJ et al (1985) Pancreatic carcinoma and hereditary nonpolyposis colorectal cancer: a family study. Br J Cancer 52:271–3

Luo J, Nordenvall C, Nyrén O, Adami HO, Permert J, Ye W (2007) The risk of pancreatic cancer in patients with gastric or duodenal ulcer disease. Int J Cancer 120:368–7

Jemal A, Seigel R, Ward E, Murray T, Xu J, Thun MJ (2007) Cancer statistics, 2007. CA Cancer J Clin 57:43–66

Jiao L, Mitrou PN, Reedy J, Graubard BI, Hollenbeck AR, Schatzkin A, Stolzenberg-Solomon R (2009b) A combined healthy lifestyle score and risk of pancreatic cancer in a large cohort study. Arch Intern Med 169:764–70

Maisonneuve P, FitzSimmons SC, Neglia JP et al (2003) Cancer risk in nontransplanted and transplanted cystic fibrosis patients: a 10-year study. J Natl Cancer Inst 95:381–7

Maitra A, Ashfaq R, Gunn CR et al (2002) Cyclooxygenase 2 expression in pancreatic adenocarcinoma and pancreatic intraepithelial neoplasia: an immunohistochemical analysis with automated cellular imaging. Am J Clin Pathol 118: 194–201

McKay CJ, Glen P, McMillan DC (2008) Chronic inflammation and pancreatic cancer. Best Pract Res Clin Gastroenterol 22:65–73

McWilliams R, Highsmith WE, Rabe KG, de Andrade M, Tordsen LA, Holtegaard LM, Petersen GM (2005) Cystic fibrosis transmembrane regulator gene carrier status is a risk factor for young onset pancreatic adenocarcinoma. Gut 54(11):1661–2

McWilliams RR, Bamlet WR, Rabe KG, Olson JE, de Andrade M, Petersen GM (2006) Association of family history of specific cancers with a younger age of onset of pancreatic adenocarcinoma. Clin Gastroenterol Hepatol 4(9):1143–7

Michaud DS, Giovannucci E, Willett WC, Colditz GA, Fuchs CS (2003) Dietary meat, dairy products, fat, and cholesterol and pancreatic cancer risk in a prospective study. Am J Epidemiol 157:1115–25

Mulder I, Hoogenveen RT, van Genugten ML (2002) Smoking cessation would substantially reduce the future incidence of pancreatic cancer in the European Union. Eur J Gastroenterol Hepatol 14:1343–53

Ojajärvi IA, Partanen TJ, Ahlbom A, Boffetta P, Hakulinen T, Jourenkova N et al (2000) Occupational exposures and pancreatic cancer: a meta-analysis. Occup Environ Med 57:316–24

Pannala R, Leirness JB, Bamlet WR, Basu A, Petersen GM, Chari ST (2008) Prevalence and clinical profile of pancreatic cancer-associated diabetes mellitus. Gastroenterology 134:981–87

Pannala R, Basu A, Petersen GM, Chari ST (2009) New-onset diabetes: a potential clue to the early diagnosis of pancreatic cancer. Lancet Oncol 10:88–95

Pezzilli R, Morselli-Labate AM, Migliori M, Manca M, Bastagli L, Gullo L (2005) Obesity and the risk of pancreatic cancer: an italian multicenter study. Pancreas 31:221–224

Pogue-Geile KL, Chen R, Bronner MP, Crnogorac-Jurcevic T, Moyes KW, Dowen S, Otey CA, Crispin DA, George RD, Whitcomb DC, Brentnall TA (2006) Palladin mutation causes familial pancreatic cancer and suggests a new cancer mechanism. PLoS Med 3(12):e516

Renehan AG, Tyson M, Egger M, Heller RF, Zwahlen M (2008) Body-mass index and incidence of cancer: a systematic review and meta-analysis of prospective observational studies. Lancet 371(9612):569–78

Rulyak SJ, Lowenfels AB, Maisonneuve P, Brentnall TA (2003) Risk factors for the development of pancreatic cancer in familial pancreatic cancer kindreds. Gastroenterology 124:1292–99

Schernhammer ES, Kang JH, Chan AT et al (2004) A prospective study of aspirin use and the risk of pancreatic cancer in women. J Natl Cancer Inst 96:22–8

Stevens RJ, Roddam AW, Beral V (2007) Pancreatic cancer in type 1 and young-onset diabetes: systematic review and meta-analysis. Br J Cancer 12(96):507–9

Stolzenberg-Solomon RZ, Blaser MJ, Limburg PJ, Perez-Perez G, Taylor PR, Virtamo J et al (2001) *Helicobacter pylori* seropositivity as a risk factor for pancreatic cancer. J Natl Cancer Inst 93:937–41

Talamini G, Falconi M, Bassi C, Sartori N, Salvia R, Caldiron E et al (1999) Incidence of cancer in the course of chronic pancreatitis. Am J Gastroenterol 92:1253–60

van Asperen CJ, Brohet RM, Meijers-Heijboer EJ et al (2005) Cancer risks in BRCA2 families: estimates for sites other than breast and ovary. J Med Genet 42:711–19

Vasen HFA, Gruis NA, Frants RR et al (2000) Risk of developing pancreatic cancer in families with familial atypical multiple mole melanoma associated with a specific19 deletion of p16 (p16-LEIDEN). Int J Cancer 87:809–11

Pathology and Genetics

Aldo Scarpa, Paola Capelli, and Ivana Cataldo

Contents

Abstract

> PDAC is an aggressive disease and early infiltrates peripancreatic tissues and adjacent organs, and gives distant metastasis and peritoneal involvement, making often surgical resection impossible. About 80% of PDACs are inoperable at the time of diagnosis. However, even if radiologically resectable, some PDAC microscopically involves the resection margins (pancreatic, retroperitoneal, or biliary, the retroperitoneal being the most important because it cannot be evaluated intraoperatorially) resulting in a non-radical excision. Local aggressiveness consists in the invasion of contiguous structures and organs (spleen, stomach, left adrenal gland, colon, and peritoneum), whereas distant metastases can occur in liver, lungs, adrenals, kidneys, bones, brain, and skin.

> Most PDACs arise in the head of the pancreas often involving and occluding the intrapancreatic biliary duct and the main pancreatic duct, typically resulting in their upstream dilation associated with jaundice and cholangitis when the former is involved, and cystic formation with a variable degree of scleroatrophy of the surrounding parenchyma when the latter is involved. PDAC can spread through the papilla of Vater and duodenal wall with or without ulceration, raising the problem of differential diagnosis with primary duodenal and ampulla of Vater carcinomas infiltrating the pancreatic parenchyma. Less frequently, PDACs occur in the tail, where they are usually larger at diagnosis, determining weaker symptoms mainly due to loco-regional invasiveness.

A. Scarpa (✉), P. Capelli, and I. Cataldo
Department of Pathology, University of Verona, Verona, Italy
e-mail: aldo.scarpa@univr.it

A. Laghi (ed.), *New Concepts in Diagnosis and Therapy of Pancreatic Adenocarcinoma*,
Medical Radiology, DOI: 10.1007/174_2010_4, © Springer-Verlag Berlin Heidelberg 2011

PDAC is an aggressive disease and early infiltrates peripancreatic tissues and adjacent organs, and gives distant metastasis and peritoneal involvement, making often surgical resection impossible. About 80% of PDACs are inoperable at the time of diagnosis. However, even if radiologically resectable, some PDAC microscopically involves the resection margins (pancreatic, retroperitoneal, or biliary, the retroperitoneal being the most important because it cannot be evaluated intraoperatorially) resulting in a nonradical excision. Local aggressiveness consists in the invasion of contiguous structures and organs (spleen, stomach, left adrenal gland, colon, and peritoneum), whereas distant metastases can occur in liver, lungs, adrenals, kidneys, bones, brain, and skin (Hamilton and Aaltonen 2000).

Most PDACs arise in the head of the pancreas often involving and occluding the intrapancreatic biliary duct and the main pancreatic duct, typically resulting in their upstream dilation associated with jaundice and cholangitis when the former is involved, and cystic formation with a variable degree of scleroatrophy of the surrounding parenchyma when the latter is involved. PDAC can spread through the papilla of Vater and duodenal wall with or without ulceration, raising the problem of differential diagnosis with primary duodenal and ampulla of Vater carcinomas infiltrating the pancreatic parenchyma. Less frequently, PDACs occur in the tail, where they are usually larger at diagnosis, determining weaker symptoms mainly due to loco-regional invasiveness (Cubilla and Fitzgerald 1984; Kloppel 1994).

1 Pathology

Macroscopically, PDACs can show a prevailing solid or, less frequently, cystic appearance. They usually present as a white firm solid mass with infiltrative vanishing borders often extending into peripancreatic structures (duodenum, ampulla of Vater, main biliary duct, retroperitoneum) (Fig. 1). Necrotic areas and, rarely, extracellular mucinous deposition can result in the formation of cystic or pseudo-cystic cavities. Peripancreatic lymph nodes can be very small and grossly undetectable, and only the extensive sampling of peripancreatic fat permits the microscopic evaluation of lymph node status and accurate staging.

Microscopically, PDACs are constituted by atypical epithelial cells arranged in glands, or singularly infiltrating, scattered in an abundant sclerotic-desmoplastic stroma (Fig. 2). Periendoneural infiltration is almost constantly present and vascular and lymphatic emboli can be detected even in major vessels (Fig. 3). The hypovascularized stromal component determines the characteristic radiological appearance of PDAC. Fibrous areas are also a feature of pancreatitis and render sometimes impossible a differential clinical radiological diagnosis between benign inflammatory disease and cancer (Zamboni et al. 2009).

Rarely, immunohistochemical markers are needed to discriminate between pancreatic ductal, nonductal, and other nonpancreatic neoplasms. The most important are MUC1, MUC3, MUC5/6, citokeratin CK19, CEA, Ca19.9, EGF, and EGFR (Westgaard et al. 2009), although these markers cannot be considered as unequivocal markers of PDACs.

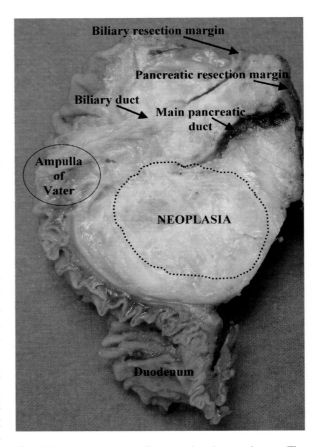

Fig. 1 Gross appearance of pancreatic adenocarcinoma. The neoplasia (*dotted line*) presents vanishing borders, infiltrates the major pancreatic duct (*square*) causing upstream dilation, and gets close to biliary duct (*star*), without macroscopically involving it. The retroperitoneal margin is posterior

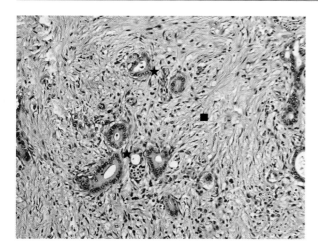

Fig. 2 Neoplastic glands (*asterisk*), intermingled to abundant fibrous stroma (*square*)

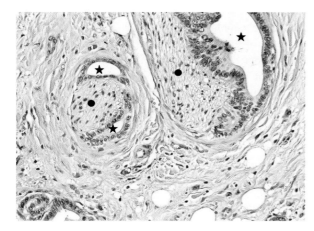

Fig. 3 Nerves (*circle*) infiltrated by adenocarcinomatous glands (*asterisk*)

2 Prognostic Parameters of Resected Adenocarcinomas

For PDACs undergoing surgical resection, the prognosis is defined by the status of the resection margins (R), grading (G), and TNM staging.

The resection margins (R) are three: pancreatic, biliary, and retroperitoneal. Biliary and pancreatic margins are usually evaluated intraoperatorially by

microscopic examination of cryostatic sections to permit enlargement of resection if they are involved. Retroperitoneal margin is constituted by adipose tissue containing the lymph nodes of the superior mesenteric artery. This is the preferential draining station for most pancreatic neoplasms. Unfortunately, the retroperitoneal margin can be evaluated only after formaline fixation, so it is the real "hot point." When involved by the neoplasm (R1), the probability that residual neoplasm causes loco-regional recurrence is high and this influences prognosis and survival.

According to the grade of nuclear atypia and glandular architecture, PDAC can be defined as well, moderately, or poorly differentiated adenocarcinomas (G1, G2, G3).

For TNM evaluation, the pathologist applies a standardized sampling procedure to assess the diameter of the neoplasia and its extension into peripancreatic structures (T). PDAC characteristically tends to form nodal micrometastasis, and it is, therefore, very important to sample and examine extensively the adipose peripancreatic tissue in which lymph nodes are contained. The assessment of lymph node status should include the evaluation of at least 15 lymph nodes and the report of the "lymph node ratio" (LNR) that is the number of involved nodes over the total number of examined nodes. In fact, LNR has been reported as one of the most powerful independent prognostic factors (Pawlik et al. 2007; Riediger et al. 2009).

3 Pancreatic Adenocarcinoma Arises from Precursor Lesions

PDACs develop through a stepwise progression model. The preinvasive microscopic lesion is the pancreatic intraepithelial neoplasia (PanIN). PanINs are classified according to the degree of cyto-architectural abnormalities. PanIN-1 are characterized by flat (1A) to papillary (1B) mucinous epithelium with minimal atypia. PanIN-2 show a more pronounced cyto-architectural atypia, pseudo-stratification, and loss of polarity (low-grade dysplasia), whereas PanIN-3 can be considered an in situ carcinoma according to their marked cellular atypia, complex papillary architecture, pronounced mitotic figures, and rarely necrosis, although they are limited within basal membrane. PanINs are variably represented within PDAC specimens, ranging from 75% for PanIN-1, 65% for PanIN-2, and 50% for PanIN-3 (Hruban et al. 2004; Ottenhof et al. 2009).

Although most frequent, PanIN lesions are not the only precursor of PDAC as it may also arise from other pancreatic lesions: intraductal papillary-mucinous tumors (IPMTs) and mucinous cystic tumors (MCTs). At variance with the more frequent PanIN lesions, these entities are clinically and radiologically relevant because they are macroscopically evident.

IPMTs are lesions constituted by proliferating epithelium arranged in papillae that grow inside the ducts and cause their dilation, leading to the formation of a clinically detectable lesion. They are classified as adenoma, border-line IPMT, or noninvasive carcinoma according to the grade of cellular atypia (Zamboni et al. 1999). IPMTs showing areas of invasive carcinoma are associated with a poorer prognosis (Furukawa et al. 2005; Sohn et al. 2004).

MCTs are cyst-forming and mucin-secreting epithelial neoplasms. MCT is usually a multilocular well-demarcated cyst, not communicating with pancreatic ducts, with focal peripheral calcifications. Its stromal cells have progesterone and estrogen receptors that are identified by immunohystochemistry, suggesting a hormone influence in the pathogenesis of MCTs (Basturk et al. 2009). As for IPMNs, a sequence adenoma-carcinoma is also recognized in MCTs, and they are classified according to the grade of epithelial atypia into adenomas, border-line tumors, or noninvasive carcinoma (Wilentz et al. 1999).

4 Benign Solid and Cystic Lesions May Mimic Malignancy

A number of benign solid and cystic lesions affecting the head or tail of the pancreas may present with clinical and radiological features fitting with the diagnosis of malignancy, and only histology can reveal the true nature of the lesion (Zamboni et al. 2000).

Autoimmune pancreatitis and *chronic obstructive pancreatitis* may mimic PDAC, because of obstructive symptoms associated with the presence of a solid, firm mass, usually involving the head of pancreas and bile ducts. These benign lesions are distinguished on histological basis from PDAC, remarking the relevance of cyto-histological preoperative diagnosis (Zamboni et al. 2009; Kloppel and Adsay 2009).

Para-duodenal pancreatitis (also referred to as *para-ampullary duodenal wall cyst* or *cystic dystrophy of the duodenal wall*) is an inflammation affecting duodenal wall mimicking an infiltration or determining its cystic dilation. Two main pathologic forms have been described: a "pure type," showing only an intraduodenal pancreatic tissue involvement; and a second type associated with chronic calcifying pancreatitis, often developing a solid mass. The solid variant has to be differentiated from common PDACs. Alternatively, rare cystic variants of PDAC can be misdiagnosed as *para-duodenal pancreatitis* (Zamboni et al. 2000, 2009).

Sometimes the presence of a PDAC of very little dimensions, not evident radiologically, can cause obstruction followed by a marked dilation of upstream pancreatic ducts, leading to a preoperative misleading diagnosis of cystic neoplasm (Klimstra et al. 2009).

Usually developing as well-circumscribed masses, endocrine neoplasms and acinar adenocarcinoma of the head of the pancreas may clinically and radiologically mimic a PDAC (Klimstra et al. 2009).

Fine needle aspiration (FNA) and biopsy are helpful in defining a correct preoperative diagnosis with a reasonable rate of adequacy (Larghi et al. 2009; Bellizzi and Stelow 2009), but in cases where it is doubtful whether the sample is representative of the entire lesion, surgery cannot be avoided and the diagnosis is warranted by the histological examination of the surgical specimen.

5 Genetics

Pancreatic cancer is a sporadic disease, although it may arise in the context of hereditary syndromes.

5.1 Hereditary Syndromes

The hereditary syndromes that have an increased risk of the development of pancreatic cancer are listed in Table 1. Of note, these syndromes are either associated with the defects of development and cellular

Table 1 Familial genetic alteration associated with an increased risk of pancreatic cancer

Individual history	Gene	Relative risk[a]	Other cancer associated
None	None	1	None
Hereditary breast-ovarian cancer (van der Heijden et al. 2003; Couch et al. 2005)	BRCA1 BRCA2	3.5–10 2	Breast, ovary, prostatic cancer
Familial atypical multiple mole melanoma (FAMMM) (Kluijt et al. 2009)	CDKN2A	20-34	Melanoma
Familial pancreatic cancer[b] (van der Heijden et al. 2003; Couch et al. 2005)	Unknown	32	Unknown
Familial pancreatitis (Hruban et al. 2007)	PRSS1	50–80	None
Peutz-Jeghers (Hruban et al. 2007)	STK11/LKB1	132	Gastroesophageal, small bowel, colorectal and breast cancer
Hereditary non polyposis colorectal cancer (HNPCC) (Yamamoto et al. 2001)	MLH1 MSH2 others	Unknown	Colorectal, endometrial, gastric, ovarian, biliary, urinary, renal and SNC cancer
Young-age-onset pancreatic cancer (van der Heijden et al. 2003; Couch et al. 2005)	FANC-C FANC-G	Unknown	unknown

[a]Relative risk is expressed as number of folds of increased risk of developing pancreatic cancer
[b]Familial pancreatic cancer: 3 or more first-degree relatives with pancreatic cancer

differentiation or with the impairment of DNA repair mechanisms. The first group includes FAMMM and Peutz-Jeghers syndromes (Kluijt et al. 2009; Hruban et al. 2007), and the second comprises HNPCC, hereditary breast-ovarian cancer, and young onset pancreatic cancer (Yamamoto et al. 2001; van der Heijden et al. 2003; Couch et al. 2005). The syndrome that bears one of the highest risks of pancreatic cancer is, however, the "Familial Pancreatitis" associated with the mutation of PRSS1, which encodes for the cationic trypsinogen (Hruban et al. 2007). Although a family history of pancreatic cancer is considered one of the most relevant risk factors (Klein et al. 2004), pancreatic cancer is not the most frequent neoplasm in any of these syndromes, and this renders difficult the identification of subjects to screen for pancreatic neoplasia in addition to those that characterize the syndrome (Goggins et al. 1996; Lynch et al. 2007; Kim et al. 2009). The knowledge of specific mutations may also be important for therapeutic choices. For example, pancreatic cancer carrying *BRCA2* mutation is more sensitive to Mitomicin C and radiation (van der Heijden et al. 2005).

5.2 Sporadic Carcinomas

The genetic aberrations associated with PDACs include anomalies in the anatomy and function of DNA. The anatomical lesions consist of chromosomal anomalies (numerical and structural) and epigenetic changes that regulate gene transcription. The third anatomical lesion of DNA is mutation in single genes. The functional genomic alterations are those found at the gene expression level and involve two main types of RNAs: protein-coding mRNAs and regulatory small RNAs known as "noncoding RNAs" (microRNAs and small noncoding RNAs or sncRNAs) (Maitra and Hruban 2008).

5.3 Chromosomal Anomalies

Sporadic PDAC characteristically contains aneuploid DNA due to a large number of complex chromosomal anomalies (Harada et al. 2008). These are responsible for the changes in copy numbers of several genes, some of which play a role in cancer development and progression of malignancy. Chromosomal deletions cause loss of genes; chromosomal gains are associated with an increase in copy number of genes with consequent overexpression of their products.

5.4 Epigenetic Changes

Epigenetic changes do not affect the sequence of the DNA, but its structure and conformation due to chemical modification of its components and consist in DNA methylation and/or acetylation of DNA-associated histonic proteins. Epigenetic modifications determine the activation or silencing of genes crucial for cell proliferation, survival, and differentiation. The most frequent epigenetic change found in PDAC is the methylation of *P16/CDKN2A* tumor suppressor gene causing its silencing at early stages of neoplastic development, but numerous other genes seem to be affected.

5.5 Mutation in Single Genes

The basic set of genetic anomalies characteristic of PDAC is represented by the activation of one oncogene and inactivation of three tumor suppressor genes by mutation of one allele and loss of the second allele. Activating mutation of the *KRAS* oncogene is found in 95% of cases. Inactivation of *P16/CDKN2A* occurs in over 80%, *P53* in about 60%, and *SMAD4* in 50% of cases. A recent report based on next generation sequencing technologies has suggested that any single case of PDAC contains an average of 63 genetic alterations. These mutations affect members of 12 cell signaling pathways and processes that are altered in 67–100% of the tumors. Six pathways are altered in 100% of cases due to mutations in variable members belonging to these pathways/processes: KRAS–MAPK pathway, Apoptosis, G1-S transition, Hedgehog, TGF, Wnt/Notch (Fig. 4).

Hedgehog and Wnt/Notch signaling pathways are developmental signaling cascade of stem cells involved in embryogenesis, maintenance of adult tissue homeostasis, and tissue repair during chronic persistent inflammation. These pathways are also activated in cancer stem cells (Lewis 2006) and result involved in almost all the PDACs (Jones et al. 2008). The cancer stem cell

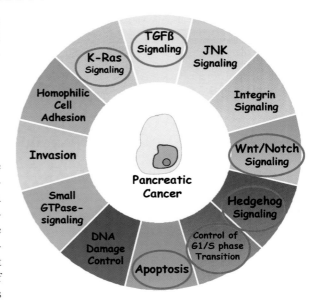

Fig. 4 Twelve signaling pathways and processes altered in pancreatic ductal adenocarcinomas. Each pathway is altered due to mutations affecting any of the genes coding for proteins involved in the signaling processes

hypothesis states the existence of a small number of neoplastic cells that acquire staminal properties and are involved in carcinogenesis and resistance to major chemotherapeutic agents (Ischenko et al. 2008). Hedgehog and notch have been demonstrated to be aberrantly activated in PDAC. They initiate neoplastic cascade by transcriptional activation of a number of downstream pathway. The presence of hedgehog and notch pathways is also described in precursor lesions of PDAC, remarking the hypothesis of their early activation in the carcinogenesis (Katoh and Katoh 2006). These two pathways may play an important role in developing new therapeutical agents for different tumor and particularly for pancreatic cancer (Wang et al. 2006).

A visual description of the different pathways and processes involved in the cell signaling, whose alterations can cause malignant transformation and cancer development, is drawn in Fig. 5 (Hanahan and Weinberg 2000).

5.6 Functional Genomic Alterations

Expression profiling studies have furnished novel databases with long lists of protein-coding genes;

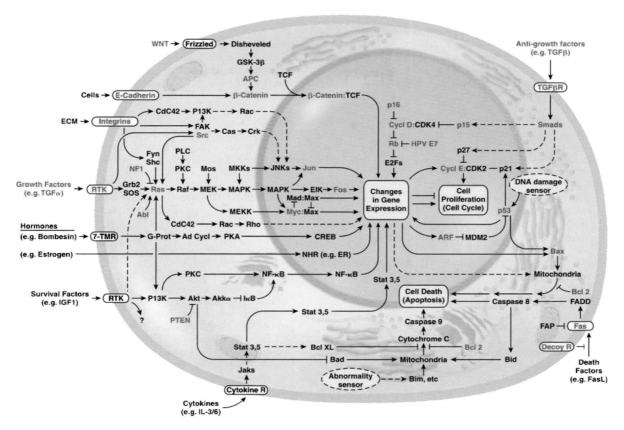

Fig. 5 Different cellular pathways and their cross-talk involved in cell growth, proliferation, differentiation, and induction of apoptosis. Some of the most important genes that are frequently altered in cancers are highlighted in *red* (from Hanahan and Weinberg (2000))

microRNAs are small noncoding RNAs that regulate gene expression, which are differentially expressed in PDAC vs. normal tissues or pancreatitis (www.moldiagpaca.eu). These differentially expressed molecules are now pieces of the fascinating puzzle of PDAC pathogenesis that awaits the discovery of keystones to be constructed.

References

Basturk O, Coban I, Adsay NV (2009) Pancreatic cysts: pathologic classification, differential diagnosis, and clinical implications. Arch Pathol Lab Med 133:423–438

Bellizzi AM, Stelow EB (2009) Pancreatic cytopathology: a practical approach and review. Arch Pathos Lab Med 133: 388–404

Couch FJ, Johnson MR, Rabe K et al (2005) Germ line Fanconi anemia complementation group C mutations and pancreatic cancer. Cancer Res 65:383–386

Cubilla A, Fitzgerald P (1984) Tumours of the exocrine pancreas – Atlas of tumor pathology. Armed Forces Institute of Pathology, Washington, D.C.

Furukawa T, Kloppel G, Volkan Adsay N et al (2005) Classification of types of intraductal papillarymucinous neoplasm of the pancreas: a consensus study. Virchows Arch 447: 794–799

Goggins M, Schutte M, Lu J et al (1996) Germline BRCA2 gene mutations in patients with apparently sporadic pancreatic carcinomas. Cancer Res 56:5360–5364

Hamilton S, Aaltonen L (2000) Pathology and genetics of tumors of the digestive system. IARC Press, Lyon

Hanahan D, Weinberg RA (2000) The hallmarks of cancer. Cell 100:57–70

Harada T, Chelala C, Bhakta V et al (2008) Genome-wide DNA copy number analysis in pancreatic cancer using high-density single nucleotide polymorphism arrays. Oncogene 27:1951–1960

Harsha HC, Kandasamy K, Ranganathan P et al (2009) A compendium of potential biomarkers of pancreatic cancer. PLoS Med 6:e1000046

Hruban RH, Takaori K, Klimstra DS et al (2004) An illustrated consensus on the classification of pancreatic intraepithelial neoplasia and intraductal papillary mucinous neoplasms. Am J Surg Pathol 28:977–987

Hruban RH, Klein AP, Eshleman JR, Axilbund JE, Goggins M (2007) Familial pancreatic cancer: from genes to improved patient care. Expert Rev Gastroenterol Hepatol 1:81–88

Ischenko I, Seeliger H, Schaffer M, Jauch KW, Bruns CJ (2008) Cancer stem cells: how can we target them? Curr Med Chem 15:3171–3184

Jones S, Zhang X, Parsons DW et al (2008) Core signaling pathways in human pancreatic cancers revealed by global genomic analyses. Science 321:1801–1806

Katoh Y, Katoh M (2006) Hedgehog signaling pathway and gastrointestinal stem cell signaling network (review). Int J Mol Med 18:1019–1023

Kim MP, Evans DB, Vu TM, Fleming JB (2009) The recognition and surgical management of heritable lesions of the pancreas. Surg Oncol Clin N Am 18:99–119; ix

Klein AP, Brune KA, Petersen GM et al (2004) Prospective risk of pancreatic cancer in familial pancreatic cancer kindreds. Cancer Res 64:2634–2638

Klimstra DS, Pitman MB, Hruban RH (2009) An algorithmic approach to the diagnosis of pancreatic neoplasms. Arch Pathol Lab Med 133:454–464

Kloppel G (1994) Pancreatic, nonendocrine tumours. In: Pancreatic pathology. Churchill Livingstone, Edinburgh

Kloppel G, Adsay NV (2009) Chronic pancreatitis and the differential diagnosis versus pancreatic cancer. Arch Pathol Lab Med 133:382–387

Kluijt I, Cats A, Fockens P, Nio Y, Gouma DJ, Bruno MJ (2009) Atypical familial presentation of FAMMM syndrome with a high incidence of pancreatic cancer: case finding of asymptomatic individuals by EUS surveillance. J Clin Gastroenterol 43:853–857

Larghi A, Verna EC, Lecca PG, Costamagna G (2009) Screening for pancreatic cancer in high-risk individuals: a call for endoscopic ultrasound. Clin Cancer Res 15:1907–1914

Lewis BC (2006) Development of the pancreas and pancreatic cancer. Endocrinol Metab Clin North Am 35:397–404; xi

Lynch HT, Fusaro RM, Lynch JF (2007) Hereditary cancer syndrome diagnosis: molecular genetic clues and cancer control. Future Oncol 3:169–181

Maitra A, Hruban RH (2008) Pancreatic cancer. Annu Rev Pathol 3:157–188

Ottenhof NA, Milne AN, Morsink FH et al (2009) Pancreatic intraepithelial neoplasia and pancreatic tumorigenesis: of mice and men. Arch Pathol Lab Med 133:375–381

Pawlik TM, Gleisner AL, Cameron JL et al (2007) Prognostic relevance of lymph node ratio following pancreaticoduodenectomy for pancreatic cancer. Surgery 141:610–618

Riediger H, Keck T, Wellner U et al (2009) The lymph node ratio is the strongest prognostic factor after resection of pancreatic cancer. J Gastrointest Surg 13:1337–1344

Sohn TA, Yeo CJ, Cameron JL et al (2004) Intraductal papillary mucinous neoplasms of the pancreas: an updated experience. Ann Surg 239:788–797; discussion 97–99

van der Heijden MS, Yeo CJ, Hruban RH, Kern SE (2003) Fanconi anemia gene mutations in young-onset pancreatic cancer. Cancer Res 63:2585–2588

van der Heijden MS, Brody JR, Dezentje DA et al (2005) In vivo therapeutic responses contingent on Fanconi anemia/BRCA2 status of the tumor. Clin Cancer Res 11:7508–7515

Wang Z, Zhang Y, Banerjee S, Li Y, Sarkar FH (2006) Notch-1 down-regulation by curcumin is associated with the inhibition of cell growth and the induction of apoptosis in pancreatic cancer cells. Cancer 106:2503–2513

Westgaard A, Schjolberg AR, Cvancarova M, Eide TJ, Clausen OP, Gladhaug IP (2009) Differentiation markers in pancreatic head adenocarcinomas: MUC1 and MUC4 expression indicates poor prognosis in pancreatobiliary differentiated tumours. Histopathology 54:337–347

Wilentz RE, Albores-Saavedra J, Zahurak M et al (1999) Pathologic examination accurately predicts prognosis in mucinous cystic neoplasms of the pancreas. Am J Surg Pathol 23:1320–1327

Yamamoto H, Itoh F, Nakamura H et al (2001) Genetic and clinical features of human pancreatic ductal adenocarcinomas with widespread microsatellite instability. Cancer Res 61:3139–3144

Zamboni G, Scarpa A, Bogina G et al (1999) Mucinous cystic tumors of the pancreas: clinicopathological features, prognosis, and relationship to other mucinous cystic tumors. Am J Surg Pathol 23:410–422

Zamboni G, Capelli P, Pesci A, Beghelli S, Luttges J, Kloppel G (2000) Pancreatic head mass: what can be done? Classification: the pathological point of view. JOP 1:77–84

Zamboni G, Capelli P, Scarpa A et al (2009) Nonneoplastic mimickers of pancreatic neoplasms. Arch Pathol Lab Med 133:439–453

Part II

Diagnosis

Ultrasound

Mirko D'Onofrio, Anna Gallotti, Enrico Martone,
Francesco Principe, and Roberto Pozzi Mucelli

Contents

Abstract

> Diagnostic imaging plays a crucial role in the management of pancreatic ductal adenocarcinoma. Conventional ultrasonography is often the first diagnostic step in the evaluation of the pancreas. The introduction of Tissue Harmonic Imaging, that reduces artifacts increasing spatial and contrast resolution, increases its accuracy. Acoustic Radiation Force Impulse imaging is a new technique able to provide numerical measurements of the tissue stiffness, improving the tissue characterization. Doppler study assesses the patency and characteristics of vessel blood flow, mainly useful to distinguish between resectable and non-resectable lesions. Intrinsic limitations tend to be overcoming since the introduction of ultrasound blood pool contrast media, that through a dynamic real-time observation and high contrast and spatial resolution, allow the evaluation of the pancreatic tumor microvasculature. In some cases a fine-needle-aspiration or a core-biopsy could be necessary to achieve a definitive diagnosis. In the last paragraph, the typical US features of pancreatic ductal adenocarcinoma are also summarized.

M. D'Onofrio (✉), A. Gallotti, E. Martone, F. Principe,
and R.M. Pozzi
Department of Radiology, GB Rossi University Hospital
Verona, University of Verona,
Piazzale LA Scuro 10, 37134, Verona, Italy
e-mail: mirko.donofrio@univr.it

1 Introduction

Diagnostic imaging plays a crucial role in the management of pancreatic ductal adenocarcinoma (Sahani et al. 2008). The major aims of imaging are the correct detection and characterization of the lesion.

A. Laghi (ed.), *New Concepts in Diagnosis and Therapy of Pancreatic Adenocarcinoma*,
Medical Radiology, DOI: 10.1007/174_2010_48, © Springer-Verlag Berlin Heidelberg 2011

Conventional ultrasonography is often the initial non-invasive imaging modality chosen for the first evaluation of the pancreas, as it is inexpensive, easy to perform, and widely available (Martinez-Noguera and D'Onofrio 2007).

Herein, we present the technical background, the examination protocols, and the new developments of ultrasound (US), currently applied in the study of pancreatic ductal adenocarcinoma. In the last paragraph, the typical US features of pancreatic ductal adenocarcinoma are summarized.

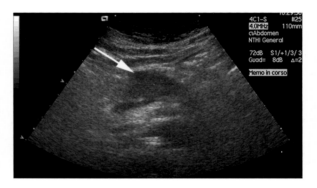

Fig. 1 Conventional ultrasound. Ductal adenocarcinoma of the pancreatic body with the typical aspect presenting as a solid hypoechoic mass (*arrow*) with infiltrative margins

2 Conventional Imaging

Conventional ultrasonography (US) is often the first diagnostic step in the evaluation of the pancreas. The more precise and accurate the initial evaluation is, the more adequate management of the patient will be. In the last decades, the introduction of new technologies that improve image quality resulted in conventional imaging of the gland with very high spatial and contrast resolution (Martinez-Noguera and D'Onofrio 2007).

By using multifrequency transducers and being based not only on the amplitude but also on the phase information of the return echo (Coherent Image Formation, Acuson, Siemens), conventional US gives images with more information and greater details. The two types of compound technology available today (frequency compounding and spatial compounding) also improve contrast resolution and border detection, by reducing speckle in the B-mode image (Martinez-Noguera and D'Onofrio 2007).

Pancreatic US examination is performed after a minimum fast of 6 h, to improve the visualization of the gland, limit bowel gas, and ensure an empty stomach. By transverse, longitudinal, and angled oblique scans, a complete visualization of all the portions of the pancreatic gland is possible. The main pancreatic duct, the common bile duct, the splenic, superior mesenteric, and portal veins, together with the celiac and superior mesenteric arteries must also be identified.

At conventional US, pancreatic ductal adenocarcinoma usually presents as a solid mass, with infiltrative margins, markedly hypoechoic (Fig. 1) to the adjacent pancreatic parenchyma due to the very low US acoustic impedance of the tumor (Martinez-Noguera and D'Onofrio 2007). Furthermore, the difference in impedance between the lesion and the pancreatic adjacent parenchyma is sometimes greater than that at CT between beam attenuation in both pre- and post-contrastographic phases (Martinez-Noguera and D'Onofrio 2007). It often determines dilatation of the upstream main pancreatic duct and, if located in the head, also of the common bile duct (double-duct sign). In highly aggressive lesions, necrosis and colliquation are common.

Although conventional US has proved its value, diagnostic difficulties have been encountered during examination (Oktar et al. 2003; Hohl et al. 2004) mainly due to the losses in lateral resolution and signal-to-noise ratio (SNR) owing to defocusing or phase displacement effects produced by inhomogeneities in biological tissues. To increase the accuracy of this method, a new approach is the tissue harmonic imaging.

3 Tissue Harmonic Imaging (THI)

THI takes advantages of non-linear harmonic frequencies generated by the propagating main US beam (Schoelgens 1998) and emitted by the transducer to correct the defocusing effects. Compared to the fundamental (f_0), harmonic overtones, which are whole numbered multiples of the f_0 frequency, have much lower amplitudes and generate contents developing only from the high amplitude pulses. Thus, this new approach extensively reduces artifacts, caused by low amplitude pulses (Hohl et al. 2007).

Two methods have been mainly implemented for the generation of harmonic images: the harmonic band filtering, realized applying a high-pass filter to the received signal and so utilizing only the higher harmonic frequency components for image creation (Shapiro et al. 1998); the phase inversion, realized applying two sequential pulses where the last is phase reversed, so removing the fundamental component and leaving only the harmonic portions of the echoes (Chapman and Lazenby 1997).

Compared to conventional B-mode US, THI can increase spatial and contrast resolution, providing an enhanced overall image quality (Shapiro et al. 1998; Desser and Jeffrey 2001), better lesion conspicuity (Hohl et al. 2004), and advantages in fluid–solid differentiation (Desser and Jeffrey 2001), so achieving a better detection of ductal adenocarcinoma (Hohl et al. 2007).

4 Acoustic Radiation Force Impulse Imaging (ARFI)

ARFI imaging is a new promising technique to assess the mechanical strain properties of deep tissues (Nightingale et al. 2001; Nightingale et al. 2002a) without a need for an external compression (Fahley et al. 2007). By short-duration acoustic radiation forces (less than 1 ms) (Zhai et al. 2008), it generates shear waves through a region of interest (ROI) (McAleavey et al. 2007; Nightingale et al. 2002b; Nightingale et al. 2003), producing localized displacements. The response is monitored with US and depends on the elastic modulus, which is mainly related to the resistance offered by the tissue to the wave propagation (Shan et al. 2008; Sumi 2008): the more elastic a tissue is, the more displacements it experiences.

Virtual Touch tissue quantification is a quantitative implementation of ARFI technology, which provides numerical measurements (wave velocity values, measured in meters per second) of the tissue stiffness: the stiffer (non-elastic) a tissue is, the greater the shear wave speed will be. Only few data are available regarding the usefulness of this technique (Gallotti et al. In press; D'Onofrio et al. In press a), so its basic features are illuminated here.

Virtual Touch tissue quantification is performed on the Siemens ACUSON S2000 ultrasound system (Siemens, Erlanger, Germany), with the preliminary selection of an anatomical location identified utilizing a target ROI on a conventional US image. An acoustic push pulse is transmitted through the tissue, inducing a shear wave immediately on the right side of the ROI. A

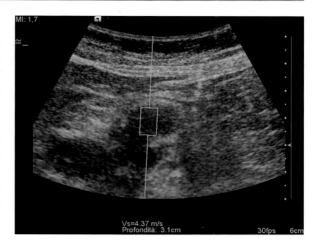

Fig. 2 ARFI imaging. Ductal adenocarcinoma of the pancreatic head with the high wave velocity value at Virtual Touch tissue quantification measured inside the lesion

numeric value, proportional to the tissue stiffness and expressing the shear wave speed (measured in meters per second), is then reported, as a result of multiple measures made for that spatial location.

Virtual Touch tissue quantification provides a numerical measurement of tissue stiffness and is potentially able to allow tissue characterization (Gallotti et al. In press). It might be a feasible alternative to invasive needle-biopsy, allowing a tissue analysis by imaging. The identification of normal wave velocity values for the healthy organs should be the first step (Gallotti et al. In press), followed by the definition of the shear wave speed for the main parenchymal lesions.

Pancreatic ductal adenocarcinoma is a firm mass, stiffer than the adjacent parenchyma, owing to the presence of fibrosis and marked desmoplasia (Seo et al. 2000). According to this, at Virtual Touch tissue quantification, the wave velocity value measured inside the lesion is higher (usually >3 m/s; Fig. 2) than that resulted in the adjacent parenchyma (mean wave velocity value in the healthy pancreas of 1.4 m/s) (Gallotti et al. In press).

5 Doppler Imaging

Further than B-mode evaluation, color and power-Doppler of the lesion and surrounding vessels integrate the conventional US study, assessing the patency and characteristics of vessel blood flow (Bertolotto et al. 2007).

By utilizing abdominal multifrequency probes, the detection of tumor vessels within the lesion often characterizes hypervascular masses (i.e., endocrine tumors), while no tumor vessels are usually detectable within hypovascular ones (Bertolotto et al. 2007; Angeli et al. 1997).

The pancreatic study must be comprehensive of the evaluation of the adjacent vascular structures, mainly to distinguish between resectable and non-resectable lesions. The preserved echogenic fatty interface between tumor and vessels or a short contiguity between them suggests the resectability of the lesion, whereas the infiltration or compression or encasement implies the unresectability (Koito et al. 2001). Localized aliasing and mosaic pattern are waveform changes due to increased flow velocities and turbulent blood flow at the site of a vascular stenosis, since the presence of a pancreatic disease (Koito et al. 2001; Ueno et al. 1997). Downstream the infiltrated tract, the flow velocity decreases, with the typical "parvus et tardus" waveform (Yassa et al. 1997).

At Doppler study, pancreatic ductal adenocarcinoma shows poor or no vascularity (Fig. 3). The vascular invasion is defined by a focal disappearance of the echogenic interface forming the vessel wall, or by a narrow lumen, with changes in blood flow velocity.

The latest-generation equipment significantly improved the diagnostic performance of color-Doppler ultrasonography, increasing sensitivity, spatial, and temporal resolution (Bertolotto et al. 2007). However, intrinsic limitations still remain and tend to be overcoming since the introduction of ultrasound contrast media.

6 Contrast-Enhanced Ultrasound Imaging

The introduction of second-generation microbubble contrast agents, characterized by harmonic responses at low mechanical index (MI <0.2) of the US beam, has improved the diagnostic accuracy of ultrasonography (D'Onofrio et al. 2007a). The application of a blood pool contrast medium (Sulfur hexafluoride contrast agent – SonoVue; Bracco, Milan, Italy), the dynamic real-time observation of the contrast-enhanced phases, and the high contrast and spatial resolution allow the evaluation of the pancreatic tumor microvasculature (D'Onofrio et al. 2007a). A microbubble-specific software filters all the background tissue signals, so that the vascular enhancement is only related to the presence of microbubbles (Cosgrove 2005).

Two technologies have been mainly introduced for enhanced US imaging: the Cadence coherent contrast imaging (Siemens-Acuson, mountain View, CA, USA), based on inversion of the phase of alternate pulses, leaving only non-linear signals; and Cadence contrast pulse sequencing (CPS; Siemens-Acuson), based on precise changes in the amplitude and phase of transmitted pulses, leaving only non-linear imaging (D'Onofrio et al. 2007a).

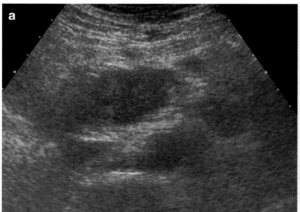 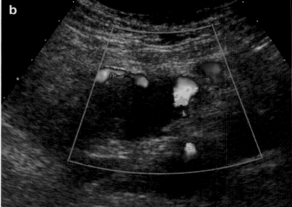

Fig. 3 Doppler ultrasound. Ductal adenocarcinoma of the pancreatic head presenting as a solid hypoechoic mass (**a**) without intratumoral vessels at Doppler (**b**). Tumor infiltration of the superior mesenteric vein is also appreciable (**b**)

One of the most interesting applications of pancreatic CEUS is the tumor characterization and local and liver staging with a single bolus (2.4 mL) injection of contrast medium. A complete dynamic evaluation of the pancreatic mass during the arterial and venous phases, with the correct identification of the contrast-enhancement pattern, is compulsory for an adequate therapy and for the immediate prognostic evaluation. In fact, association between intratumoral microvessel density and tumor aggressiveness has been already proved (D'Onofrio et al. In press b; Klöppel and Schlüter 1999). Moreover, the judgment of the relation between tumor and adjacent vessels is mandatory for the depiction of tumoral margins (Faccioli et al. 2008) and, together with the liver study during the late phase, so to exclude the presence of metastases (D'Onofrio et al. 2006), is crucial to define the resectability or unresectability of the pancreatic lesion.

At CEUS examination, pancreatic ductal adenocarcinoma usually presents as an ill-defined mass, showing poor enhancement (Fig. 4) in all dynamic phases (D'Onofrio et al. 2005). The finding of a poorly vascularized lesion could suggest its undifferentiated grade (Numata et al. 2005) and is related to intratumoral fibrosis and necrosis, and to reduction in the microvascular density and in perfusion (D'Onofrio et al. 2007a; Nagase et al. 2003). Moreover, CEUS can be helpful in confirming vascular infiltration and liver involvement (D'Onofrio et al. 2007a).

7 Ultrasound-Guided Interventional Procedures

The identification of an unresectable pancreatic mass, or of a resectable lesion with uncertain diagnosis at imaging, or of a suspected rare or metastatic malignancy requires a pathological confirmation (Zamboni et al. 2009). Fine-needle-aspiration (FNA) under US-guidance is the procedure of choice if available, because it is sensitive, safe, and accurate for tissue sampling of focal pancreatic lesions (Zamboni et al. 2009).

Depending on the site of the lesion, probes with lateral or central support may be used (Fig. 5). The entry point has to be chosen avoiding important structures such as gallbladder, common bile duct, and main peri-pancreatic arteries and veins. Transcolonic passage is avoided, while transgastric passage is not (D'Onofrio et al. 2007b). After local anesthesia in the abdominal wall at the chosen entry point, the pancreatic lesion is reached, and the needle subtly moved in and out. FNA procedure is performed with fine needles (22–20-G caliber), and the material rises due to capillarity or aspiration. When a histopathological evaluation is required, a core-biopsy is performed: a core of the pancreatic lesion is taken with a suction or guillotine mechanism, by using a Menghini-type or a Trucut-type needle, respectively (22–16-G).

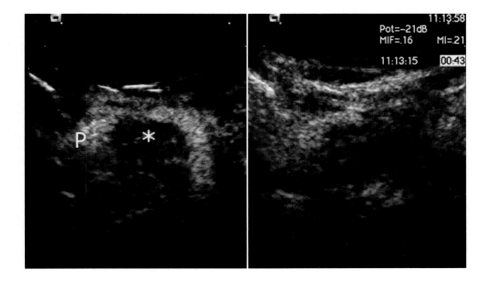

Fig. 4 CEUS. Ductal adenocarcinoma of the pancreatic head with the typical aspect presenting as a solid hypovascular mass (*asterisk*) in respect to the adjacent pancreatic parenchyma (P)

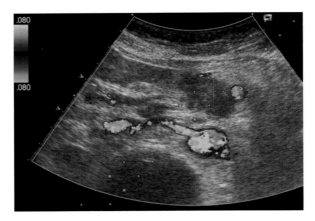

Fig. 5 FNAC. Doppler US-guidance of fine-needle-aspiration of a ductal adenocarcinoma infiltrating the superior mesenteric artery

8 Typical Features of Pancreatic Ductal Adenocarcinoma

At conventional US, pancreatic ductal adenocarcinoma usually presents as a solid mass, hypoechoic to the adjacent pancreatic parenchyma, with infiltrative margins. It often determines dilatation of the upstream main pancreatic duct and, if located in the head, also of the common bile duct (double-duct sign). In highly aggressive lesions, necrosis and colliquation are common (Martinez-Noguera and D'Onofrio 2007). The tumor may be better detected by using THI, that increases the lesion conspicuity, because of its superior soft tissue differentiation (Hohl et al. 2007).

At ARFI imaging, the wave velocity value measured inside the pancreatic ductal adenocarcinoma is higher (usually >3 m/s) than that resulted in the adjacent parenchyma (mean wave velocity value of 1.4 m/s) (Gallotti et al. 2010) owing to the presence of marked desmoplasia (Seo et al. 2000).

At Doppler study, pancreatic ductal adenocarcinoma shows poor or no vascularity (Bertolotto et al. 2007). The vascular invasion is defined by a focal disappearance of the echogenic interface forming the vessel wall, or by a narrow lumen, with changes in blood flow velocity (Koito et al. 2001; Ueno et al. 1997; Yassa et al. 1997). In these cases or if liver metastases are detected (usually in the late phase of CEUS study, as hypovascular lesions) (D'Onofrio et al. 2006), the

tissue pathological characterization is required (Zamboni et al. 2009), before starting a palliative therapy.

At CEUS examination, pancreatic ductal adenocarcinoma usually shows poor enhancement in all dynamic phases (D'Onofrio et al. 2005). The evidence of a poorly vascularized lesion, related to intratumoral fibrosis and necrosis with reduction of tumoral mean vascular density and perfusion (D'Onofrio et al. 2007a; Nagase et al. 2003), could suggest the undifferentiated grade (Numata et al. 2005). CEUS can be also helpful in the evaluation of vascular infiltration and liver involvement (D'Onofrio et al. 2007a).

References

Angeli E, Venturini M, Vanzulli A et al (1997) Color-Doppler imaging in the assessment of vascular involvement by pancreatic carcinoma. AJR 168:193–197

Bertolotto M, D'Onofrio M, Martone E et al (2007) Ultrasonography of the pancreas. 3. Doppler imaging. Abdom Imaging 32(2):161–170

Chapman CS, Lazenby JC (1997) Ultrasound imaging system employing phase inversion subtraction to enhance the image. US patent 5,632,277

Cosgrove D (2005) Advances in contrast agent imaging using Cadence contrast pulse sequencing technology (CPS) and SonoVue. Eur Rad 14(Suppl 8):P1–P3

D'Onofrio M, Malagò R, Zamboni G et al (2005) Contrast-enhanced ultrasonography better identifies pancreatic tumor vascularization than helical CT. Pancreatology 5(4–5):398–402

D'Onofrio M, Martone E, Faccioli N et al (2006) Focal liver lesions: sinusoidal phase of CEUS. Abdom Imaging 31(5):529–536

D'Onofrio M, Zamboni G, Faccioli N et al (2007a) Ultrasonography of the pancreas. 4. Contrast-enhanced imaging. Abdom Imaging 32:171–181

D'Onofrio M, Malagò R, Zamboni G et al (2007b) Ultrasonography of the pancreas. 5. Interventional procedures. Abdom Imaging 32(2):182–190

D'Onofrio M, Gallotti A, Martone E et al (2009) Solid appearance of serous cystadenoma diagnosed as cystic at ultrasound acoustic radiation force impulse imaging. JOP 10(5):543–546

D'Onofrio M, Zamboni G, Malagò R et al (2009) Resectable pancreatic adenocarcinoma: is the enhancement pattern at Contrast-enhanced ultrasonography a pre-operative prognostic factor? Ultrasound Med Biol 35(12):1929–1937

Desser TS, Jeffrey RB (2001) Tissue harmonic imaging techniques: physical principles and clinical applications. Semin Ultrasound CT MR 22:1–10

Faccioli N, D'Onofrio M, Zamboni G et al (2008) Resectable pancreatic adenocarcinoma: depiction of tumoral margins at contrast-enhanced ultrasonography. Pancreas 37(3):265–268

Fahley BJ, Palmeri ML, Trahey GE (2007) The impact of physiological motion on tissue tracking during radiation force imaging. Ultrasound Med Biol 33:1149–1166

Gallotti A, D'Onofrio M, Pozzi Mucelli R (2010) Acoustic radiation force impulse (ARFI) technique in the ultrasound study with Virtual Touch tissue quantification of the superior abdomen. Radiol Med [Epub ahead of print]

Hohl C, Schmidt T, Haage P et al (2004) Phase-inversion tissue harmonic imaging compared with conventional B-mode ultrasound in the evaluation of pancreatic lesions. Eur Radiol 14:1109–1117

Hohl C, Schmidt T, Honnef D et al (2007) Ultrasonography of the pancreas. 2. Harmonic imaging. Abdom Imaging 32(2):150–160, Review

Klöppel G, Schlüter E (1999) Pathology of the pancreas. In: Baert AL, Delorme G, Van Hoe L (eds) Radiology of the pancreas, 2nd edn. Springer-Verlag, Berlin, pp 69–100

Koito K, Namieno T, Nagakawa T et al (2001) Pancreas: imaging diagnosis with color/power-Doppler ultrasonography, endoscopic ultrasonography, and intraductal ultrasonography. Eur J Radiol 38:94–104

Martinez-Noguera A, D'Onofrio M (2007) Ultrasonography of the pancreas. 1. Conventional imaging. Abdom Imaging 32:136–149

McAleavey SA, Menon M, Orszulak J (2007) Shear-modulus estimation by application of spatially-modulated impulsive acoustic radiation force. Ultrason Imaging 29(2):87–104

Nagase M, Furuse J, Ishii H et al (2003) Evaluation of contrast enhancement patterns in pancreatic tumors by coded harmonic sonographic imaging with a microbubble contrast agent. J Ultrasound Med 22(8):789–795

Nightingale KR, Palmeri ML, Nightingale RW et al (2001) On the feasibility of remote palpation using acoustic radiation force. J Acoustic Soc Am 110(1):625–634

Nightingale KR, Bentley R, Trahey G (2002a) Observations of tissue response to acoustic radiation force: opportunities for imaging. Ultrason Imaging 24(3):129–138

Nightingale K, Soo MS, Nightingale R et al (2002b) Acoustic radiation force impulse imaging: in vivo demonstration of clinical feasibility. Ultrasound Med Biol 28(2):227–235

Nightingale K, McAleavey SA, Trahey G (2003) Shear-wave generation using acoustic radiation force: in vivo and ex vivo results. Ultrasound Med Biol 29(12):1715–1723

Numata K, Ozawa Y, Kobayashi N et al (2005) Contrast-enhanced sonography of pancreatic carcinoma: correlations with pathological findings. J Gastroenterol 40:631–640

Oktar SO, Yucel C, Ozdemir H et al (2003) Comparison of conventional sonography, real-time compound sonography, tissue harmonic sonography, and tissue harmonic compound sonography of abdominal and pelvic lesions. AJR 181:1341–1347

Sahani DV, Shan ZK, Catalano OA et al (2008) Radiology of pancreatic adenocarcinoma: current status of imaging. J Gastroenterol Hepatol 23(1):23–33, Review

Schoelgens C (1998) Native tissue harmonic imaging. Radiology 38:420–423

Seo Y, Baba H, Fukuda T et al (2000) High expression of vascular endothelial growth factor is associated with liver metastasis and poor prognosis for patients with ductal adenocarcinoma. Cancer 88:2239–2245

Shan B, Pelegri AA, Maleke C et al (2008) A mechanical model to compute elastic modulus of tissue for harmonic motion imaging. J Biomech 41(10):2150–2158

Shapiro RS, Wagreich J, Parsons RB et al (1998) Tissue harmonic imaging sonography: evaluation of image quality compared with conventional sonography. AJR 171:1203–1206

Sumi C (2008) Regularization of tissue shear modulus reconstruction using strain variance. IEEE Trans Ultrason Ferroelectr Freq Control 55(2):297–307

Ueno N, Tomiyama T, Tano S et al (1997) Color-Doppler ultrasonography in the diagnosis of portal vein invasion in patients with pancreatic cancer. J Ultrasound Med 16:825–830

Yassa NA, Yang J, Stein S et al (1997) Gray-scale and color flow sonography of pancreatic ductal adenocarcinoma. J Clin Ultrasound 25:473–480

Zamboni GA, D'Onofrio M, Principe F et al (2010) Focal pancreatic lesions: accuracy and complications of US-guided fine-needle aspiration cytology. Abdom Imaging 35(3):362–366

Zhai L, Palmeri ML, Bouchard RR et al (2008) An integrated indenter-ARFI imaging system for tissue stiffness quantification. Ultrason Imaging 30(2):95–111

The Case for MDCT

Carlo Nicola De Cecco, Franco Iafrate, Marco Rengo,
Saif Ramman, and Andrea Laghi

Contents

C.N. De Cecco
Department of Radiological Sciences,
University of Rome "Sapienza" – Polo Pontino,
Via Franco Faggiana, 34, 04100 Latina, Italy and
Department of Radiological Sciences,
University of Rome "Sapienza" – St. Andrea Hospital,
Via di Grottarossa, 1035, 00189 Rome, Italy

F. Iafrate, M. Rengo, and A. Laghi (✉)
Department of Radiological Sciences,
University of Rome "Sapienza" – Polo Pontino,
Via Franco Faggiana, 34, 04100 Latina, Italy
e-mail: andrea.laghi@uniroma1.it

S. Ramman
University of Glasgow, University Avenue,
Glasgow G12 8QQ, UK

Abstract

> Multidetector CT (MDCT) examination with multiphasic acquisition should be advocated as routine study in patient investigated for pancreatic adenocarcinoma. The application of a biphasic protocol gives the best results, using a pancreatic phase for tumor identification and arterial infiltration, and portal phase for the assement of venous infiltration and liver metastasis. Pancreatic adenocarcinoma is classically visualized as an ill-defined solid mass, not capsulated, isodense to the pancreatic parenchyma in pre-contrast scan and hypo-attenuating in the pancreatic-portal phases. Ancillary signs can be helpful in the diagnosis of small tumors (< 2 cm) and isoattenuating adenocarcinoma. Several benign and malignant condition can mimick adenocarcinoma, in this case magnetic resonance and endoscopic ultrasonography biopsy can be helpful in diagnosis. MDCT enables an accurate tumor staging and presents a positive predictive values for unresectability between 89% to 100%; it also allows a complete preoperative planning and presents high accuracy both in surgical complications and tumor recurrence detection.

A. Laghi (ed.), *New Concepts in Diagnosis and Therapy of Pancreatic Adenocarcinoma*,
Medical Radiology, DOI: 10.1007/174_2010_49, © Springer-Verlag Berlin Heidelberg 2011

1 Introduction

Multidetector computed tomography (MDCT) has been introduced in 1998 and it has changed the way to do imaging. Compared with single-detector helical CT, MDCT improves spatial resolution with a decrease in image acquisition time and tube heating. The high examination speed enables defined perfusion phases to be obtained that enhance tumor detection. Submillimetric acquisition leads to voxel isotrophy and it has opened the way to multiparametric analysis and postprocessing technique which improve tumor assessment and staging. This also means a better delineation of tumor relationship with adjacent structures without volume averaging problems.

The advent of MDCT changed the diagnostic approach to pancreatic adenocarcinoma improving tumor detection and early assessment. Nowadays, multiphasic imaging of the pancreas should be advocated as routine examination in patient investigated for pancreatic adenocarcinoma. The application of a biphasic protocol gives the best results, using a pancreatic phase for tumor identification and arterial infiltration, and portal phase for the assessment of venous infiltration and liver metastasis. Shorter volume acquisition and faster scan time also allow better contrast enhancement of vessels and pancreatic Parenchyma, in addition to a reduction in respiratory artifacts. As a matter of fact, there are different examination and reconstruction protocols available for different multidetector technology (Table 1).

Moreover, the data set obtained could be easily analyzed with several postprocessing algorithms, which can improve tumor detection, staging, and follow-up.

2 Study Protocol

2.1 Patient Preparation

The administration of 500–1,000 mL of water as an oral contrast agent improves delineation of the pancreatic gland and could be useful for evaluation of gastric or duodenal wall infiltration. Positive contrast agents are not suitable for vascular delineation and can mask bile duct stones. A spasmolytic drug can also be administered in order to improve bowel distensibility.

2.2 Precontrast Scan

A precontrast scan of upper abdomen should be acquired from diaphragmatic dome to iliac crest in order to evaluate abdominal Parenchyma and in particular to show bile duct stones, blood clots, or pancreatic calcifications as sign of chronic pancreatitis (Tunaci 2004). Precontrast scan is also important to set the postcontrast phases acquisition.

Table 1 MDCT study protocols

Channels	4		8		16		64	
	Pancreatic phase	Portal phase	Pancreatic phase	Portal phase	Pancreatic phase	Portal phase	Pancreatic phase	Portal phase
Collimation (mm)	4×1.25	4×2.5	8×1.25	8×2.5	16×1.25	16×1.25	64×0.625	64×0.625
Slice thickness (mm)	1.25	2.5	1.25	2.5	1.25	1.25	0.625	0.625
Rotation time (s)	0.5	0.5	0.8	0.8	0.8	0.8	0.8	0.8
Kvp	120	120	120	120	120	120	120	120
mAs	200–240	200–240	360	360	Automatic	Automatic	Automatic	Automatic
Scan delay	40	70	40	70	BT	BT	BT	BT
Scan direction	Craniocaudal	Craniocaudal	Craniocaudal	Craniocaudal	Craniocaudal	Craniocaudal	Craniocaudal	Craniocaudal

2.3 Early Arterial Phase

Early arterial phase starts about 15–20 s after contrast administration or using a bolus tracking technique 3 s after abdominal aorta peak enhancement at 150 HU, which allows to obtain a perfect vascular depiction (CT Angiography) without parenchymal enhancement (Shioyama et al. 2001). In the absence of specific indications, this phase can be avoided in pancreatic evaluation because we have the same vascular information with a pancreatic phase, reducing patient radiation exposure especially in young subjects.

2.4 Pancreatic Phase

Pancreatic phase is a term coined by Lu et al. (1996) and starts about 35–40 s after contrast administration or using a bolus tracking technique 15–20 s after an aortic peak of 50 HU (Kondo et al. 2007), corresponding to a late arterial phase. During the pancreatic phase we obtain the higher parenchyma contrast impregnation and have a better delineation of pancreatic adenocarcinoma, which is an ipovascular lesion due to its stromal tissue. Pancreatic phase is also more reliable in tumor measurement providing a more accurate evaluation, instead of portal phase in which we have an underestimation of tumor dimension due to vascularized peripheral tumor tissue. Pancreatic phase should be considered mandatory in tumor extension evaluation because it improves the tumor conspicuity when compared with portal phase (Fig. 1).

2.5 Portal Venous Phase

The venous phase starts about 70 s after contrast administration and provides a better opacification of superior mesenteric vein and portal vein. In this phase we can evaluate the presence of vascular involvement and assess the extension of infiltration. It is also necessary to detect liver metastasis.

2.6 Late Phase

In late venous phase we have a pancreatic wash out with a reduction in mean pancreatic density. Persistence of high density area can be suggestive of pathological process, such as fibrosis. This phase could also be implemented in liver metastasis evaluation.

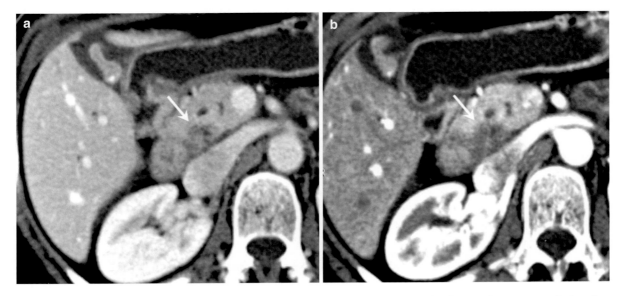

Fig. 1 In pancreatic phase (**b**) there is a better delineation of pancreatic adenocarcinoma and an increase in tumor conspicuity when compared with portal phase (**a**) (*arrows*)

In summary, the following should be performed for a complete pancreatic study: (1) precontrast scan of upper abdomen; (2) pancreatic phase, for tumor conspicuity assessment and arterial delineation; (3) portal phase for superior mesenteric vein and portal vein involvement, and for liver metastasis evaluation.

3 Image Postprocessing

MDCT volumetric acquisition with isotropic voxel permits several postprocessing techniques which can improve tumor detectability, peripancreatic invasion, and vascular infiltration assessment (Raptopoulos et al. 1997; Prokesch et al. 2002a; Baek et al. 2001; Nino-Murcia et al. 2001).

Multiplanar reconstruction (MPR) is useful to define the spatial relationship of the tumor with the peripancreatic structures such as duodenum, stomach, spleen, omentum, and mesocolon. Maximum Intensity Projection (MIP) contributes to additional information regarding vessels enhancement and invasion. Curved reformat can be useful for a better analysis of the relationship between the tumor and curved structures like common biliary duct, pancreatic ducts, and vessels. Minimum Intensity Projection (Min-IP) can easily detect postoperative aerobilia and it clearly visualizes biliary morphology and late complications such as stenosis of hepaticojejunal anastomosis. Volume rendering (VR) technique could be useful in vascular assessment enhancing vessels distortion and stenosis (Fig. 2). The application of postprocessing techniques increases tumor diagnosis and permits also an accurate preoperative staging.

4 Pancreatic Ductal Adenocarcinoma: Signs and Pitfalls

4.1 MDCT Tumor Identification

Pancreatic adenocarcinoma is classically visualized as an ill-defined solid mass, not capsulated, isodense to the pancreatic Parenchyma in precontrast scan and hypoattenuating in the pancreatic-portal phases. Hypoattenuation is due to the low tumor vascularization with the presence of flourish extracellular matrix, often associated with small necrotic foci (Schima et al. 2007; Freeny et al. 1988). At the MDCT diagnosis, tumor often presents with a small dimension (<2 cm) if localized in the head or uncinate process than if it is localized into the body-tail (5–7 cm). Usually calcifications are not present (Warshaw et al. 1992) (Fig. 3).

Small tumors (<2 cm) can be difficult to recognize at CT and radiologists should pay attention to secondary signs. Ancillary signs can be helpful in the diagnosis of pancreatic tumors. Any distortion to the normal glandular lobulated outline associated with a mass effect (adjacent structures displacement) should alert the radiologist, in particular if there is also an observed pancreatic atrophy distal to the mass, which is suggestive of chronic obstructive pancreatitis. The presence of both pancreatic and biliary duct dilation (double duct sign) associated with their abrupt interruption (interrupted duct sign) is also suggestive of a pancreatic mass (Fig. 4). Small tumor can also be hidden from associated pathological conditions such as acute pancreatitis and chronic obstructive pancreatitis. In the first case, a small lesion can determine the rupture of the pancreatic duct instead of its occlusion, with the onset of an acute focal inflammation.

The presence of a chronic pancreatitis represents a risk factor for the development of adenocarcinoma and can also mask the tumor. The diffuse parenchymal atrophy associated with ductal dilatation and diffuse calcification can make it difficult to assess small lesions. Also in this condition, the presence of ancillary signs should be recognized, such as the mass effect of the calcification with a peripheral dislocation and the presence of an area with difference in tissue texture. MDCT cannot always differentiate this confounding conditions and other imaging technique should be applied.

4.2 Isoattenuating Adenocarcinoma

Some tumors show remarkably little attenuation difference compared with the normal pancreas basing their recognition only on ancillary signs. Isoattenuating

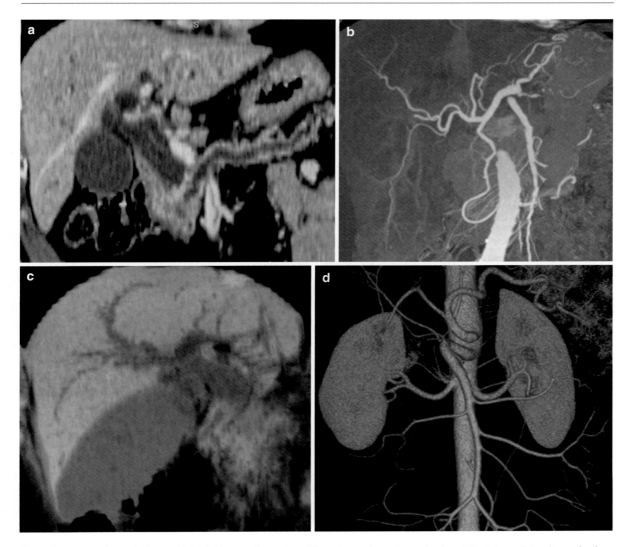

Fig. 2 Postprocessing techniques. (**a**) Multiplanar reformation; (**b**) maximum intensity projection; (**c**) minimum intensity projection; (**d**) volume rendering

pancreatic adenocarcinoma represents a well-differentiated pancreatic carcinoma with a higher number of microvessels as opposed to hypovascular adenocarcinoma (Wang et al. 2003; Zhongqiu et al. 2004). This tumor has an incidence of about 10% (Prokesch et al. 2002b) and the mean size is significantly smaller than of hypoattenuating tumor at the diagnosis (Ishigami et al. 2009). The combined presence of interrupted duct sign with mass effect should alert the radiologist. Also, the evidence of atrophy of pancreatic parenchyma distal to the mass can be useful. In this case secretine study with MRI could help make the diagnosis by showing the "penetrating duct" sign (Fig. 5). Endoscopic Ultrasound (EUS) and biopsy are fundamental in order to obtain a diagnosis.

Since pancreatic adenocarcinoma contains fibrotic tissue, as reported by Ishigami et al. (2009), isoattenuating adenocarcinoma could be detected with a delayed phase as a slightly hyperattenuating tumor such as is described in the case of intrahepatic cholangiocarcinoma. If an "interrupted duct" sign is detected without the evidence of any mass, a delayed acquisition should be performed in order to visualize a small hyperenhanced lesion.

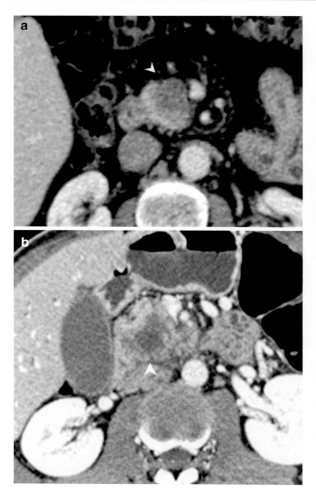

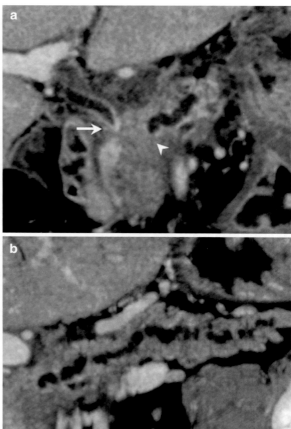

Fig. 3 Typical pancreatic adenocarcinoma presentation. (**a**) An ill-defined solid mass of pancreatic head hypodense to the pancreatic parenchyma (*arrowhead*) in portal phase; (**b**) An head tumor with central necrosis (*arrowhead*)

Fig. 4 Ancillary signs. (**a**) Double duct sign, consisting in common bile duct (*arrow*) and main pancreatic duct (*arrowhead*) dilatation. (**b**) Interrupted duct sign, abrupt interruption of the main pancreatic duct

4.3 Tumors Mimicking Adenocarcinoma

Several other neoplastic conditions can mimic pancreatic adenocarcinoma. Papillary adenocarcinoma is a rare tumor associated with ductal dilatation and distal pancreatitis, but with a better prognosis than ductal adenocarcinoma. It is visualized as a papillary mass with an extrapancreatic growth protruding into duodenal lumen; it also presents a slight hypervascularization in pancreatic phase. Both neoplastic diseases have the same surgical treatment (Kim et al. 2007).

Pancreatic lymphoma is a very rare condition represented by a large hypoattenuating pancreatic mass. Imaging differentiation between the two condition is difficult. Other signs suggestive of lymphoma are the presence of diffuse adenopathy, secondary localization in kidney and spleen, and a larger extension unusual for a typical adenocarcinoma.

Nonfunctional neuroendocrine tumor represents 30% of neuroendocrine neoplasia and has a better prognosis than adenocarcinoma. It is visualized as hypovascular solid lesion with a greater dimension (5–6 cm) and clear margins for the presence of capsular structure (Fig. 6). Mucinous cystic tumor may present a rare microcystic pattern which appears as a solid mass indistinguishable from pancreatic adenocarcinoma (Visser et al. 2004).

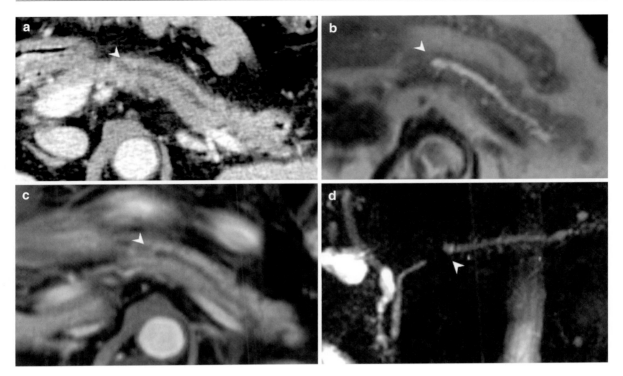

Fig. 5 Isoattenuating adenocarcinoma. (**a**) Dilatation of the main pancreatic duct with interruption at the body level (*arrowhead*) without evidence of any pancreatic mass; (**b, c**) MR examination confirmed CT findings both in T1- and T2-weighted images (*arrowheads*); (**d**) Cholangiopancreatic MR study with secretin stimulus revealed the lack of the "penetrating duct sign" (*arrowhead*), confirming the presence of a isoattenuating pancreatic mass

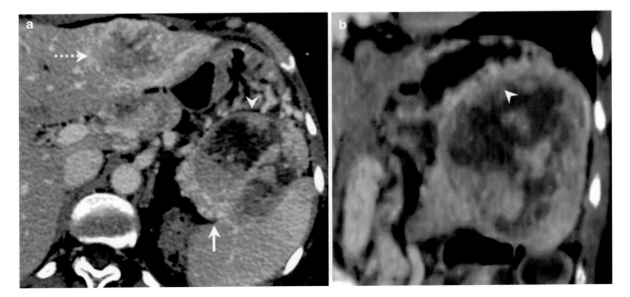

Fig. 6 Nonfunctional neuroendocrine tumor. (**a, b**) A cystic lesion (*arrow*) in pancreatic tail with necrotic foci and clear margins for the presence of a capsular structure (*arrowhead*); a liver metastasis was also noticed (*dashed-arrow*)

Pancreatic metastasis from other tumors is infrequent. However, CT patterns can mimic adenocarcinoma and the knowledge of a primitive neoplasia is fundamental to the diagnosis. Pancreatic adenocarcinoma with extensive intratumoral necrosis and hemorrhagic area can also mimic other pancreatic tumors such as cystic, anaplastic, small cell, and giant cell types (Ichikawa et al. 2000). A CT differential diagnosis of this conditions could not be easily obtained, and as a result, the final diagnosis is often obtained with EUS biopsy or FNAB (fine needle aspiration biopsy) (Brugge 1998).

4.4 Benign Conditions Mimicking Adenocarcinoma

The pancreatic region contains several structures with complex anatomic relationships that represent a diagnostic challenge. Several benign conditions can mimic pancreatic adenocarcinoma (To'o et al. 2005; Lawler et al. 2003).

Anatomic variants represent a common confounding problem in pancreas evaluation. Duodenal diverticula and duplications may be misinterpreted as pancreatic masses, especially cystic tumors, due to their fluid content. Duodenal duplications are usually found on the mesenteric side of the second duodenal portion and are typically noncommunicating with the lumen. Diverticulum is easily differentiated because of its communication with duodenal lumen and the appearance of an air-fluid level with ingested material. Barium studies can help to distinguish these conditions demonstrating the lumen communication. Also, choledocal cysts can appear as fusiform cystic masses located in the pancreatic head. MR cholangiopancreatography allows confirmation of the diagnosis.

Both focal acute pancreatitis and adenocarcinoma appear hypoattenuating on CT making it difficult to assess masses. In this case it is possible to observe the so-called "black and white" sign where we have clear delimitation in pancreatic phase between the hypoattenuating area containing the tumor with the inflammation and a proximal normal area of pancreatic enhancement.

Severe acute pancreatitis with a heterogeneous presentation due to hemorrhagic area can also mimic a pancreatic tumor. Clinical presentation and follow-up can be useful in the diagnosis.

Chronic pancreatitis is normally associated with a wide range of pancreatic abnormalities. Approximately 20% of patients with chronic pancreatitis develop a focal inflammatory mass, which may closely simulate pancreatic adenocarcinoma (Boll and Merkle 2003). Another uncommon inflammatory condition is represented by groove pancreatitis. The presence of ectopic pancreatic stroma in duodenal wall can induce a micro- or macrocystic pattern which can mimic both a cystic tumor or a solid mass. Patient history is important since patients usually are middle-age men with a history of alcohol abuse (Procacci et al. 1997).

Focal pancreatitis could be indistinguishable from adenocarcinoma on the basis of morphological features and enhancement pattern. MR imaging with secretin can be useful in the demonstration of a "penetrating duct" sign which is characteristic of benign conditions (Ichikawa et al. 2001). When the MRI is not resolutive, a strict follow-up or FNAB is mandatory (Fig. 7).

In autoimmune pacreatitis a diffuse glandular enlargement is observed with a typical peripancreatic hypodense rim representing inflammatory exudation and the absence of calcification or vascular encasement. Other typical features are represented by multiple biliary strictures and diffuse irregular narrowing of the main pancreatic duct. These findings are frequently observed in young women with a coexisting autoimmune diseases (Wakabashi et al. 2003).

5 Tumor Staging

5.1 T Parameter

Multidetector CT with multiplanar reformation is highly sensitive for assessment of T stage. T1 stage is defined as tumor <2 cm in the largest diameter and entirely confined to the pancreas. T2 stage is defined as tumor >2 cm, still confined to the pancreatic gland. In stage T3 there is a local invasion as extension into the peripancreatic soft tissue and/or invasion of the tumor into the duodenum or common bile duct. The infiltration of surrounding organs, such as spleen, stomach, or transverse colon, is defined as stage T4; also the infiltration of the peripancreatic vessels such as superior mesenteric vein and artery, portal vein, hepatic artery, or celiac trunk is

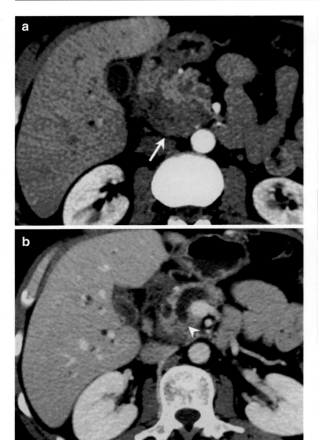

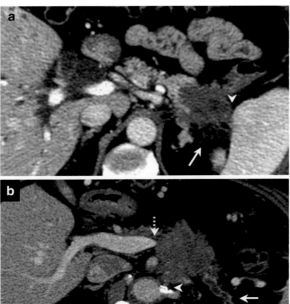

Fig. 8 Stage T4. (**a**) Tail tumor with an invasion into the peripancreatic fat tissue (*arrow*) and splenic ilium (*arrowhead*). (**b**) Body tumor occluding splenic vena (*dashed-arrow*) and infiltrating the anterior pararenal fascia (*arrowhead*); there is also a focal pancreatitis of the tail (*arrow*)

Fig. 7 An hypodense lesion in pancreatic head (**a**) (*arrow*) causing a double duct sign (**b**) (*arrowhead*) was misinterpreted as pancreatic tumor. MRI and FNAB revealed a focal pancreatitis

classified as T4 (Fig. 8). T3 tumors are potentially resectable, but pancreatic tumor infiltrates lymphatic vessels earlier producing a perivascular cuff of soft tissue, which can be underestimated in the radiological assessment. The infiltration of adjacent organs and the invasion of peripancreatic vessels is a contraindication against surgical resection. A limited invasion into the superior mesenteric vein or the portal vein, typically less than 2 cm, is considered a relative contraindication to the surgical approach with vascular reconstruction, although it has been shown that survival is not improved (Park et al. 2001) (Table 2 and Fig. 9).

MDCT permits an accurate evaluation of vascular involvement, in fact the possibility to obtain curved multiplanar reformations better displaying the tumor relationship with the adjacent vessels. Vargas et al. (2004) reported an accuracy of 99% with a negative

predictive value of 100%. A grading system of vascular invasion probability based on the circumferential contiguity of tumor to vessel has been proposed by Lu et al. (Lu DSK, Reber HA et al 1997. Am J Roentgenol 168), which found that when more than 50% of the vessel circumference is in contact with a vessel the tumor would not be resectable (Table 3 and Figs. 10–12).

Although loss of the fat plane does not automatically mean vascular involvement, it can also be surrounded by fibrous tissue or inflammatory stranding (Nakayama et al. 2001). Tumor thrombus, vascular occlusion or changes in vessel caliber, or the so-called teardrop sign (Hough et al. 1999) of the superior mesenteric vein represent reliable signs of vascular invasion.

5.2 N Parameter

MDCT is not accurate in the assessment of nodal involvement with an overall accuracy of 58% (Zeman et al. 1997), since it is based purely on dimensional and

Table 2 TNM staging of pancreatic adenocarcinoma

TNM	Definition
Tumor	
Tis	Carcinoma in situ
T1	Tumor limited to pancreas, <2 cm in any direction
T2	Tumor limited to pancreas, <2 cm in any direction
T3	Infiltration into peripancreatic tissues, duodenum, and/or common bile duct
T4	Infiltration into peripancreatic vessels, stomach, spleen, large bowel
Lymph nodes	
N0	No lymph node metastasis
N1	Metastasis in peripancreatic lymph nodes
Nx	Unknown
Distant metastasis	
M0	No distant metastases
M1	Distant metastases present
Mx	Unknown

morphological criteria. A lymph node with a greater diameter than 1 cm in short axis is usually described as significant. But normal-sized nodes may be involved and some enlarged nodes can be inflammatory. Hence, CT cannot accurately predict nodal metastasis, and preoperative evaluation should include an accurate description of visualized nodes. MPR images represent a power tool also in nodal distribution analysis. The name-based classification AJCC-UICC of the lymph nodes distribution allows an accurate intraoperative guide for the surgeon and for the subsequent pathological dissection. AJCC-UICC system divides lymph nodes into four groups: (1) superior to the body and head of the pancreas; (2) anterior, including anterior pancreaticoduodenal, pyloric, and proximal mesenteric; (3) inferior to the body and head of the pancreas; (4) posterior, including posterior pancreaticoduodenal, common bile duct, and proximal mesenteric. Other lymph nodes metastases distant from peripancreatic sites are defined as stage M1. Another classification has been created by the Japanese Pancreatic Society which identifies 18 different sites, but this approach does not improve lymph nodes yield.

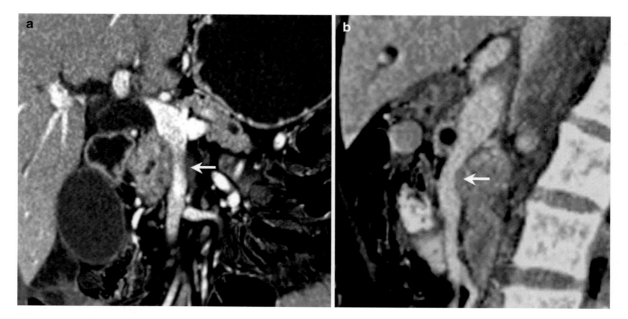

Fig. 9 Venous infiltration. (**a**) Head tumor infiltrating the superior mesenteric vein more than 2 cm (*arrow*); (**b**) Body tumor infiltrating the superior mesenteric vein less than 2 cm (*arrow*)

Table 3 Vascular invasion criteria

Degree of contiguity (%)	Resectability
0	Resectable
<25	Resectable
25–50	Resectable
50–75	Unresectable
>75	Unresectable

5.3 M Parameter

The commonest causes of CT understaging are small liver and peritoneal metastasis. MDCT permits a high resolution whole-body examination for the assessment of distal tumor involvement. The submillimetric liver assessment associated with multiphasic imaging increases detection rate of small hepatic lesions (Catalano et al. 2003) (Fig. 13). However, CT remains limited in peritoneal localization which can upstage patient to stage IV; for this reason, laparoscopic assessment is often performed prior to laparotomy in order to evaluate peritoneum (Fig. 14).

5.4 Resectability Criteria

MDCT presents positive predictive values for unresectability between 89 and 100%, with accuracies of 85–95% (Lu et al. 1997; Freeny et al. 1993). However, we have a lower positive predictive values for resectability that range between 45 and 79% (Freeny et al. 1993; Bluemque et al. 1995; Tabuchi et al. 1999).

Absolute criteria of unresectability are the presence of metastases, lymphadenopathy beyond the peripancreatic chain, malignant ascites or pleural effusion, peritoneal deposits, arterial invasion, and extensive venous involvement (>2 cm) (Table 4).

Contiguous invasion of the duodenum, stomach, right colon, or regional lymph nodes is not a contraindication to surgery (Alexakis et al. 2004). However, a positive retroperitoneal margin, that is the soft tissue to the right of proximal superior mesenteric artery, represents a relative contraindication to surgery since the median survival after pancreatic resection in patients with a positive margin is not significantly different from those who undergo palliative therapy (Neoptolemos et al. 2001).

In some condition equivocal findings are present and it is not possible to clearly evaluate the tumor

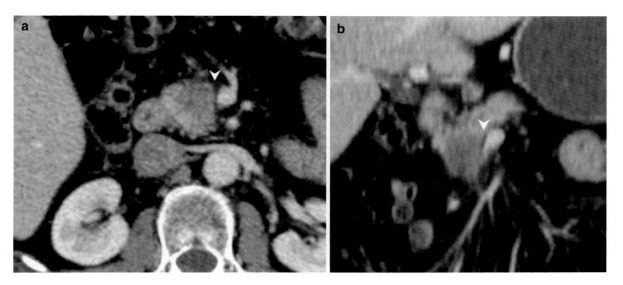

Fig. 10 (**a–b**) The presence of a preserved fat plane (*arrowheads*) between tumor and vessel with a contiguity less than 180° is suggestive of vascular sparing

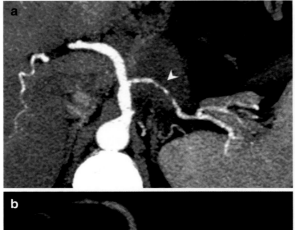

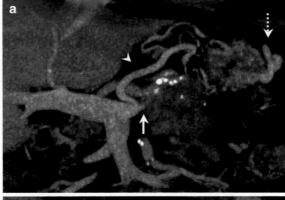

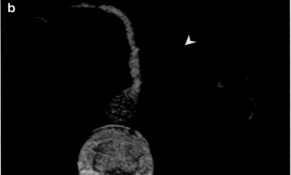

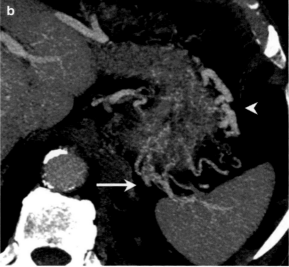

Fig. 11 (**a–b**) A circumferential vessel enchasement with lumen narrowing (*arrowheads*) is indicative of vascular infiltration

extension, in particular when the tumor is greater than 3 cm, there is a contiguity between tumor and vessel between 25 and 50% and a stranding of the perivascular fat plane is present (Cameron et al. 1991).

Fig. 12 Collateral circulation. (**a**) Body tumor occluding the splenic vena (*arrow*) with hypertrophic short gastric veins (*dashed-arrow*) and left gastric vein (*arrowhead*). (**b**) Compensatory hypertrophy of short gastric veins (*arrow*) and collateral vessels along the great gastric curvature (*arrowhead*)

6 Perioperative Findings

6.1 Preoperative Planning

MDCT allows a complete preoperative planning in patients who underwent curative or palliative surgery. CT angiography provides precious information to the surgeon of normal vascular anatomy or variant relevant to the Whipple procedure. Also, the knowledge of variant anatomy of arteries and veins is important in considering resectability. The presence of multiple jejunal branches with a high insertion on the superior mesenteric vein near the portal confluence may make vein

reconstruction difficult or impossible. Arterial anatomic variants that make resection impossible include a replaced common hepatic artery from SMA (Fig. 15). For this reason it is important to differentiate a replaced artery from an accessory that can be ligated during resection without liver inflow impairment. Anatomical variants may also make resection more likely, for example, the presence of a common hepatic artery arising separately from the aorta with the celiac artery only supplying splenic or gastroduodenal arteries (Lall et al. 2007). MDCT angiography demonstrated a perfect depiction of abdominal arterial anatomy and high accuracy in aberrant hepatic arteries recognition (Ferrari et al. 2007; De Cecco et al. 2009).

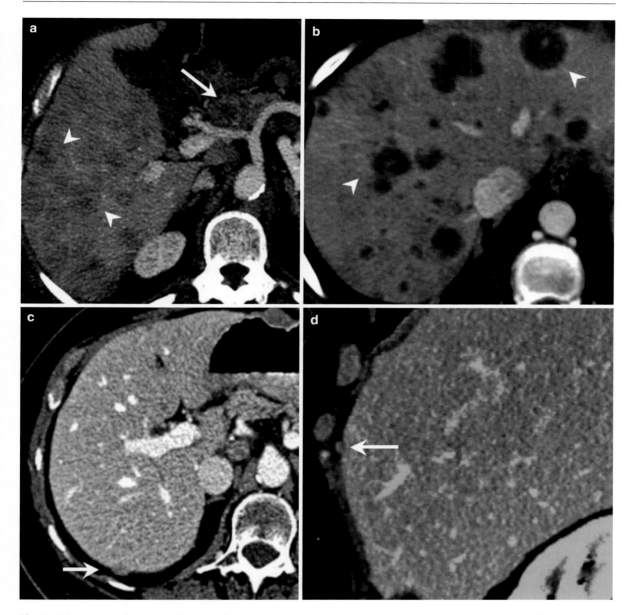

Fig. 13 Liver metastasis. (**a**) Head tumor adjacent to the common hepatic artery (*arrow*) with extensive liver involvement (*arrowheads*); (**b**) Multiple hepatic metastasis with ring enhancement (*arrowheads*). (**c–d**) Small subglissonian metastasis (*arrows*)

6.2 Postoperative Complications and Tumor Recurrence

MDCT enables to recognize both early and late surgical complications. Early complications include pancreatic fistula, anastomotic leakage (pancreatic, biliary, and intestinal anastomosis), hemorrhage, acute pancreatitis, fluid collections, abscess, biloma, cholangitis, and peritonitis (Scialpi et al. 2005).

Retroperitoneal abscess represents the most common early complication and it is visualized as a fluid collection which can present gas bubble inside. In the suspect of retoperitonal abscess, oral contrast should be administrated in order to distinguish between infected fluid collection and unopacified anastomotic bowel loop; for this reason the suspect should be administrated oral contrast. MDCT permits also a good anatomical delineation of fluid collection and relationship assessment,

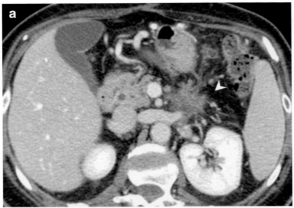

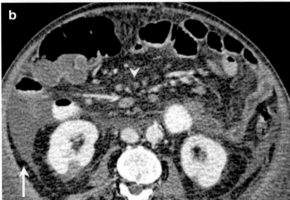

Fig. 14 (**a**) Pancreatic tumor recurrence as a solid ill-defined mass into the mesenteric root (*arrowhead*). (**b**) Malignant ascites (*arrow*) with associated multiple mesenteric lymph nodes (*arrowhead*)

Table 4 Resectability criteria

Irresectability	Equivocal findings
Metastasis	Tumor >3 cm
Distal lymph nodes	Contiguity 25–50% between tumor and vessels
Malignant ascites	Venous invasion >2 cm
Peritoneal implants	Stranding of perivascular fat planes
Arterial vessels contiguity >50% or signs of vascular invasion (thrombosis/occlusion)	

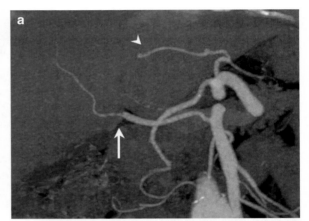

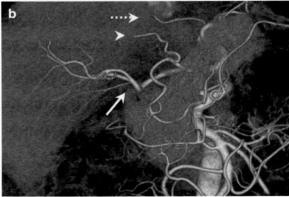

Fig. 15 Preoperative planning. (**a**) Replaced right hepatic artery from SMA (*arrow*) and replaced left hepatic artery from gastric artery (*arrowhead*); (**b**) Replaced right hepatic artery from SMA (*arrow*), left hepatic artery (*arrowhead*), and accessory left hepatic artery from left gastric artery (*dashed-arrow*)

fundamental in the planning of percutaneous drainage, especially for the identification of multiloculated abscesses that are not suitable of drainage.

Another frequent complication after Whipple procedure is the pancreatico-jejunal fistula, defined as concentration of amylase and lipase in the drainage fluid than three times the serum concentration and drainage volume of more than 500 mL per day. MDCT is important in the exclusion of infected fluid collection and in delineating complex fistulous tracts.

Anastomotic leakage occurs in the first 1–2 weeks after surgery and it is involved more frequently in pacreaticojejunal anastomosis (Pessaux et al. 2001). MDCT could be useful in leak identification, especially with the administration of positive contrast into the drainage with the opacification of the perianastomotic collection.

Late complications include chronic fistula, aneurysm, perianastomotic ulcers, and stenosis of hepaticojejunostomy. Arterial aneurisms are caused by enzymatic arterial wall destruction and represent a threatening life

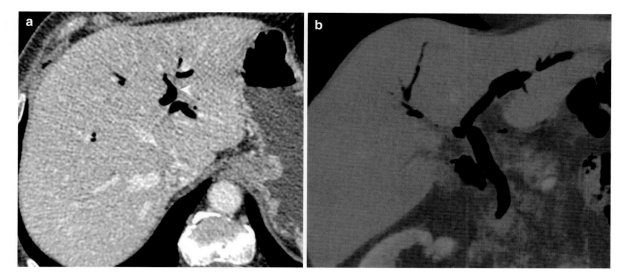

Fig. 16 (**a–b**) Extensive aerobilia (*arrowhead*) after ampullectomy

condition; MDCT angiography allows an excellent delineation also of small distal aneurisms and a preoperative planning. Biliary stenosis represents a frequent complication; MDCT is accurate in its detection with postprocessing technique such as MinIP.

Pneumobilia is considered a normal postoperative finding in pancreatic head surgery, given that it is present in 67–80% of the cases on postoperative CT examination (Bluemke et al. 1992; Mortelè et al. 2000) (Fig. 16).

MDCT permits an accurate evaluation of local and distant recurrences. Local recurrence presents an incidence of 60%. The accuracy of CT for the detection of disease recurrence is 93.5% (Mortelè et al. 2000; Dalla Valle et al. 2006). The knowledge of tumor recurrence is important to assess patient prognosis and response to adjuvant therapy. In early postoperative period the evidence of hyperplastic lymph nodes and perivascular fibrosis could represent a confusing factor that may simulate recurrent disease. The pancreatic bed is a common site of recurrence (Cameron et al. 1991; Johnson et al. 2002), in particular the area around the common hepatic arteries and proximal superior mesenteric artery. A gastric and jejunal loops opacification is also important to differentiate recurrent or residual tumor from unopacified anastomotic bowel loops in the surgical bed (Coombs et al. 1990). Also, the presence of surgical clips for vascular ligature can obscure the bed of the pancreatic head making difficult the detection of recurrence (Mortelè et al. 2000). Perivascular soft tissue around these vessels may create a diagnostic challenge when distinguishing postoperative change from recurrent disease. As reported by Ishigami et al. (2008), patients with a perivascular cuff of soft tissue should be monitored for at least two years to exclude recurrence, since size and enhancement criteria would not be helpful in distinguishing the two conditions.

Patients who underwent adjuvant chemo or radiotherapy frequently present fibrosis which appears as a hypovascular mass and represents a confounding problem. The knowledge of tumor marker CA 19–9 serum level is useful in discriminating between recurrence and postoperative changes (Bluemke et al. 1997); CT-PET examination can recognize the metabolic activity of hypovascular tissue permitting to differentiate the two conditions (Ruf et al. 2005).

References

Alexakis N, Halloran C, Raraty M, Ghaneh P, Sutton R (2004) Current standards of surgery for pancreatic cancer. Br J Surg 91:1410–1427

Baek SY, Sheafor DH, Keogan MT et al (2001) Two-dimensional multiplanar and three-dimensional volume-rendered vascular CT in pancreatic cancer: interobserver agreement and comparison with standard helical techniques. Am J Roentgenol 176:1467–1473

Bluemke DA, Fishman EK, Kuhlman J (1992) CT evaluation following Whipple procedure: potential pitfalls in interpretation. J Comput Assist Tomogr 16:704–708

Bluemke DA, Abrams RA, Yeo CJ, Cameron JL, Fishman EK (1997) Recurrent pancreatic adenocarcinoma: spiral CT evaluation following the Whipple procedure. Radiographics 17:303–313

Bluemque DA, Cameron JL, Hruban RH et al (1995) Potentially resectable pancreatic adenocarcinoma: spiral CT assessment with surgical and pathologic correlation. Radiology 197: 381–385

Boll DT, Merkle EM (2003) Differentiating a chronic hyperplastic mass from pancreatic cancer: a challenge remaining in multidetector CT of the pancreas. Eur Radiol 13:M42–M49

Brugge WR (1998) Fine needle aspiratiion of pancreatic masses: results of a multicenter study. Am J Gastroenterol 93:1329–1333

Cameron JL, Crist DW, Sitzman JV et al (1991) Factors influencing survival after pancreaticoduodenectomy for pancreatic cancer. Am J Surg 161:120–124

Catalano C, Laghi A, Fraioli F et al (2003) Pancreatic carcinoma: the role of high resolution multislice spiral CT in the diagnosis and assessment of resectability. Eur Radiol 13:149–156

Coombs RJ, Zeiss J, Howard JM, Thomford NR, Merrick HW (1990) CT of the abdomen after the Whipple procedure: value in depicting postoperative anatomy, surgical complications, and tumor recurrence. Am J Roentgenol 154:1011–1014

Dalla Valle R, Mancini C, Crafa P et al (2006) Pancreatic carcinoma recurrence in the remnant pancreas after a pancreaticoduodenectomy. JOP 7:473–477

De Cecco CN, Ferrari R, Rengo M, Paolantonio P, Vecchietti F, Laghi A (2009) Anatomic variations of the hepatic arteries in 250 patients studied with 64-row CT angiography. Eur Radiol; doi: 10.1007/s00330-009-1458-7

Ferrari R, De Cecco CN, Iafrate F, Paolantonio P, Rengo M, Laghi A (2007) Anatomical variations of the coeliac trunk and the mesenteric arteries evaluated with 64-row CT angiography. Radiol Med 112:988–998

Freeny PC, Marks WM, Ryan JA et al (1988) Pancreatic duct adenocarcinoma: diagnosis and staging with dynamic CT. Radiology 166:125–133

Freeny PC, Traverso LW, Ryan JA (1993) Diagnosis and staging of pancreatic adenocarcinoma with dynamic computed tomography. Am J Surg 165:600–606

Hough TJ, Raptopoulos V, Siewert B, Matthews JB (1999) Teardrop superior mesenteric vein: CT sign of unresectable carcinoma of the pancreas. Am J Roentgenol 173:1509–1512

Ichikawa T, Federle MP, Ohba S et al (2000) Atypical exocrine and endocrine pancreatic tumors (anaplastic, small cell, and giant cell types): CT and pathological features in 14 patients. Abdom Imaging 25:409–419

Ichikawa T, Sou H, Araki T et al (2001) Duct-penetrating sign at MRCP: usefulness for differentiating inflammatory pancreatic mass from pancreatic carcinomas. Radiology 221: 107–116

Ishigami K, Yoshimitsu K, Irie H, Tajima T, Asayama Y, Hirakawa M et al (2008) Significance of perivascular soft tissue around the common hepatic and proximal superior mesenteric arteries arising after pancreaticoduodenectomy: evaluation with serial MDCT. Abdom Imaging 33:654–661

Ishigami K, Yoshimitsu K, Irie H, Tajima T, Asayama Y, Nishie A, Hirakawa M et al (2009) Diagnostic value of the delayed phase image for iso-attenuating pancreatic carcinomas in the pancreatic parenchymal phase on multidetector computed tomography. Eur J Radiol 69:139–146

Johnson PT, Curry CA, Urban BA, Fishman EK (2002) Spiral CT following the Whipple procedures: distinguish normal postoperative findings from complications. J Comput Assist Tomogr 26:956–961

Kim S, Lee NK, Lee JW, Won C et al (2007) CT evaluation of the bulging papilla with endoscopic correlation. RadioGraphics 27:1023–1038

Kondo H, Kanematsu M, Goshima S, Miyoshi T, Shiratori Y, Onozuka M, Moriyama N, Bae KT (2007) MDCT of the pancreas: optimizing scanning delay with a bolus-tracking technique for pancreatic, peripancreatic vascular, and hepatic contrast enhancement. Am J Roentgenol 188:751–756

Lall CG, Howard TJ, Skandaraja A, DeWitt JM, Aisen AM, Sandrasegaran K (2007) New concepts in staging and treatment of locally advanced pancreatic head cancer. Am J Roentgenol 189:1044–1050

Lawler LP, Horton KM, Fishman EK (2003) Peripancreatic masses that simulate pancreatic disease: spectrum of disease and role of CT. Radiographics 23:1117–1131

Lu DSK, Vedantham S, Krasny RM, Kadell B, Berger WL, Reber HA (1996) Two-phase helical CT for pancreatic tumors: pancreatic versus hepatic phase enhancement of tumor, pancreas and vascular structures. Radiology 199:697–701

Lu DSK, Reber HA, Krasny RM, Kadell BM, Sayre J (1997) Local staging of pancreatic cancer: criteria for unresectability of major vessels as revealed by pancreatic-phase, thin section helical CT. Am J Roentgenol 168:1439–1443

Mortelè KJ, Lemmerling M, de Hemptinne B et al (2000) Postoperative findings following the Whipple procedure: determination of prevalence and morphologic abdominal CT features. Eur Radiol 10:123–128

Nakayama Y, Yamashita Y, Kadota M et al (2001) Vascular encasement by pancreatic cancer: correlation of CT findings with surgical and pathological results. J Comput Assist Tomogr 25:337–342

Neoptolemos JP, Stocken DD, Dunn JA et al (2001) Influence of resection margins on survival for patients with pancreatic cancer treated by adjuvant chemoradiation and/or chemotherapy in the ESPAC-1 randomized controlled trial. Ann Surg 234:758–768

Nino-Murcia M, Jeffrey RB, Beualieau CF et al (2001) Multidetector CT of the ppancreas and bile duct system: value of curved planar. Am J Roentgenol 176:689–693

Park DI, Lee JK, kim J-E et al (2001) The analysis of resectability and survival in pancreatic cancer with vascular invasion. J Clin Gastroenterol 31:231–234

Pessaux P, Tuech JJ, Arnaud JP (2001) Prevention of pancreatic fistulas after surgical resection. A decade of clinical trials. Presse Méd 30:1359–1563

Procacci C, Graziani R, Zamboni G et al (1997) Cystic dystrophy of the duodenal wall: radiologic findings. Radiology 205:741–747

Prokesch RW, Chow LC, Beaulieu CF et al (2002a) Local staging of pancreatic carcinoma with multi-detector row CT: use of curved planar reformations-initial experience. Radiography 225:759–765

Prokesch RW, Chow LC, Beaulieu CF, Bammer R, Jeffrey RB (2002b) Isoattenuating pancreatic adenocarcinoma at multi–detector row CT: secondary signs. Radiology 224:764–768

Raptopoulos V, Steer ML, Sheiman RG et al (1997) The use of helical CT and CT angiography to predict vascular involvement from pancreatic cancer: correlation with findings at surgery. Am J Roentgenol 168:971–977

Ruf J, Lopez Hanninen E, Oettle H et al (2005) Detection of recurrent pancreatic cancer: comparison of FDG-PET with CT/MRI. Pancreatology 5:266–272

Schima W, Ba-Ssalamah A, Kolblinger C, Kulinna-Cosentini C et al (2007) Pancreatic adenocarcinoma. Eur Radiol 17: 638–649

Scialpi M, Scaglione M, Volterrani L, Lupattelli L, Ragozzino A, Romano S, Rotondo A (2005) Imaging evaluation of post pancreatic surgery. Eur J Radiol 53:417–424

Shioyama Y, Kimura M, Horihata K et al (2001) Peripancreatic arteries in thin section multislice helicall CT. Abdom Imaging 26:234–242

Tabuchi T, Itoh K, Ohshio G et al (1999) Tumor staging of pancreatic adenocarcinoma using early and late-phase helical CT. Am J Roentgenol 173:375–380

To'o KJ, Raman SS, Yu NC et al (2005) Pancreatic and peripancreatic diseases mimicking primary pancreatic neoplasia. Radiographics 25:949–965

Tunaci M (2004) Multidetector row CT of the pancreas. Eur J Radiol 52:18–30

Vargas R, Nino-Murcia M, Trueblood W, Jeffrey RB (2004) MDCT in pancreatic adenocarcinoma: prediction of vascular invasion and resectability using a multiphasic technique wiith curved planar reformations. Am J Roentgenol 182: 419–425

Visser BC, Muthusamay VR, Mulvihill SJ, Coakley F (2004) Diagnostic imaging of cystic pancreatic neoplasms. Surg Oncol 13:27–39

Wakabashi T, Kawaura Y, Satomura Y et al (2003) Clinical and imaging features of autoimmune pancreatitis with focal pancreatic swelling or mass formation: comparison with so-called tumor-forming pancreatitis and pancreatic adenocarcinoma. Am J Gastroenterol 98:2679–2687

Wang ZQ, Li JS, Lu GM, Zhang XH, Chen ZQ, Meng K (2003) Correlation of CT enhancement, tumor angiogenesis and pathologic grading of pancreatic carcinoma. World J Gastroenterol 9:2100–2104

Warshaw AL, Gu Z, Fernandez-del Castillo C (1992) Pancreatic carcinoma. N Engl J Med 326:455–465

Zeman RK, Cooper C, Zeiberg AS et al (1997) TNM staging of pancreatic carcinoma using helical CT. Am J Roentgenol 169:459–464

Zhongqiu W, Guangming L, Jieshou L, Xinhua Z, Ziqian C, Kui M (2004) The comparative study of tumor angiogenesis and CT enhancement in pancre-atic carcinoma. Eur J Radiol 49:274–280

The Case for MRI

Giovanni Morana, Raffaella Pozzi Mucelli, Giuseppe Granieri, and Christian Cugini

Contents

Abstract

> Recently MRI has gained an increased importance in the evaluation of pancreatic pathology and especially pancreatic tumors thanks to its capacity for noninvasively exploring the pancreatic parenchyma, ducts and vascular structures.

> The past limits due to movements artifacts, high acquisition time for T2w sequences and poor quality dynamic imaging are now swept away by several innovations, as rapid sequences, respiratory trigger compensation, fast high resolution sequences for dynamic imaging with contrast agent, 2D or 3D cholangio-pancreatography sequences with or without the use of secretin.

> State of the art MRI equipment with high field magnets, powerful and fast gradients, phased-array surface coils and dedicated sequences provides detailed information about a suspicious pancreatic mass, differentiating it from benign conditions.   MR-cholangiopancreatography sequence, with or without secretin, delineates its relations with the main pancreatic duct and the biliary tree, as well as the dynamic findings after secretin injection, useful in the differential diagnosis between benign and malignant strictures. Dynamic imaging with contrast agent allows staging of the tumor and, similarly to CT, determines if it is resectable or not.

> In this chapter these aspects will be extensively analyzed to provide a valid help to understand all the issues of this pathology and to obtain all the information, fundamental for the surgeon and the patient, from a complex examination as MRI seems to be.

G. Morana (✉), R. P. Mucelli, G. Granieri, and C. Cugini
Radiological Department, General Hospital Ca' Foncello,
Piazza Ospedale 1, 31100 Treviso, Italy
email: gmorana@ulss.tv.it

A. Laghi (ed.), *New Concepts in Diagnosis and Therapy of Pancreatic Adenocarcinoma*,
Medical Radiology, DOI: 10.1007/174_2010_52, © Springer-Verlag Berlin Heidelberg 2011

1 Introduction

MR Imaging has gained a leading role in the imaging of the pancreas thanks to most recent technical innovations with either breath hold T1 and T2 weighted images and respiratory triggered T2 weighted images, as well as dynamic imaging after injection of contrast material and with the use of secretin, allowing a great capacity for noninvasive exploration of the pancreatic ducts and pancreatic parenchyma, and imaging of the pancreatic vessels.

2 MR Technique

Actual MR Imaging of the pancreas requires the use of high-magnetic-field magnets, powerful and fast gradients, phased array surface coil, parallel imaging technology, and adapted sequences. The pancreas is explored both in T2- and T1-weighted sequences, in axial and coronal planes. MR imaging of the pancreas is able to provide multiple informations on pancreatic diseases, from morphology to signal intensity to vascularization to water diffusion, as well as ductal imaging with functional informations after secretin injection. With state of the art MR equipment a complete study of a pancreatic lesion can be conducted in about 30–40 min (Figs. 1–5).

2.1 T2-Weighted Sequences

2.1.1 Fast Spin-Echo (HASTE, RARE) Sequence

These are single-shot turbo spin-echo sequence with half acquisition of the K space with a short echo time (40–80 ms) and long echo time, in axial and coronal views. Each slice is acquired in approximately 1 s. Main features of this sequence are a low sensitivity to movement artifacts, which makes it suitable in non cooperative patients. Moreover, it has a great sensitivity to fluids, which appear highly hyperintense, either in the pancreas (pancreatic duct, cystic lesions) as well as around it (stomach and duodenal content; peripancreatic fluid collections). Its main disadvantages are a signal-to-noise ratio lower than the fast multishot spin-

echo sequence and slight blurring, which explains the lower sensitivity in detection of small, low-contrast solid lesions. The signal of the normal pancreas is equal to the liver signal or higher, whereas the ducts (biliary and pancreatic) appear highly hyperintense.

2.1.2 Conventional T2-Weighted Fast Spin-Echo Sequence

The most recent sequences are acquired with fat suppression and respiratory compensation. They clearly show liquid infiltrations in acute pancreatitis, but they are not really useful in the study of focal solid or cystic pancreatic lesions.

2.2 T1-Weighted Sequences

2.2.1 GRE T1-Weighted 2D Sequence with Fat Saturation

In the unenhanced imaging of the pancreas this is the sequence which best differentiates between normal and affected pancreas: the normal pancreas appears as homogeneously hyperintense. This behavior is attributed to the presence of large quantities of aqueous protein in the acini of the pancreas, the abundance of endoplasmic reticulum in the acinus cells, and the paramagnetic ion-rich content, notably manganese (Pamuklar and Semelka 2005; Hakimé et al. 2007). Fatty infiltration and fibrosis reduces the high signal of the pancreas. Focal or diffuse pancreatic disease appears as hypointense areas (Fig. 1b). Thus this sequence can be considered very sensitive to pancreatic diseases, but with a low capacity to differentiate between lesions (Figs. 1b and 5b).

2.2.2 GRE T1-Weighted 3D Sequence with Small Flip Angle, Interpolation, and Fat Saturation

This sequence has been suggested in the dynamic imaging after injection of gadolinium chelates; thanks to its excellent contrast after bolus injection of contrast agent and thin slices, it is possible to reconstruct the

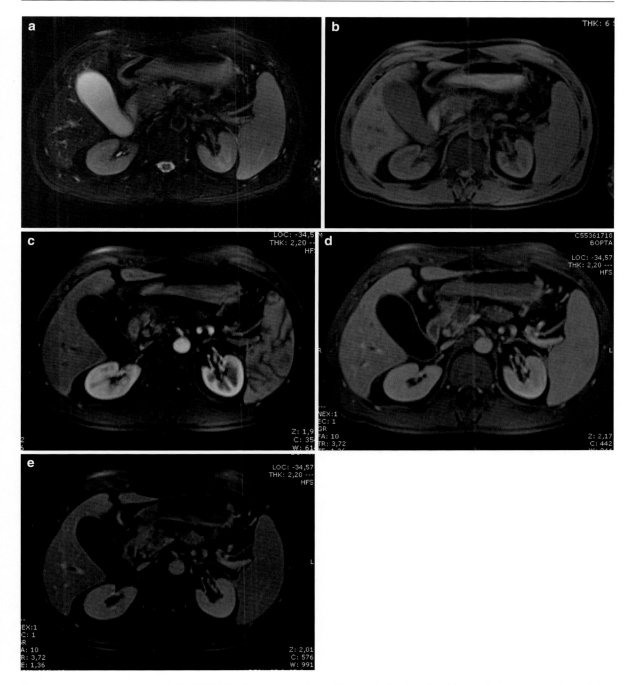

Fig. 1 Pancreatic carcinoma. (**a**) On TSE T2w fat suppressed image the pancreatic tumor appears as a slightly hypointense mass in the pancreatic head with irregular margins. (**b**) On T1w fat suppressed image the pancreatic tumor appears hypointense with irregular borders. (**c–e**) Dynamic imaging after bolus injection of paramagnetic contrast agent. The tumor appears hypointense either in the arterial phase (**c**), as well as in the venous (**d**), and distribution phase (**e**)

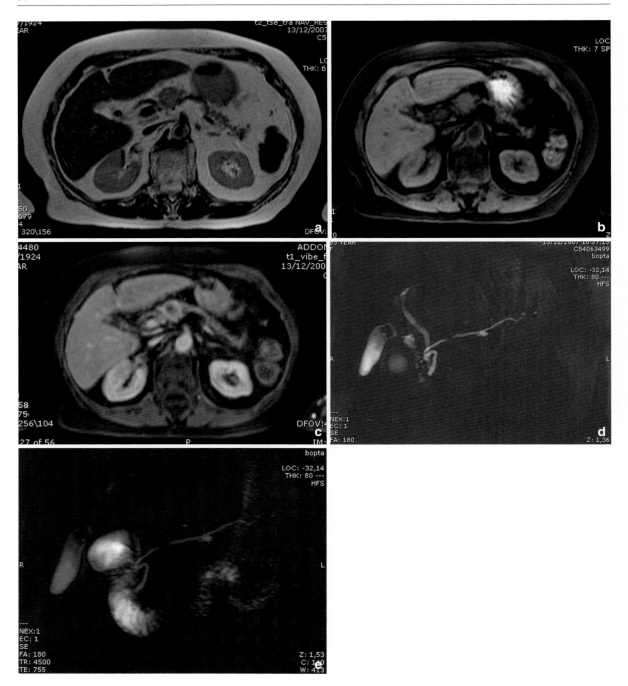

Fig. 2 Pancreatic carcinoma. (**a**) On TSE T2w image a small isointense pancreatic lesion in the pancreatic neck with slightly irregular borders can be appreciated. (**b**) On T1w fat saturated image the lesion appear hypointense. (**c**) After bolus injection of paramagnetic contrast agent the tumor appears hypointense with rim enhancement. (**d**) MRCP shows an abrupt stenosis of the MPD, highly suspicious for malignancy. (**e**) After secretin injection the stenosis of the MPD persists (negative duct penetrating sign), highly suspicious for malignancy

vessels with MIP or VR techniques. These sequences have been suggested to combine parenchyma and vascular imaging.

Dynamic imaging of the pancreas is necessary in the study of solid or cystic pancreatic lesions. After a test bolus in order to evaluate the correct timing of acquisition, an arterial, pancreatic (late arterial), venous and delayed sequences are consecutively acquired (Fig. 1c–e). Arterial phase (15–20 s after injection of contrast medium) is useful in the post processing, in order to evaluate the arterial tree in the pancreatic region, and in the evaluation of solid hypervascular lesions. In this phase pancreatic enhancement is greater than liver enhancement. The pancreatic phase is usually obtained about 15 s after the peak bolus in the

abdominal aorta (Kanematsu et al. 2000) and is useful in the identification of solid pancreatic lesions, as well as the venous phase (45 s after the injection of contrast medium). When looking for fibrous material (such as in groove pancreatitis), a delayed sequence can be added 10 min after injection of the contrast.

2.3 Diffusion Weighted Imaging (DWI)

DWI measures change in the microscopic diffusion of water due to Brownian motion. DW images are acquired with the single-shot echoplanar technique (SE-EPI-SSh), a spin-echo sequence to which two

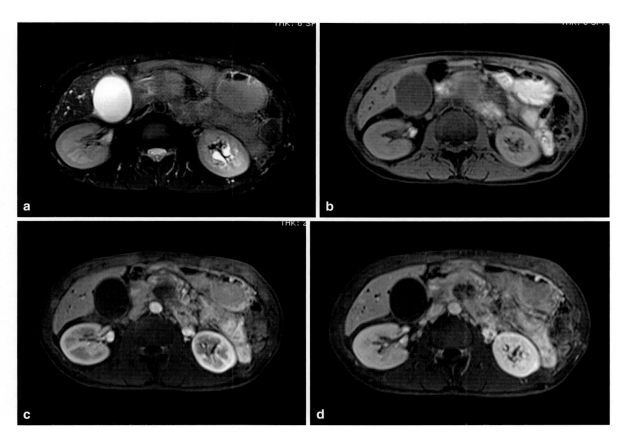

Fig. 3 Pancreatic carcinoma. (**a**) On TSE T2w fat suppressed image a large slightly hyperintense pancreatic lesion is appreciated in the body of the pancreas. (**b**) On T1w fat saturated sequence the lesion appear hypointense. (**c, d**) Dynamic imaging after bolus injection of paramagnetic contrast agent. The tumor appears hypointense either in the arterial phase (c) as well as in the venous (d) phase. (**e**) At MRCP an abrupt stenosis with upstream dilatation of both MPD and biliary duct ("double duct sign"), with atrophy of the pancreatic gland upstream and dilation of the main pancreatic duct. F-H. DWI at b0 (**f**), b 800 (**g**) and ADC map (**h**). The tumor appears highly hyperintense at high b-value (b = 800 s/mm^2) due to restricted free water molecules motions because of its high cellularity. The ADC map shows low values of the focal lesion in comparison to the normal pancreatic gland

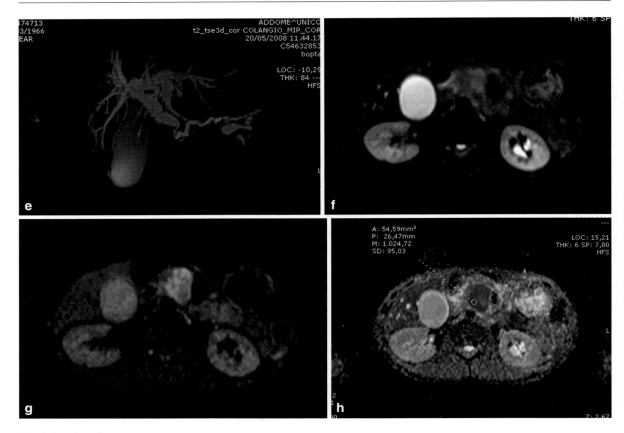

Fig. 3 (continued)

additional equal gradients but opposite in direction are added immediately before and after the 180° impulse. The amount of breadth and duration of the diffusion gradients influences the diffusion weighting of the sequence, defined by the factor b and expressed in seconds per millimeters squared (s/mm^2) (Colagrande et al. 2008). The sequence is generally repeated for various b values, resulting in the acquisition of different Diffusion Weight for each section of image. Finally, the different DW images are used to obtain the respective ADC maps which allow a quantitative analysis of the signal by positioning a ROI on the structure being studied.

DWI has been proposed as a diagnostic tool in neoplastic diseases based on the principle that malignant lesions have a denser cellularity with larger volume, with a reduction of the extracellular space leading to restriction of the free movement of water particles. This condition results in a lower ADC values and hyperintensity on diffusion-weighted (DW) images with high b values. On the contrary, benign lesions (such as benign tumors or inflammatory lesions) are characterized by an increase of the extracellular space, with conservation of the diffusion of water molecules, which is displayed as high ADC values and hypointensity on DW images with high b values.

Till recently DWI of the pancreas as well as upper abdomen has been of limited utility due to the presence of bulky physiologic motions: respiration movements, bowel peristalsis and blood flow hindered the application of the sequence due the long acquisition time. The recent application of parallel imaging as well as respiratory triggering has made the application of DWI in the upper abdomen part of the routine in the state of the art MR equipments (Kartalis et al. 2009).

However, some drawbacks have to be well known: the long TR of the acquisition gives to the sequences a T2 weight with low b value (0–50), which tends to disappear increasing the b value (>400), but still considerable even at higher b value, thus still giving a high

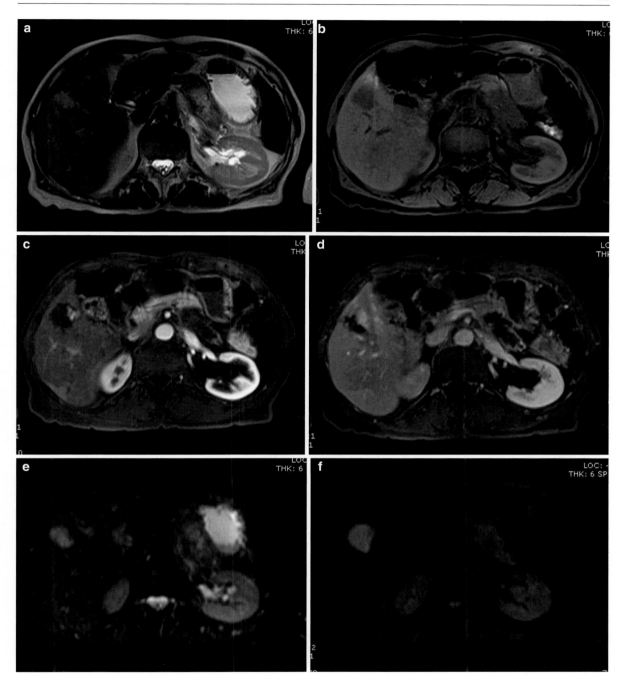

Fig. 4 Pancreatic carcinoma with necrotic changes. (**a**) On TSE T2w image a large oval irregularly shaped lesion with inhomogeneous high signal intensity is depicted in the pancreatic tail. (**b**) On unenhanced T1w fat suppressed image the lesion is homogeneously hypointense. (**c**, **d**) Dynamic imaging after bolus injection of paramagnetic contrast agent. The tumor appears hypointense either in the arterial phase (c), and markedly hypointense in the venous phase (d) due to the presence of necrosis. DWI at b0 (e), b 800 (f) and ADC map (g). The tumor appears highly hyperintense at high b-value (b = 800 s/mm²) due to restricted free water molecules motions because of its high cellularity. The ADC map shows low values of the focal lesion in comparison to the normal pancreatic gland

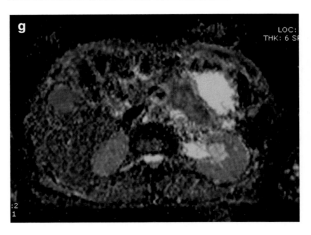

Fig. 4 (continued)

signal to water even in unrestricted conditions with high b values (T2 shine through).

Moreover with low b values, the signal is also dependent to capillary perfusion, while the importance of water diffusion increases with high b values (Colagrande et al. 2008). Thus, ADC represents microcirculation of blood (perfusion) as well as molecular diffusion of water, and some Authors suggest to calculate pure diffusion by using two high b values (500–1,000), thus eliminating the quota of perfusion (Lee at al. 2008). Normal pancreas on DWI shows a signal intensity similar to that of the liver in the different b values (Fig. 6). ADC value of normal pancreas has been reported to be higher than those of pancreatic cancer and mass-forming pancreatitis (Lee et al. 2008; Matsuki et al. 2007).

2.4 MR Cholangiopancreatography (MRCP)

Highly T2-weighted sequences render static fluid or slow-flow structures very hyperintense with a very low signal from solid structures. Different and complementary approaches are used: 2D T2w single shot fast spin echo, thick and/or thin multi-slice sequences, and 3D T2w.

2D T2w thick-slab sequence has usually a width of 40–70 mm in order to comprise all the pancreatic duct. It can be obtained in all planes although it is generally acquired in the coronal plane and only requires a less than 3-s breath hold. It provides excellent biliary and

pancreatic mapping, with no respiratory artifacts and few susceptibility artifacts and good planar resolution. Better quality of the images are obtained after oral administration of superparamagnetic contrast agent, such as true contrast agent (1 mL gadolinium chelate in 250 mL water) or fruit juice (pineapple, blueberry, cranberry, etc.), which lower the signal of the fluid content of the stomach and duodenum (Fig. 7a, b). The IV administration of paramagnetic contrast agent gives a superior image quality of MRCP thanks to the T2* effect of gadolinium, which suppresses the overlapping vessel signals as well as the signal from liquids in the interstitial compartment of the pancreatic gland, while the signal from the ducts is unaffected (Fig. 7c) (Takahashi et al. 2000).

2D T2w thin-slab sequence is the HASTE sequence described above, consisting in a series of 4- to 6-mm contiguous slices acquired with a shorter echo time and echo train than thicker slices. This sequence therefore visualizes not only the ducts, but also the solid organs.

Moreover, 3D T2w techniques have been implemented with respiratory triggering and free breathing, which provide a very high spatial resolution and a isotropic voxel, allowing a multi view approach thanks to multiplanar and postprocessing capabilities of the acquired slices; images are of superior quality and give better delineation of pancreaticobiliary anatomy than conventional 2D images (Zhang et al. 2006).

2.5 Secretin MRCP (S-MRCP)

Administration of secretin stimulates the production of fluid and bicarbonate by the exocrine pancreas with an increase of the flow rate of the pancreas almost immediately and for a few minutes after. At the same time an increase in Oddi's sphincter (SO) tone is appreciated. In normal subjects, an increase in the main duct pressure is observed after 1 min with an almost complete return to baseline values after 5 min, after reversion of SO contraction (Matos et al. 2002). The rise in the fluid volume of the main pancreatic duct (MPD) makes it more clearly visualized at MRCP. Serial acquisition of pancreatic duct with 2D thick slab sequence with a time interval of 30″–60″ for 15 min after IV administration of 1 mL/kg bw secretin gives a dynamic visualization of the pancreatic response to secretin (Manfredi et al. 2000; Akisik et al. 2006; Fukukura et al. 2002).

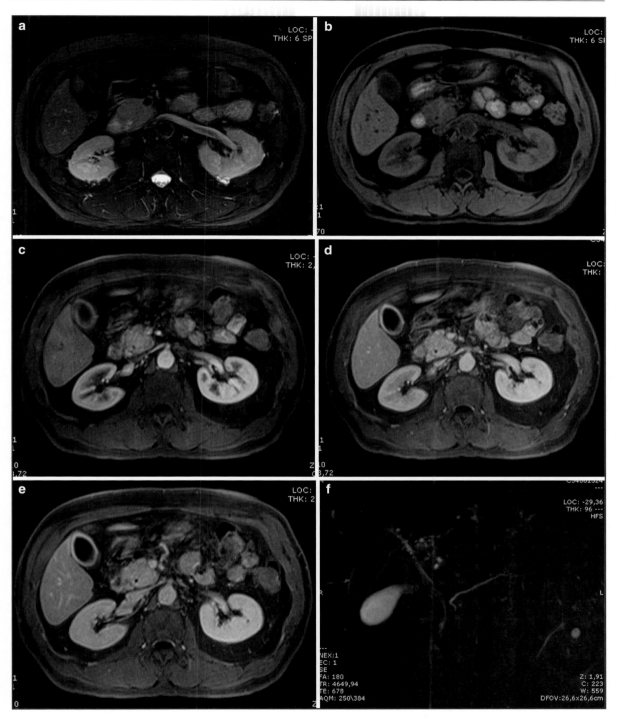

Fig. 5 Chronic sclerosing pancreatitis of the head of the pancreas. (**a**) On TSE T2w image a large lesion with low signal intensity can be appreciated in the head of the pancreas. (**b**) On unenhanced T1w fat suppressed image the lesion is homogeneously hypointense. (**c–e**) Dynamic imaging after bolus injection of paramagnetic contrast agent. The lesion shows progressive contrast enhancement in the arterial (c), venous (d) and distribution phase (e). At MRCP (**f**) the Wirsung's duct cannot be appreciated at the level of the lesion, with upstream dilation. DWI at b0 (**g**), b 800 (**h**) and ADC map (**i, l**). The lesion does not show significant hyperintensity at high b-value (b = 800 s/mm²) due to fibrous component. However the ADC map (i) shows low values of the focal lesion in comparison to the normal pancreatic gland (l), which shows normal signal intensity at unenhanced T1w fat suppressed image (**m**)

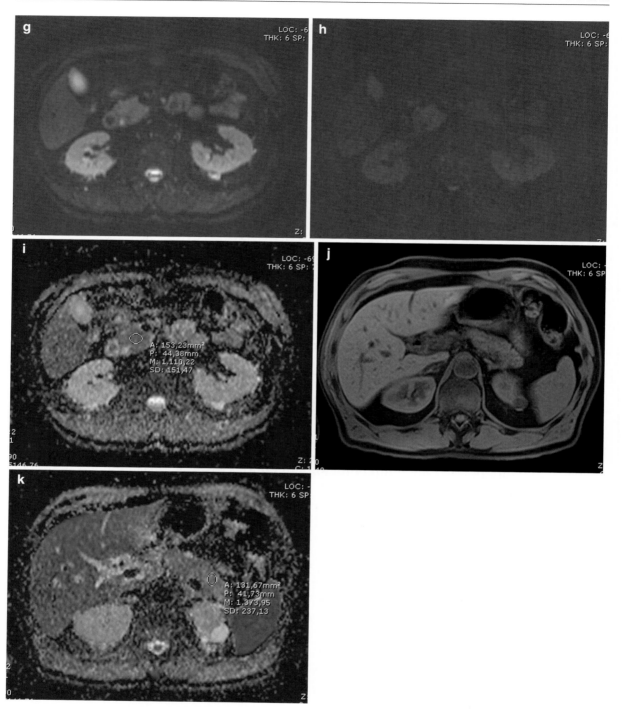

Fig. 5 (continued)

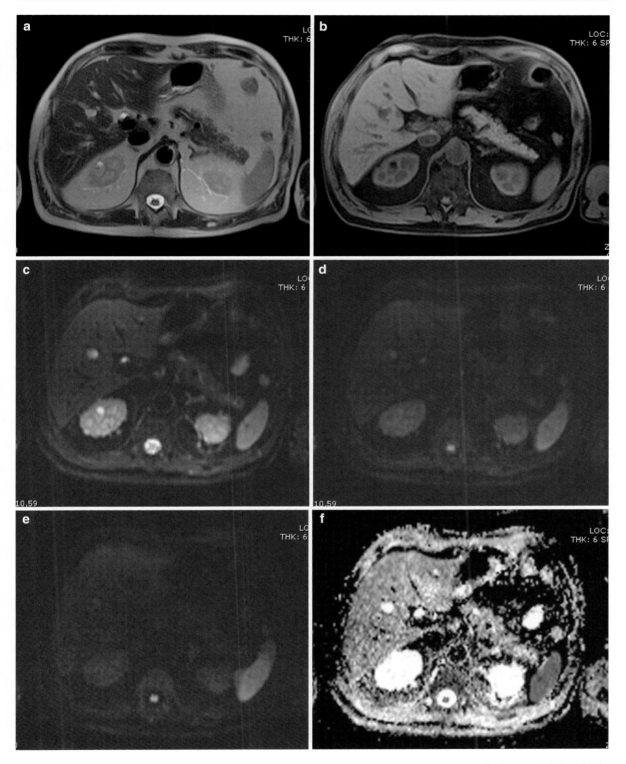

Fig. 6 Normal pancreas. The pancreas show a signal intensity similar to that of the liver either on TSE T2w image (**a**), T1w with fat saturation (**b**), DWI b0 (**c**), DWI b 400 (**d**), DWI b 800 (**e**) and ADC map (**f**). In the liver an hemangioma can be appreciated

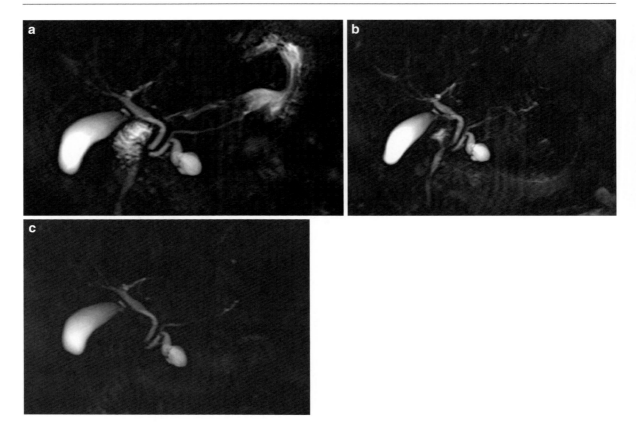

Fig. 7 MCRP with 2D T2w thick-slab sequence provides an excellent evaluation of biliary and pancreatic ducts anatomy, without respiratory artifacts (**a**); the administration of oral superparamagnetic contras agent (such as pineapple juice) improves the quality of the image, as it lowers the signal of the fluid content of stomach and duodenum (**b**). The intravenous administration of paramagnetic contrast agent allows superior image quality of MRCP (**c**). A large IPMT of the secondary duct in the uncinate process can be appreciated

The advantages of secretin MRI are therefore both morphological and functional:

Morphological: better visualization of the MPD, easier detection of the anatomical variants, such as pancreas divisum; clear depiction of obstruction, stenosis, dilatation and irregular contours of the duct. As a whole secretin MRCP increases the negative predictive value of MR imaging of the pancreas (Hellerhoff et al. 2002).

Functional: visualization of side branches at body-tail after secretin is a sign of early chronic pancreatitis; an abnormally prolonged dilatation of the MPD (>3 mm 10 min after secretin injection) indicates a deficit of pancreatic juice outflow; the parenchymogram (parenchymal enhancement) is a sign of recurrent acute pancreatitis; a reduced duodenal filling suggests a decrease of pancreatic exocrine reserve.

3 MR Features of Pancreatic Carcinoma

3.1 Identification

The gross pathological features of pancreatic carcinoma are represented by a mass with irregular ill-defined contour with a significant fibrous component, and less frequently necrotic changes. Lack of capsule is responsible for early spread of the lesion to the surrounding structures, with special regard to vascular and neural infiltration.

On unenhanced MR imaging, pancreatic carcinoma shows a slightly different signal on T2w images from the surrounding pancreas, from minimally hypointense (Fig. 1a) to isointense (Fig. 2a) to slightly hyperintense

(Fig. 3a), making it difficult to be identified when small. In case of necrotic or cystic degeneration of the lesion, these can be easily identified due to their hyperintensity on T2w images (Fig. 4a) (Balci and Semelka 2001). T2w images with fat saturation are considered useful in the staging of the lesion, for the evaluation of lymph node and peritoneal or hepatic metastases (Zhong et al. 2007), where MRI is considered more sensitive in comparison to MDCT (Schima et al. 2007; Miller et al. 2006).

With MRCP the stenosis of the MPD can be easily identified with dilation upstream (Fig. 8) (Sahani et al. 2008; Miller et al. 2006; Matos et al. 2002); in case of tumor in the head of the pancreas, a stenosis of the intrapancreatic biliary duct can be seen, with dilation upstream as well as the stenosis of both biliary and pancreatic duct ("double duct sign": Figs. 3e and 9) (Lopez Hänninen et al. 2002).

However, stenosis of the biliary duct and MPD can be appreciated also in case of chronic pancreatitis or inflammatory duodenal lesions (Manfredi et al. 2000). An abrupt stenosis with sharp margins is indicative of a malignant stenosis (Fig. 2d), while an irregular shape with severe dilation, mural irregularity and obstructions is more indicative for a chronic inflammation of the pancreas (Fig. 10). Moreover, secondary duct dilation is more frequently seen in case of pancreatic carcinoma instead of other tumors in the periampullary region (Kim et al. 2002).

On T1w images pancreatic carcinoma usually appears as a mass of low signal in comparison to the normal pancreas (Figs. 1b, 2b, 3b, and 4b). Moreover, the obstruction of the MPD is responsible for a chronic obstructive pancreatitis of the pancreatic gland upstream, which has the same low signal on T1w imaging, masquerading the real extension of the tumor making it indiscernible from the pancreatic tumor on T2w and especially on T1w images (Hakimé et al. 2007). Later, the obstruction of the MPD is responsible for the dilation of the duct and the atrophy of the pancreatic gland upstream (Fig. 3e).

On dynamic imaging after injection of paramagnetic contrast agent, the presence of an abundant fibrous stroma within the tumor makes the tumor hypovascular, thus appearing hypointense to the surrounding parenchyma (Figs. 1c–e, 2c, and 3c, d), but it can be responsible for a delayed enhancement with secondary isointensity of the lesion (Fig. 8c, d) (Miller et al. 2006). Isointensity of the tumor to the surrounding parenchyma as well as coexisting or secondary chronic pancreatitis upstream can make the identification of the tumor as well as differential diagnosis with chronic pancreatitis difficult (Birchard et al. 2005; Zins et al. 2005). Some Authors suggest that time-intensity curve of the lesion is useful for the differential diagnosis between the pancreatic carcinoma and mass-forming pancreatitis (Tajima et al. 2007). Hata and Colleagues have correlated the enhancement pattern on CT with the vessel density and the amount of fibrous stroma; results of the study suggest a direct correlation between vessel density and fibrous content and the amount of enhancement (Hata et al. 2010). Same results were obtained by Johnson et al. (1999) with MR.

Diffusion Weighted Imaging: ADC values of the tissues are dependent on the cellularity and amount of tissue fibrosis. Pancreatic carcinoma in most papers shows a restricted diffusion of free water with high (>500) b values, thus appearing hyperintense on DW images at high b value (Figs. 3g and 9f). ADC maps show low values of the tumor in comparison to normal pancreatic parenchyma (Figs. 3h and 9g) (Fattahi et al. 2009). However, similar findings have been described also with benign inflammatory lesions (Fig. 5i). The low ADC value of pancreatic cancer and mass-forming pancreatitis may stem from its high cellularity and abundant fibrosis, common histopathological features of pancreatic cancer and mass-forming pancreatitis (Lee et al. 2008). In chronic pancreatitis, fibrosis and chronic inflammation lead to destruction and permanent loss of exocrine pancreatic tissue, with replacement of normal pancreatic parenchyma with fibrous tissue which may reduce the diffusion of tissue water and result in decreased measured ADCs (Akisik et al. 2009). In autoimmune pancreatitis, the lymphocytic infiltration of the pancreatic gland cause a restriction of the movement of free water, with a signal on DW images and ADC maps similar to pancreatic carcinoma (Fig. 11). Lee et al. (2008) reported a significantly lower ADC values for mass-forming pancreatitis compared with those for pancreatic cancer. High b values (up to 1,000) are requested in order to obtain a good differentiation between benign and malignant solid lesions (Tsushima et al. 2007), although with high b value there is a decrease in signal-to-noise ratio. However, still doubt remains about the reproducibility of these results (Braithwaite et al. 2009). Moreover, the overall diagnostic performance of these parameters in differentiating pancreatic cancer

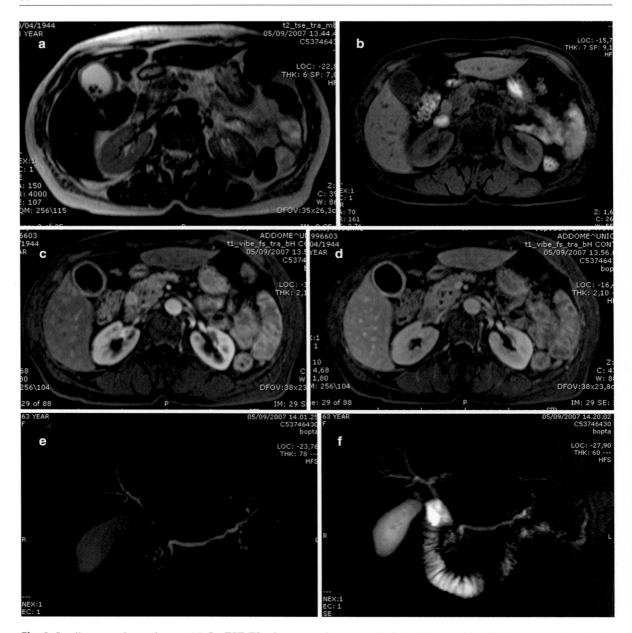

Fig. 8 Small pancreatic carcinoma. (**a**) On TSE T2w image a small lesion with high signal intensity can be appreciated in the head of the pancreas. (**b**) On unenhanced T1w fat suppressed image the lesion is homogeneously hypointense. (**c, d**) Dynamic imaging after bolus injection of paramagnetic contrast agent. The lesion is hypointense in the arterial phase (c), to become isointense in the venous phase (d). During arterial phase a round hypervascular lesion is appreciated in the groove region, due to normal pancreatic parenchyma whose drainage is not hampered by the Wirsung's stenosis (via Santorini duct). At MRCP (**e**) the Wirsung's duct cannot be appreciated at the level of the lesion, with upstream dilation. After injection of Secretin the stenosis of the Wirsung's duct still persists (**f**)

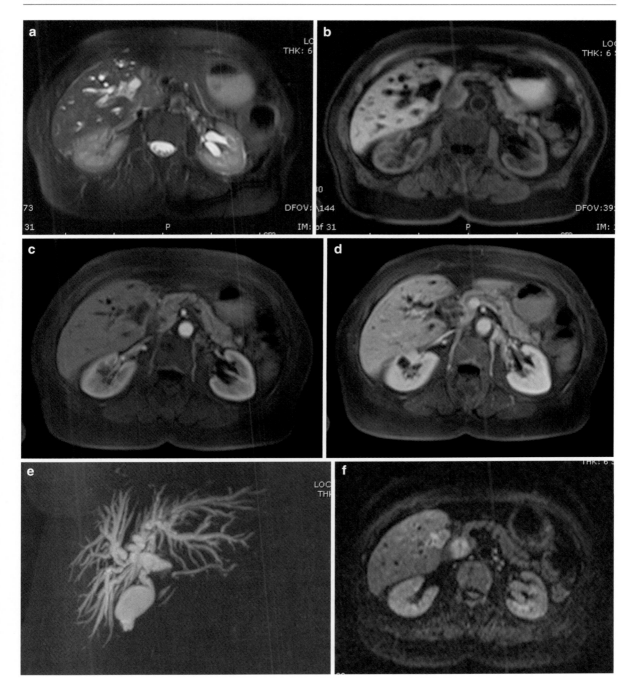

Fig. 9 Pancreatic carcinoma. (**a**) On TSE T2w image an isointense lesion can be appreciated in the head of the pancreas. (**b**) On unenhanced T1w fat suppressed image the lesion is homogeneously hypointense. (**c, d**) Dynamic imaging after bolus injection of paramagnetic contrast agent. The lesion is hypointense either in the arterial (c) as well as in the venous phase (d). At MRCP (**e**) a "double duct" sign can be appreciated, with upstream dilation of both the choledocus and Wirsung's duct. DWI at b 800 (**f**) and ADC map (**g**). The lesion shows significant hyperintensity at high b-value due to high cellularity. The ADC map shows low values of the focal lesion in comparison to the normal pancreatic gland at the level of the tail

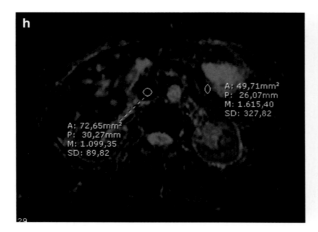

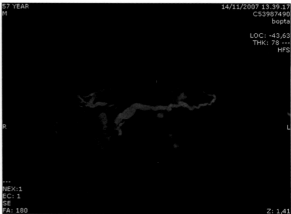

Fig. 9 (continued)

Fig. 10 Chronic pancreatitis. MRCP image depicts a highly dilated MPD with "corona di rosario" appearance, suggestive for benign chronic inflammation

from mass-forming pancreatitis was similar to or slightly inferior to those of various diagnostic examinations reported in previous studies, with sensitivities ranging from 72.3% to 87.2% and specificities from 61.5% to 76.9%. Further study is required to evaluate the actual additional values of the quantitative analysis of DWI for differentiating pancreatic cancer from mass-forming pancreatitis compared with the values of conventional anatomic imaging studies (Lee et al. 2009).

3.2 Differential Diagnosis

A variety of non-neoplastic and neoplastic abnormalities may mimic pancreatic adenocarcinoma. A lesion whose location suggests a pancreatic origin requires a correct differential diagnosis (To'o et al. 2005). The complex structure of the pancreas and the anatomical relationship between the gland and surrounding organs and structures, is often a diagnostic challenge in differentiating between a primary pancreatic neoplastic process, a flogistic lesion and a peripancreatic abnormality.

3.2.1 Focal Chronic Pancreatitis

The most common mass-like lesion that simulates a pancreatic adenocarcinoma is a focal chronic pancreatitis.

Chronic pancreatitis is a rare disease (7–10 persons/100,000/year) (Kawaguchi et al. 1991), characterized

by fibro-inflammatory changes to the pancreatic tissue. It may develop in association with alcohol abuse, smoking, gene mutations, autoimmune syndromes, metabolic disturbances, environmental conditions and anatomical abnormalities. The largest number of patients is found in industrialized countries and approximately 80% of them are alcoholics. Patients with this disease have an increased risk of developing a pancreatic cancer later in life, especially if they have an hereditary form of chronic pancreatitis that starts very early in life.

The pathology of chronic pancreatitis was considered to be uniform, but currently it is more seen as varying according to the etiology of the disease. The rather vague term of "chronic sclerosing pancreatitis" should be replaced by etiologically derived terms such as "alcoholic chronic pancreatitis," "hereditary chronic pancreatitis," "obstructive chronic pancreatitis," "autoimmune pancreatitis," "paraduodenal pancreatitis" (groove pancreatitis, cystic dystrophy of heterotopic pancreas) (Klöppel 2007).

For the pathogenesis it is important to note that alcoholic chronic pancreatitis, hereditary chronic pancreatitis and paraduodenal pancreatitis evolve from recurrent acute pancreatitis.

Chronic pancreatitis can be associated with a range of anatomic abnormalities of the pancreas, including atrophy or enlargement of the organ, ductal dilatation and calcifications.

Approximately 20% of patients with chronic pancreatitis develop a focal inflammatory mass (Schima et al. 2007), which may closely mimic a pancreatic

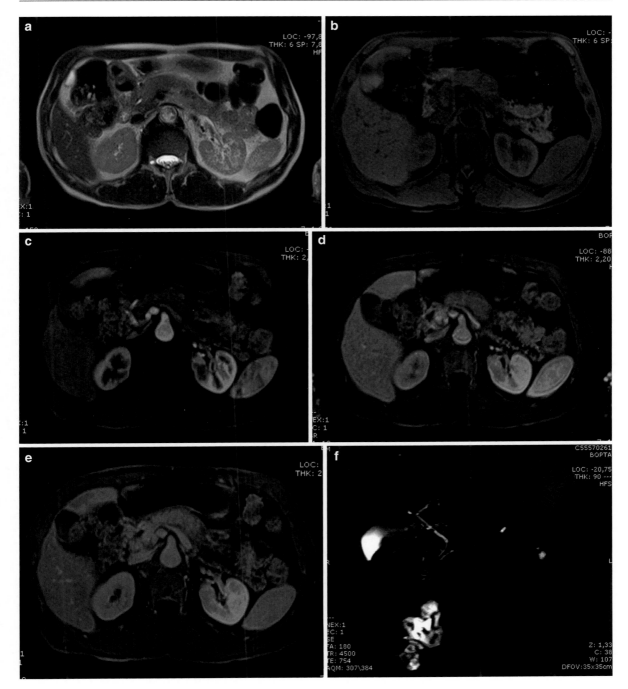

Fig. 11 Autoimmune pancreatitis. (**a**) On TSE T2w image a large lesion with intermediate signal intensity can be appreciated in the body of the pancreas. (**b**) On unenhanced T1w fat suppressed image the lesion is homogeneously hypointense. (**c–e**) Dynamic imaging after bolus injection of paramagnetic contrast agent. The lesion shows progressive contrast enhancement in the arterial (**c**), venous (**d**), and distribution phase (**e**). At MRCP (**f**) the Wirsung's duct is markedly narrowed with irregular shape, even if it penetrates the mass. DWI at b 600 (**g**) and ADC map (**h, i**). The lesion shows significant hyperintensity at high b-value due to high cellularity. The ADC map shows low values of the focal lesion (**h**) in comparison to the normal pancreatic gland (**i**), which shows normal signal intensity at unenhanced T1w fat suppressed image (**l**)

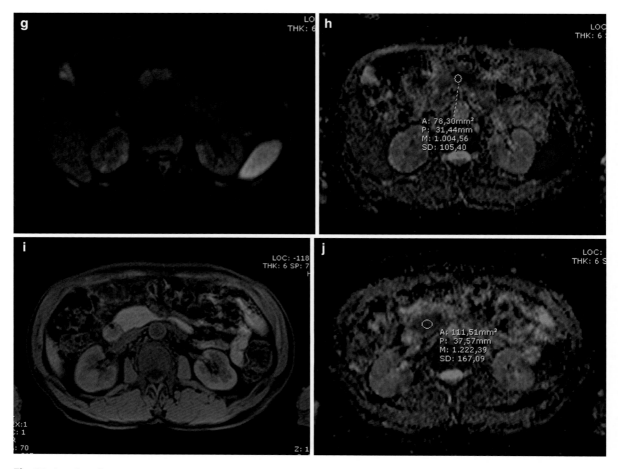

Fig. 11 (continued)

cancer (Fig. 20). In this case the differential diagnosis becomes an important diagnostic challenge for the radiologist because of its clinical relevance: firstly, patients with chronic pancreatitis have higher risk of developing pancreatic adenocarcinoma; secondly, subjects with pancreatic adenocarcinoma often develop chronic pancreatitis related to duct obstruction by the neoplastic mass, even a small one.

These two entities may be virtually indistinguishable on the basis of morphologic features or enhancement pattern at MR; both of them show hypointensity on unenhanced T1-weighted fat-suppressed images, hypovascularity in pancreatic arterial phase and delayed enhancement with isointensity in venous and equilibrium phases, due to the presence of an abundant fibrous stroma both in adenocarcinoma and in focal pancreatitis (Fig. 20) (Miller et al. 2006).

In chronic pancreatitis, there are often calcifications that are rarely present in adenocarcinoma, even if the detection of calcifications, especially if tiny, can be hard on MRI, as they appear as signal voids.

Furthermore, inflammatory changes in chronic pancreatitis may result in local lymphadenopathy, peripancreatic fat stranding and vessel involvement.

Some authors have proposed the use of Mangafodipir trisodium (Mn-DPDP) in the evaluation of focal pancreatic lesion. Mn-DPDP is a contrast agent that after intravenous infusion is uptaken by functioning hepatocytes and has also a significant uptake into the pancreatic gland. It shortens the T1 relaxation time, leading to an increase in signal intensity of targeting tissues on T1-weighted images. Signal intensity enhancement lasts for several hours. The rational of its use in pancreatic lesions assessing is that there is a very little uptake of the agent into pancreatic tumors compared to the normal pancreatic tissue, but it was shown that in the differentiation between focal pancreatitis and adenocarcinoma this contrast agent could not be conclusive, as the inflammatory alterations may results in lack of Mn-DPDP uptake, mimicking a tumor (Schima et al. 2002). Furthermore at the time in which this chapter was written, the production of Mn-DPDP was suspended and it is not anymore available for the clinical use.

MRCP is an important tool in the differentiation of most of these pancreatic lesions. Morphologic change of the MPD may be one of the most useful factor for distinguishing a focal chronic pancreatitis from an adenocarcinoma. The most characteristic findings for cancer, derived from ERCP semeiotic, are complete obstruction of the MPD and dilatation of the upper stream of the MPD (Fig. 2d). In contrast, a non obstructed MPD penetrates the mass more frequently in focal chronic pancreatitis and this sign is called "duct penetrating sign" (Fig. 11f), although stenotic change of the intralesional portion of the MPD, dilatation of its upper stream and obstruction of small side branches may not be rare (Fig. 5f).

Even in case of complete obstruction of Wirsung's duct, after injection of secretin, the "duct penetrating sign" on MRCP images is more frequently observed in a focal inflammatory lesion (Fig. 12) than in cancer (Figs. 2d, e), with a sensitivity of 85% and specificity of 96%; if the "duct penetrating sign" is defined as only normal MPD penetrating the mass, the specificity raises to 100%, although the sensitivity is 36% (Ichikawa et al. 2001). However, overlapping between benign and malignant stenosis can be observed (Fig. 11).

DWI sequences may be an additional tool in the evaluation of a pancreatic mass and in its differential diagnosis, with most of pancreatic cancers having high signal intensity respect to low signal intensity of mass-forming chronic pancreatitis on high b-value DWI images. Significantly different ADC values, higher for pancreatic cancer have been reported (Takeuchi et al. 2008), although overlap can be observed (Figs. 3h, 5i, and 9g).

3.2.2 Groove Pancreatitis (Paraduodenal Pancreatitis, Cystic Dystrophy of Heterotopic Pancreas)

Clinically this rare type of pancreatitis is found predominantly in male patients (40–50 years) with a history of alcohol abuse. The clinical setting is similar to the usual form of chronic pancreatitis, but recurrent vomiting, due to duodenal stenosis and impaired motility, tends to be more pronounced in groove pancreatitis. Jaundice is not usual and if present often fluctuates. Amylase serum levels may be elevated (Blasbalg et al. 2007).

Histologically, there is thickening and scarring of the duodenal wall, particularly in the area corresponding to the minor papilla, that extend to the adjacent pancreatic tissue and/or cystic changes in the duodenal wall. The cysts contain clear fluid but sometimes granular white material and even stones can be found. Occasionally, some of the cysts may have diameter of several centimeters. The fibrotic tissue that develops in the duodenal wall also involves the groove between the duodenum and the pancreatic head, which may compress and indent the common bile duct.

Even if alcohol abuse appears as an important risk factor, the location of the inflammatory process, that resides in the duodenal submucosa, in the duodenal wall and in the adjacent pancreatic tissue, suggests that there may be some anatomic variation in the region of the minor papilla that makes this area particularly susceptible to alcohol injury. It is conceivable that the fluids outflow may be obstructed at the level of the minor papilla, as in some cases of "pancreas divisum." The frequent presence of the so-called heterotopic pancreatic tissue in the duodenal wall may reflect the incomplete involution of the dorsal pancreas in this region and contribute to an obstruction of the outflow in this area (Klöppel 2007).

Groove pancreatitis is usually classified into pure and segmental forms (Stolte et al. 1982). The pure form affects exclusively the groove; the segmental form extends to the pancreatic head despite a clear predominance in the groove.

The most characteristic finding on MRI is a sheet-like mass between the head of pancreas and the C-loop of duodenum (the so-called groove). The mass is hypointense to pancreatic parenchyma on T1-weighted images and can be hypo-, iso- or slightly hyperintense on T2-weighted images (Fig. 13). This variation in T2 signal can be attributed to the time of onset of the disease because subacute disease shows brighter T2 images due to edema, while chronic disease has a lower signal due to fibrosis (Blasbalg et al. 2007). Fat-suppressed T1-weighted images reveal the best delineation of the pancreatic head (normal hyperintensity, if the pancreatic head is spared as in the pure form) from the hypointense mass in the pancreatico-duodenal groove (Fig. 13b) (Castell-Monsalve et al. 2008).

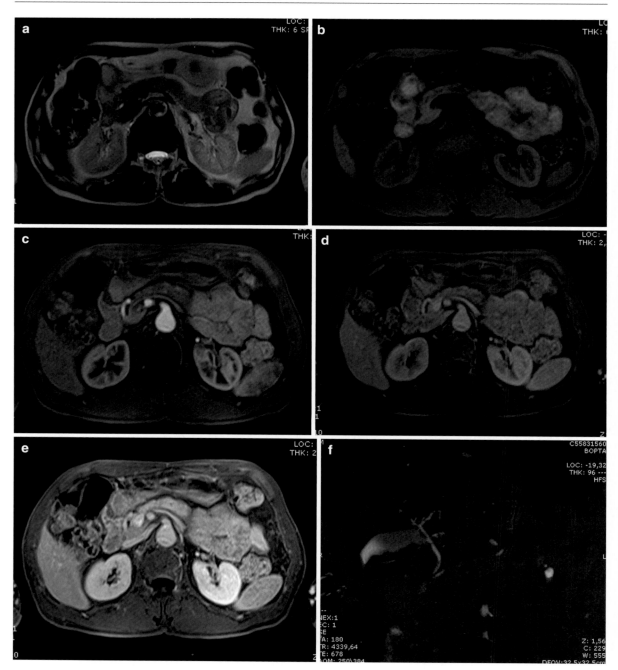

Fig. 12 Autoimmune pancreatitis, same patient of Fig. 11, 6 months after steroid therapy. (**a**) On TSE T2w image the lesion is smaller with normal signal intensity. (**b**) On unenhanced T1w fat suppressed image the lesion is slightly hypointense. (**c–e**) Dynamic imaging after bolus injection of paramagnetic contrast agent. The lesion shows progressive contrast enhancement in the arterial (**c**), venous (**d**), and distribution phase (**e**). At MRCP (**f**) the Wirsung's duct is still markedly narrowed; however after secretin injection (**g**) the duct shows a good response with enlargement at the level of the lesion ("duct penetrating sign"). DWI at b 600 (**h**) and ADC map (**i**). The lesion shows isointensity at high b-value. The ADC map shows high values of the focal lesion (i) in comparison to the normal pancreatic gland

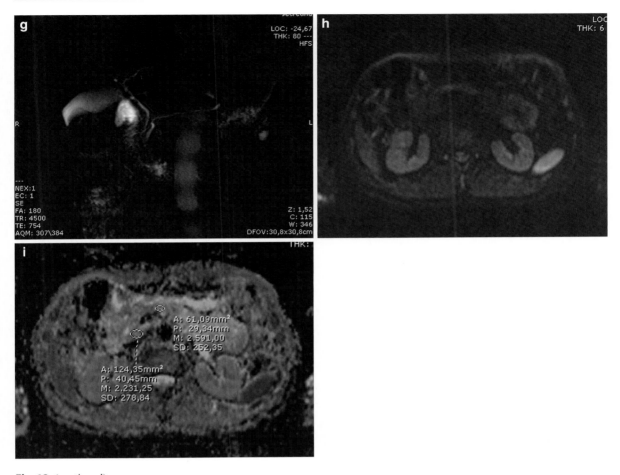

Fig. 12 (continued)

Contrast-enhanced dynamic images show a delayed and progressive enhancement in the late phase that reflects the fibrous nature of the tissue (Fig. 13c, d).

When pancreatic head or the entire gland is involved, hypointensity on T1-weighted images is observed; in groove pancreatitis usually the MPD is normal. A ductal dilatation with secondary ducts ectasia is seen in some patients, when groove pancreatitis and diffuse chronic inflammatory disease are both present (Fig. 13e). Some patients may present with focal enlargement of the pancreatic head.

Cystic lesions are well depicted in the groove or in the duodenal wall, especially in T2-weighted images (Fig. 13e). MRCP helps to show the relationship between the ductal system and the cystic changes.

Usually the duodenal wall is thickened and this sign should be carefully searched, as it is not commonly associated with tumors in the pancreatic head.

Sometimes the common bile duct appears stenotic, but this tapering is characteristically regular in contrast to the abrupt aspect of stenosis in pancreatic cancer (Fig. 13e) (Blasbalg et al. 2007).

An important differentiating point is the absence of vascular encasement in groove pancreatitis, with leftward vascular (gastroduodenal artery) displacement without obstruction (Fig. 13c); pancreatic carcinoma extending to the groove or duodenal wall invades along peripancreatic vessels (Castell-Monsalve et al. 2008).

3.2.3 Autoimmune Pancreatitis

Autoimmune pancreatitis is a special type of chronic pancreatitis. It is a relatively new entity and it has been increasingly recognized. It has a prevalence of 1–6%

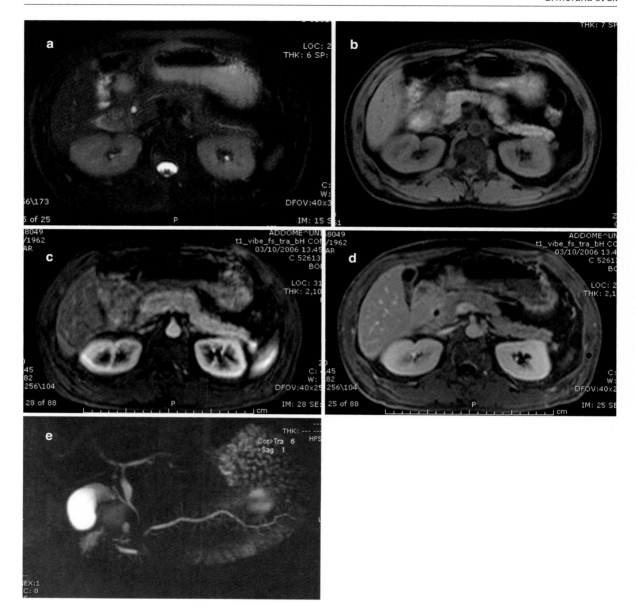

Fig. 13 Groove pancreatitis. (**a**) HASTE image shows a small cyst in the head of the pancreas. (**b**) On unenhanced T1w fat suppressed image a "sheet-like" mass with regular borders between the pancreatic head and the C-loop of the duodenum can be appreciated. (**c, d**) dynamic imaging after bolus injection of paramagnetic contrast agent. The lesion shows progressive contrast enhancement in the arterial (c) to distribution phase (d). At MRCP (**e**) the Wirsung's duct is markedly narrowed with dilation upstream also of the secondary ducts, sign of obstructive chronic pancreatitis

of cases of chronic pancreatitis (Pearson et al. 2003). Most of the affected patients are 40–60 years old, with a strong male preponderance. There is an association between autoimmune pancreatitis and other autoimmune disorders such as Crohn's disease, Sjögren's syndrome, rheumatoid arthritis, primary sclerosing cholangitis, primary biliary cirrhosis, ulcerative colitis, systemic lupus erythematous and retroperitoneal fibrosis (Okazaki and Chiba 2002).

Clinical symptoms are nonspecific and include abdominal pain, weight loss, anorexia, recent-onset diabetes, absence of alcohol excess and jaundice. Jaundice is caused by direct involvement of the bile duct by the fibro-inflammatory process and occurs in about 75–80% of the cases (Klöppel 2007). Recently it has been observed that IgG4 levels are commonly elevated in patients with autoimmune pancreatitis. A good response to steroid therapy has been described (Kuroiwa et al. 2002).

The pathologic gross appearance of autoimmune pancreatitis mimics pancreatic ductal adenocarcinoma because the inflammatory process commonly focuses on the head of the pancreas and leads to a gray to yellowish-white induration of the affected tissue with loss of its normal lobular structure. The involved portion may be enlarged. These changes cause obstruction of the MPD and usually also of the distal bile duct, including the papilla. In a minority of cases, body or tail of the pancreas are involved. Diffuse involvement of the pancreas may also be seen. In contrast to other types of pancreatitis, there are no pseudocysts. The hallmark of the histological changes is an intense inflammatory cell infiltration

of lymphocytes, plasma cells, some macrophages and eosinophilic granulocytes. Frequently there is a vasculitis affecting the small veins; less commonly there is an obliterative arteritis (Klöppel 2007). Pancreatic calcifications are absent in AIP (Klöppel 2007), although pancreatic stone formation in some patients with AIP has been seen, suggesting that autoimmune pancreatitis has the potential of being a progressive disease with pancreatic stones (Takayama et al. 2004).

At MR imaging there is an enlargement of the pancreas, which is usually diffuse ("sausage shape": Figs. 14 a, b) but can be focal (Fig. 11), with a hypointense capsule-like rim that is smooth and well-defined due to peripancreatic inflammation and fibrosis (Fig. 14a). In some cases a minimal peripancreatic fat stranding can be seen (Sahani et al. 2004). On T2-weighted images the pancreas shows an increased signal intensity compared with the signal intensity of

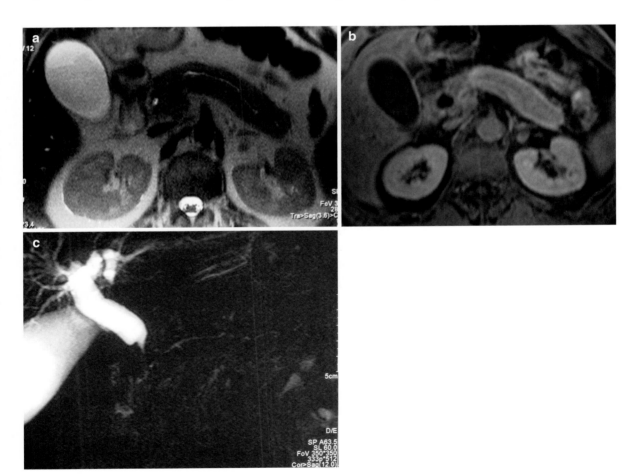

Fig. 14 Diffuse autoimmune pancreatitis. (**a**) HASTE image shows a diffuse enlargement of the pancreas with "sausage shape." (**b**) Dynamic imaging after bolus injection of paramagnetic contrast agent, venous phase. The pancreas show reduced enhancement with a capsule-like rim enhancement. (**c**) MRCP demonstrates a stenosis of the intrapancreatic common bile duct with the upstream biliary tree dilation due to inflammatory cellular infiltration associated to a diffuse narrowing of the MPD

the liver, with the hypointense capsule-like rim usually best demonstrated (Fig. 14a) (Albaraz et al. 2009; Morana et al. 2005; Wakabayashi et al. 2003). A narrowing of the intrapancreatic common bile duct with dilatation of the upstream biliary tree may be observed, due to inflammatory cellular infiltrate causing thickening of the duct wall. Thus, the MPD appears non-dilated or diffusely narrowed, where narrowing is usually longer than the stenosis of the MPD in pancreatic cancer (Fig. 14c). Mild dilatation of the MPD upstream the affected area may occur.

On T1-weighted images the affected pancreas shows a decreased signal intensity compared with the signal intensity of the liver, due to pancreatic fibrosis, with distinctive reduction in signal on fat saturated sequences. Contrast enhancement of the affected pancreatic parenchyma is usually reduced, with a delayed contrast enhancement of the capsule-like rim (Fig. 14b).

The invasion of vessels, vascular encasement, mass effect, and fluid collections are absent (Fig. 11d) (Sahani et al. 2004).

After steroid therapy abnormal signal intensity of the pancreas improves to isointensity with that of the liver both in T1 and T2 weighted images; pancreas returns to normal size or becomes atrophic, the capsule-like rim disappears and stenosis of lower common bile duct improves with subsequent decompression of the biliary tree ad well as of the pancreatic duct (Fig. 12) (Albaraz et al. 2009; Morana et al. 2005).

The role of Diffusion Weighted images (DWI) is not well established yet. Lee et al. (2008) report statistically different ADC values between autoimmune pancreatitis and pancreatic cancer both at b 500 and b 1,000, thus helping in the differential diagnosis. Moreover, some Authors propose this sequence in the evaluation of autoimmune pancreatitis especially in its follow-up after steroids therapy (Taniguchi et al. 2009). In this study, autoimmune pancreatitis showed high signal intensity on DWI, which improved after steroid treatment (Figs. 11g and 12h). The Authors demonstrated that ADCs of the affected pancreas and IgG4 index were significantly inversely correlated, thus suggesting that ADCs reflected disease activity (Figs. 11h and 12i). However, DW signal and ADC map are similar to pancreatic carcinoma (Figs. 3h and 11h), making the differential diagnosis difficult. The clinical finding of the existence of an autoimmune disorder is an important clue to suspect an autoimmune pancreatitis, although this finding is reported only in about 50% of the cases.

4 Staging

Surgical resection is the only curative treatment of pancreatic carcinoma. Unfortunately, at surgical exploration only 5–30% of the tumors are amenable to resection (Cooperman et al. 2000; Wray et al. 2005). Even in expert hands, Whipple's procedure has a mortality up to 4% while exploratory laparotomy has a morbidity up to 25% (Birkmeyer et al. 2002). Therefore, the principle goal of preoperative staging is to identify all resectable diseases to avoid surgical exploration to those patients with unresectable disease.

Staging of pancreatic carcinoma is based on the TNM classification, thus on dimensions and extensions of primitive tumor (T), presence or absence of metastatic lymph nodes (N), presence or absence of distant metastases (M) (Tamm et al. 2003; Liu and Traverso 2005).

Based on TNM, the most used classification of the extension of the pancreatic cancer are that of the Union Internationale Contre le Cancer (Sobin and Wittekind 2002), the AJCC (Greene et al. 2002) and of the Japan Pancreas Society (Pancreatic Cancer Registration Committee in Japan Pancreas Society 2003) (Seiki et al. 2004; Isaji et al. 2004). As a whole, according to the different stages of T, N and M, pancreatic cancer is classified as locally resectable, locally unresectable and unresectable for distant metastases.

As concern the T parameter, last changes in TNM classification have extended the number of patients amenable to surgical resection, as T4 now is considered only the tumor which infiltrates either the celiac axis or the superior mesenteric artery, while a limited superior mesenteric vein infiltration is now considered resectable thanks to venous interposition grafts, thus downstaging the tumor to T3 (Wolff et al. 2000).

Contrast-enhanced techniques both at CT or MRI, combined with MPR and MIP post-processing, have improved the capability to identify and stage the extent of the tumor, the extra-pancreatic involvement, (Brennan et al. 2007), especially the vascular arterial and venous infiltration, with an accuracy for resectability of about 90% both for CT and MRI in a direct comparison (Arslan et al. 2001; Grenacher et al. 2004).

The degree of circumferential vessel involvement by tumor as shown by CT/MRI is useful in predicting which patients will have surgically unresectable tumors. Involvement of vessel to tumor that exceeds one-half circumference of the vessel is highly specific for unresectable tumor (O'Malley et al. 1999; Lu et al. 1997), both for arteries and veins. CT/MRI with vascular reconstructions allows higher degree of recognition than axials alone (Figs. 15a, b and 16) (Lepanto et al. 2002). However, in a direct comparison of CT and MRI for detection and resectability of pancreatic carcinoma with two independent readers, Kappa analysis of interobserver agreement showed a good correlation for

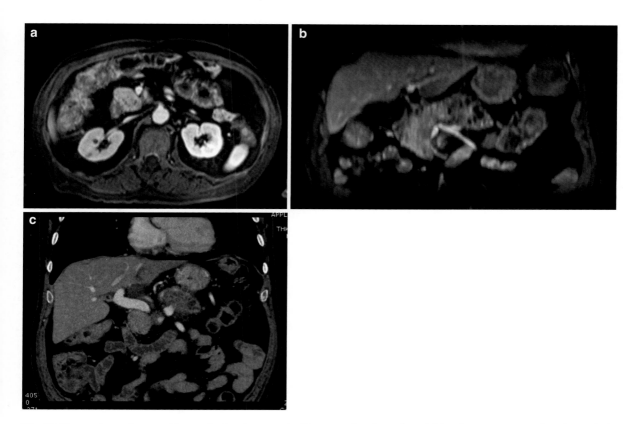

Fig. 15 Pancreatic carcinoma with vascular involvement. (**a, b**) Dynamic imaging after bolus injection of paramagnetic contrast agent, venous phase, axial image (**a**) and coronal reconstruction (**b**). The coronal reconstructions allow a better delineation of vascular circumferential involvement compared to the analysis of the axial image alone. (**c**) Coronal reconstruction of venous phase after iodinated contrast agent in multislice CT. The vascular infiltration is more clearly recognizable

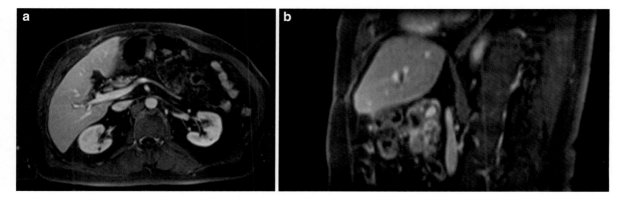

Fig. 16 Pancreatic carcinoma with vascular involvement. (**a, b**) Dynamic imaging after bolus injection of paramagnetic contrast agent, venous phase, axial image (**a**) and sagittal reconstruction (**b**). The sagittal reconstructions allow a better delineation of portal vein involvement compared to the analysis of the axial image alone

CT (0.71) and a moderate correlation of both groups for MRI (0.49) (Fig. 15b, c) (Grenacher et al. 2004).

Specific sign of venous involvement are the reduction of the diameter of the superior mesenteric vein (SMV), the "teardrop" shape of SMV (Fig. 17) (Hough et al. 1999; Sahani et al. 2008), and the dilatation of SMV tributaries (Hommeyer et al. 1995; Kanematsu et al. 2000) especially the enlargement of postero-superior pancreatico-duodenal vein (PDV)(Mori et al. 1991), and the visualization of inferior PDV (Yamada et al. 2000), while the enlargement of gastro-colic trunk is not conclusive (O'Malley et al. 1999). Attention must be paid to vascular infiltration, as fibrosis and chronic inflammation can modify the shape of the vessel, simulating an infiltration, especially in case of a venous vessel (Michl et al. 2006; Zhong et al. 2005). Moreover, due to the different strategies of revascularization, it is important to evaluate all others venous structures, such as the inferior mesenteric vein, the first venous duodenal branch, and their distances from the tumor and the spleno-portal confluence (Brennan et al. 2007; Kanematsu et al. 2000).

The location of the tumor in the pancreas determines its route of spread and the nodal groups involved. Lymph node involvement has a significant impact on the survival of patients with pancreatic cancer (Kayahara et al. 1999). However, lymph node involvement in the peri-pancreatic area does not impact surgical planning, because they are removed with the surgical specimen; it is more important to recognize nodal metastases in the celiac node, common hepatic artery (CHA) node and para-aortic node, because metastases to these nodes would preclude patients from surgery, especially for the tumor of the head of the pancreas (Maithel et al. 2007). Nodal involvement in the para-aortic region does not indicate regional invasion but is a statistically independent predictor of early recurrence, and considerably affects survival (Sai et al. 2008).

T2 weighted fat-suppressed sequences are the most sensitive in order to evaluate lymph nodes, which appear as moderately hyperintense. The size threshold in order to suspect a nodal involvement is 1 cm in the short axis (Roche et al. 2003); however, although with 1 cm threshold specificity is quite good (85%) (Roche et al. 2003), its sensitivity is very low (14%) (Roche et al. 2003), as up to 36% of lymph nodes of 5–10 mm in short axis have been found with tumoral involvement, even in less than 5 mm lymph nodes (Roche et al. 2003), while lymph nodes >10 mm can also be inflammatory (Doi et al. 2007).

The presence of distant metastases preclude the surgical resection and is therefore fundamental their correct identification and characterization. 60% of patients who present with pancreatic ductal adenocarcinoma have advanced disease (Douglass et al. 1997). The liver and peritoneum are the most common sites of distant metastases. To date, no definite decision on the best technique for the staging of abdominal metastases can be given, with MRI and laparoscopy as the most performant techniques, with similar results (Schneider et al. 2003).

MR of the liver is affected by the in-plane motion (anterior-posterior chest motion due to respiration); Propeller or BLADE technique with radial acquisition of the k space reduces the sensitivity to various sources of image artifacts (e.g., motion artifacts, field inhomogeneity). It can be used with GE and TSE in a wide range of applications. The liver is also affected by through-plane diaphragm motion artifacts which can be corrected using a prospective motion correction with navigator echo (PACE) that detects the diaphragm movement. MRI has the best sensitivity to liver metastases, thanks to its high contrast: both T2w (especially fat saturated) and GRE T1w (especially 3D with thin slices after administration of paramagnetic contrast agent) and the use of liver specific contrast agent have greatly improved the sensitivity of the technique.

Hepatic metastases from pancreatic carcinoma are usually multiple (Gabata et al. 2008) and their size range

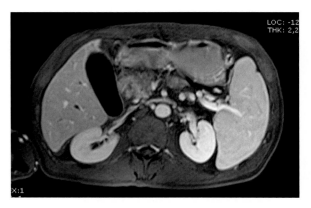

Fig. 17 Pancreatic carcinoma with vascular involvement. Dynamic imaging after bolus injection of paramagnetic contrast agent, venous phase. Tethering of the superior mesenteric vein ("teardrop sign") determined by the pancreatic mass

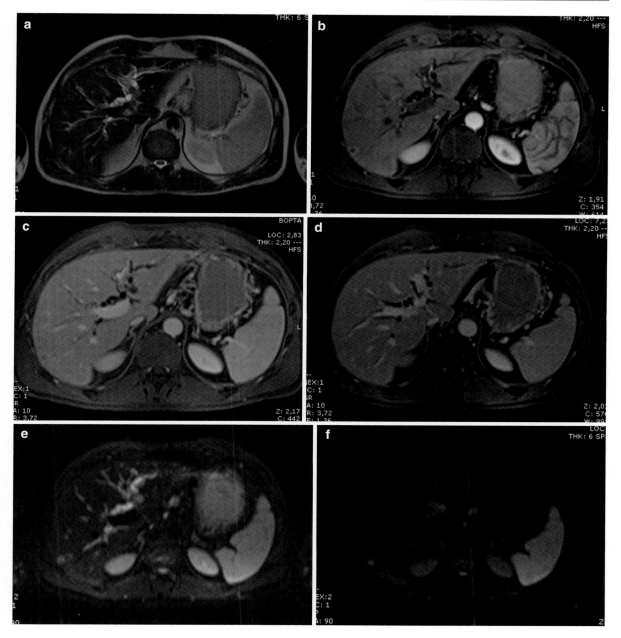

Fig. 18 Small liver metastasis from pancreatic carcinoma. (**a**) On TSE T2w image a small lesion slightly hyperintense can be appreciated in the seventh segment. (**b–d**) Dynamic imaging after bolus injection of paramagnetic contrast agent. The lesion shows ring enhancement in the arterial (b), venous (c), and dis- tribution phase (d). A dilation of the intrahepatic biliary ducts can be appreciated. (**e, f**) DWI at b 50 (**e**) and b 600 (**f**). The lesion shows significant hyperintensity both at low and high b-value due to high cellularity

from few millimeters (Fig. 18) to some centimeters (Fig. 19) (Danet et al. 2003). They appear hypointense on T1 and moderately hyperintense on T2 and DWI, with frequently a capsular based distribution.

DWI is a promising technique for the identification of small hepatic metastases: respiratory triggering and a value of b 50 give a high quality image, with a high SNR and suppression of signal from vessels, thus

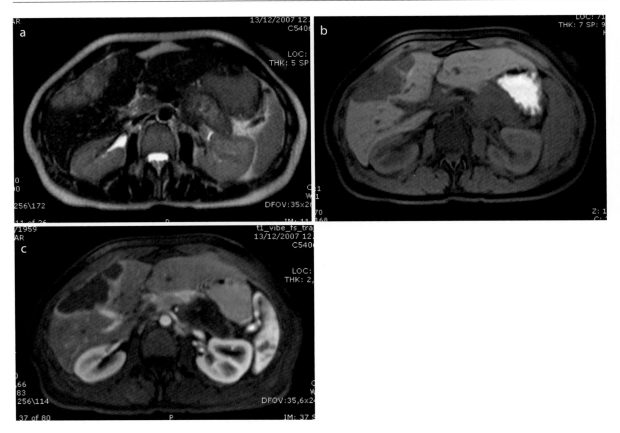

Fig. 19 Large liver metastasis from pancreatic carcinoma. (**a**) On TSE T2w image a large hyperintense lesion can be appreciated in the right lobo and a large lesion in the tail of the pancreas. (**b, c**) It appears inhomogenously hypointense on GRE T1w fat sat image (**b**) with peripheral enhancement after contrast agent injection (**c**)

allowing an easy detection of the lesion from the nearby intrahepatic vessels (Fig. 18f) (Bruegel and Rummeny 2009). According to many Authors, lesion detection with DWI is significantly higher for DWI than for T2w images, with more significant results for small metastases (<10 mm) (Bruegel and Rummeny 2009).

During dynamic imaging after injection of paramagnetic contrast agent they usually appear hypointense with a perilesional enhancement in more than 50% of the patients (Danet et al. 2003), with either ring perilesional enhancement (Fig. 18b) or wedge-shaped perilesional enhancement (Fig. 20c) (Gabata et al. 2008). Occasionally pancreatic liver metastases have been misdiagnosed as pseudolesions because they initially emerged as arterioportal shunts on dynamic CT/MR imaging (Gabata et al. 2008). The etiology of this transient enhancement related with liver metastases from pancreatic cancer is unknown. Gabata and Colleagues supposed that the etiology of

transient hepatic enhancement of liver metastasis from pancreatic carcinomas may be correlated with the tumor invasion of portal tract and tumor thrombi of portal venules which causes decreased portal flow and increased hepatic arterial blood flow (Gabata et al. 2008). Delayed contrast enhancement of the central portion of the lesion can be observed (Fig. 20e), due to desmoplastic reaction secondary to the stimulation of hepatic stellate cells (Tien et al. 2009).

Dynamic imaging after injection of paramagnetic liver specific contrast agent (MultiHance, Bracco SpA, Milano, Italy; Primovist, Bayer Schering, Berlin, Germany), is superimposable to that obtained with conventional extravascular-extracellular gadolinium-based contrast agents (Fig. 20), while in the hepatobiliary phase the lesions do not show significant enhancement, as they are not able to uptake the CM (Fig. 20h) (Petersein et al. 2000; Reimer et al. 1997).

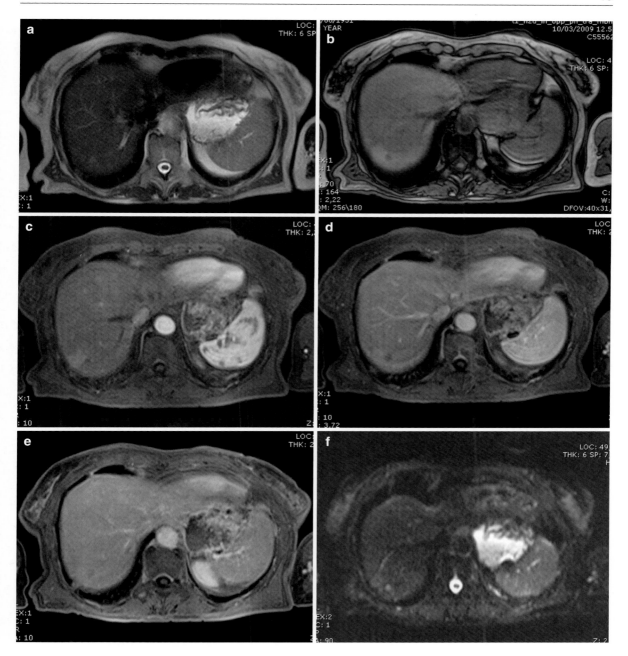

Fig. 20 Small liver metastasis from pancreatic carcinoma. (**a**) On HASTE image a small lesion slightly hyperintense can be appreciated in the seventh segment. (**b**) On GRE T1w out of phase image, the lesion is hypointense within a focal sparing area in comparison to the remaining liver parenchyma, which appear slightly hypointense due to steatosis. (**c–e**) Dynamic imaging after bolus injection of paramagnetic liver specific contrast agent gadobenate dimeglumine (MultiHance; Bracco SpA, Milan, Italy). During arterial phase (**c**) a wedge shaped perilesional enhancement can be observed. During the venous (**d**) and distribution phase (**e**) the lesion appear hypovascular; at the distribution phase a central dot of enhancement can be observed. (**f, g**) DWI at b 50 (**f**) and b 600 (**g**). The lesion shows significant hyperintensity both at low and high b-value due to high cellularity. (**h**) GRE T1w image 2 h after the injection of MultiHance. The lesion appears hypointense due to the lack of active uptake

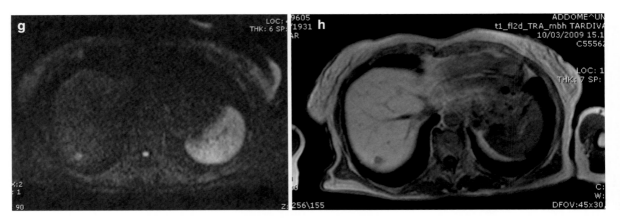

Fig. 20 (continued)

After mangafodipir trisodium (Teslascan, GE Health) there is an increase of the liver-to-lesion contrast-to-noise ratio due to the lack of contrast uptake (Schima et al. 2002). Metastases do not contain RES cells, thus after SPIO injection the liver-metastasis CNR is improved with increased lesion conspicuity and detection when compared to non-enhanced T2-weihted images (Seneterre et al. 1996; Ward et al. 1999, Oudkerk et al. 1997).

4.1 Differential Diagnosis

Attention must be paid to small (<1 cm) solid focal liver lesions, as even in oncologic patients they are benign (Jones et al. 1992; Mueller et al. 2003; Schwartz et al. 1999). The size and margins of the lesions can be helpful in making a correct differential diagnosis, and small size (<5 mm) with sharp margins has only 6% of possibility to be a metastasis at CT (Robinson et al. 2003).

Intrahepatic cholangitis can be observed in patients with obstructive jaundice secondary to pancreatic head carcinoma and it also shows transient inhomogeneous wedge-shaped enhancement on dynamic imaging, difficult to differentiate from that of hepatic metastases of pancreatic carcinomas, although it disappear or decrease in size after treatment of cholangitis like hepatic abscesses (Arai et al. 2003). So, follow-up by dynamic imaging can be useful to differentiate intrahepatic cholangitis from pancreatic hepatic metastasis.

Biliary hamartomas are composed of cystic spaces and fibrous stroma; their size ranges from 0.5 to 1.5 cm. They can be either solitary or more often numerous. Lesions show low signal on T1-weighted images and high signal on T2-weighted images with well defined margins (Fig. 21); after injection of paramagnetic contrast agent they demonstrate thin rim enhancement on early images that persisted on late images (Fig. 21), which at histopathology is correlated with compression of the liver parenchyma surrounding the lesions. No appreciable central enhancement of the lesions is observed (Semelka et al. 1999), a feature which helps in distinguishing it from small pancreatic carcinoma metastases, which often show delayed central dot enhancement in the desmoplastic component of the lesion (Fig. 20d). With DWI a correct characterization of focal liver lesions can be obtained by the analysis of ADC map after high b values, where benign lesions such as hemangiomas have a higher ADC value in comparison to metastases, although some overlap has been reported (Bruegel and Rummeny 2009). Small hemangiomas (Fig. 22) can still maintain high signal at DWI images with high b value ; in this attempt ADC maps after DWI are rarely useful as the small size of the lesions does not allow their correct visualization at ADC map. A combination of DWI and contrast-enhanced images are helpful to reach the correct diagnosis. Small cysts are easily recognized with HASTE sequences, as well as show a significant decrease of the signal intensity with DWI at high b values (>500) (Fig. 23).

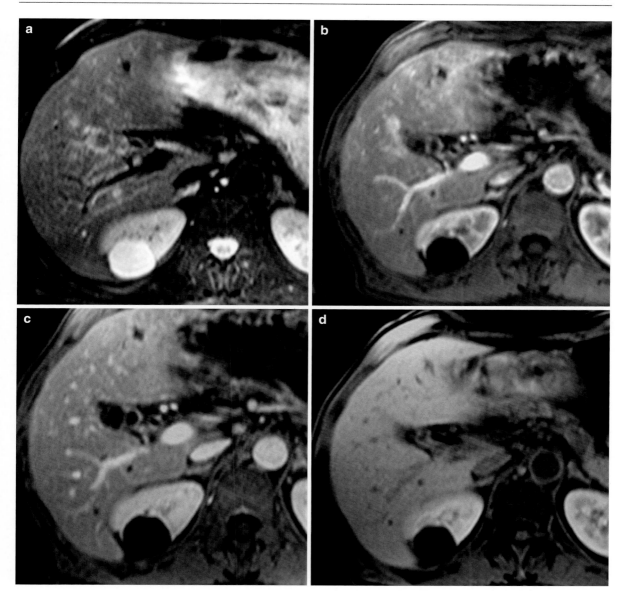

Fig. 21 Biliary hamartomas in a patient with pancreatic carcinoma. (**a**) On TSE T2w image two small lesions slightly hyperintense can be appreciated in the sixth segment. (**b**, **c**) dynamic imaging after bolus injection of paramagnetic liver specific contrast agent gadobenate dimeglumine (MultiHance; Bracco SpA, Milan, Italy). The lesion shows sharp margins with ring enhancement in the arterial (**d**) and venous phase (**c**). (**d**) GRE T1w image 2 h after the injection of MultiHance. The lesions appear markedly hypointense due to the lack of active uptake

5 Post-treatment Evaluation

Imaging has an important role in assessing treatment response in patients who are undergoing neoadjuvant therapy for presumed resectable disease, in order to decide whether use a different protocol if disease progresses or to stop the treatment if disease has progressed to the point that it is no longer resectable.

More radical treatment, whether surgery or treatment with radiation therapy and chemotherapy, can be followed by imaging to detect postoperative complications, local recurrence, local disease progression

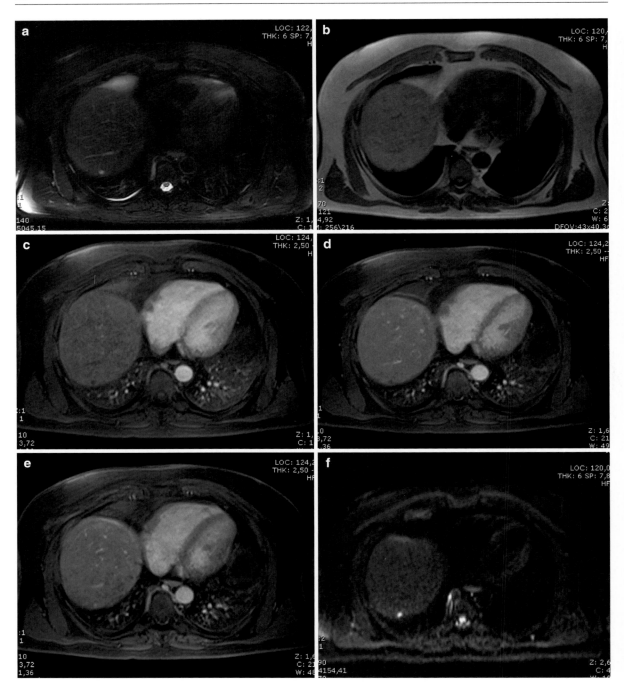

Fig. 22 Small hemangioma. (**a**) On TSE T2w image a small lesion with high signal intensity can be appreciated in the seventh segment. (**b**) On unenhanced GRE T1w image the lesion is homogeneously hypointense. (**c–e**) Dynamic imaging after bolus injection of paramagnetic contrast agent. The lesion does not show significant enhancement in the arterial (**c**) and venous (**d**) phase. During distribution phase (**e**) complete fill in of the lesion can be observed. (**f–h**) DWI at b 50 (**f**), b 800 (**g**), and ADC map (**h**). The lesion shows a decrease of signal intensity from low- to high b value. The ADC map shows high signal of the focal lesion (*arrow* in **h**) due to non restricted diffusion

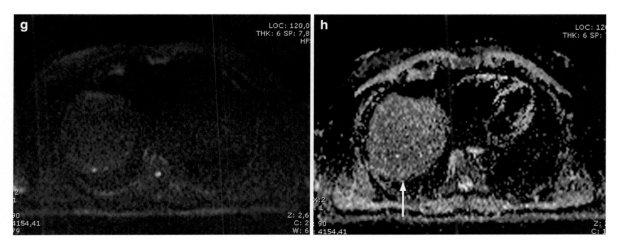

Fig. 22 (continued)

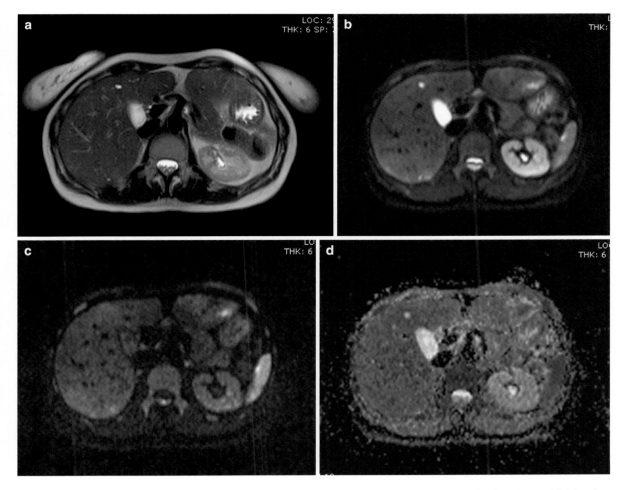

Fig. 23 Small simple hepatic cyst. (**a**) HASTE image perfectly identifies a small well-defined highly hyperintense lesion. (**b–d**) DWI at b 50 (**b**), b 800 (**c**), and ADC map (**d**). The lesion shows a marked decrease of signal intensity from low- to high b value. The ADC map shows high signal of the focal lesion due to non restricted diffusion

or distant metastases. Due to local changes after therapy it can be difficult to distinguish them from recurrent tumor: to follow these patients it is important a close follow-up compared with an initial baseline postoperative examination.

References

Akisik MF, Sandrasegaran K, Aisen AA, Maglinte DD, Sherman S, Lehman GA (2006) Dynamic secretin-enhanced MR cholangiopancreatography. Radiographics 26:665–677

Akisik MF, Aisen AM, Sandrasegaran K, Jennings SG, Lin C, Sherman S, Lin JA, Rydberg M (2009) Assessment of chronic pancreatitis: utility of diffusion-weighted MR imaging with secretin enhancement. Radiology 250:103–109

Albaraz R et al. (2009) Autoimmune pancreatitis: MR features before and after steroid therapy. E-Poster P-281 EPOSTM Online, System; ESGAR

Arai K, Kawai K, Kohda W, Tatsu H, Matsui O, Nakahama T (2003) Dynamic CT of acute cholangitis; early inhomogeneous enhancement of the liver. AJR AM J Roentgenol 181:115–118

Arslan A, Buanes T, Geitung JT (2001) Pancreatic carcinoma: MR, MR angiography and dynamic helical CT in the evaluation of vascular invasion. Eur J Radiol 38:151–159

Balci NC, Semelka RC (2001) Radiologic diagnosis and staging of pancreatic ductal adenocarcinoma. Eur J Rad 38:105–112

Birchard KR, Semelka RC, Hyslop WB, Brown A, Armao D, Firat Z, Vaidean G (2005) Suspected pancreatic cancer: evaluation by dynamic gadolinium-enhanced 3D gradient-echo MRI. AJR Am J Roentgenol 185:700–703

Birkmeyer JD, Siewers AE, Finlayson EV, Stukel TA, Lucas FL, Batista I, Welch HG, Wennberg DE (2002) Hospital volume and surgical mortality in the United States. N Engl J Med 11(346):1128–1137

Blasbalg R, Baroni RH, Costa DN, Machado MC (2007) MRI features of groove pancreatitis. AJR Am J Roentgenol 189:73–80

Braithwaite AC, Dale BM, Boll DT, Merkle EM (2009) Short- and midterm reproducibility of apparent diffusion coefficient measurements at 3.0-T diffusion-weighted imaging of the abdomen. Radiology 250:459–465

Brennan DD, Zamboni GA, Raptopoulos VD, Kruskal JB (2007) Comprehensive preoperative assessment of pancreatic adenocarcinoma with 64-section volumetric CT. Radiographics 27:1653–1666

Bruegel M, Rummeny EJ (2010) Hepatic metastases: use of diffusion-weighted echo-planar imaging. Abdom Imaging 35: 454–61

Castell-Monsalve FJ, Sousa-Martin JM, Carranza-Carranza A (2008) Groove pancreatitis: MRI and pathologic findings. Abdom Imaging 33:342–348

Colagrande S, Belli G, Politi LS, Mannelli L, Pasquinelli F, Villari N (2008) The influence of diffusion- and relaxation-related factors on signal intensity: an introductive guide to magnetic resonance diffusion-weighted imaging studies. J Comput Assist Tomogr 32:463–474

Cooperman AM, Kini S, Snady H, Bruckner H, Chamberlain RS (2000) Current surgical therapy for carcinoma of the pancreas. J Clin Gastroenterol 31:107–113

Danet IM, Semelka RC, Nagase LL, Woosely JT, Leonardou P, Armao D (2003) Liver metastases from pancreatic adenocarcinoma: MR imaging characteristics. J Magn Reson Imaging 18:181–188

Doi R, Kami K, Ito D, Fujimoto K, Kawaguchi Y, Wada M, Kogire M, Hosotani R, Imamura M, Uemoto S (2007) Prognostic implication of para-aortic lymph node metastasis in resectable pancreatic cancer. World J Surg 31:147–154

Douglass HJ, Kim S, Meropol N (1997) Neoplasms of the exocrine pancreas. In: Holland J, Frei EI, Bast RJ, Kufe DW, Morton DL, Weichselbaum RR (eds) Cancer medicine, 4th edn. Williams & Wilkins, Baltimore, pp 1989–2018

Fattahi R, Balci NC, Perman WH, Hsueh EC, Alkaade S, Havlioglu N, Burton FR (2009) Pancreatic diffusion-weighted imaging (DWI): comparison between mass-forming focal pancreatitis (FP), pancreatic cancer (PC), and normal pancreas. J Magn Reson Imaging 29:350–356

Fukukura Y, Fujiyoshi F, Sasaki M, Nakajo M (2002) Pancreatic duct: morphologic evaluation with MR cholangiopancreatography after secretin stimulation. Radiology 222: 674–680

Gabata T, Matsui O, Terayama N, Kobayashi S, Sanada J (2008) Imaging diagnosis of hepatic metastases of pancreatic carcinomas: significance of transient wedge-shaped contrast enhancement mimicking arterioportal shunt. Abdom Imaging 33:437–443

Greene FL, Page DL, Fleming ID et al (2002) Exocrine pancreas. In: Greene FL, Page DL, Fleming ID et al (eds) AJCC cancer staging manual, vol 6. Springer, New York, pp 157–164

Grenacher L, Klauss M, Dukic L, Delorme S, Knaebel HP, Dux M, Kauczor HU, Buchler MW, Kauffmann GW, Richter GM (2004) Diagnosis and staging of pancreatic carcinoma: MRI versus MSCT – a prospective study. Rofo 176:1624–1633

Hakimé A, Giraud M, Vullierme MP, Vilgrain V (2007) MR imaging of the pancreas. J Radiol 88:11–25

Hata H, Mori H, Matsumoto S, Yamada Y, Kiyosue H, Tanoue S, Hongo N, Kashima K (2010). Fibrous stroma and vascularity of pancreatic carcinoma: correlation with enhancement patterns on CT. Abdom Imaging. 35:172–80

Hellerhoff KJ, Helmberger H 3rd, Rösch T, Settles MR, Link TM, Rummeny EJ (2002) Dynamic MR pancreatography after secretin administration: image quality and diagnostic accuracy. AJR Am J Roentgenol 179:121–129

Hommeyer SC, Freeny PC, Crabo LG (1995) Carcinoma of the head of the pancreas: evaluation of the pancreaticoduodenal veins with dynamic CT–potential for improved accuracy in staging. Radiology 196:233–238

Hough TJ, Raptopoulos V, Siewert B, Matthews JB (1999) Teardrop superior mesenteric vein: CT sign for unresectable carcinoma of the pancreas. AJR Am J Roentgenol 173: 1509–1512

Ichikawa T, Sou H, Araki T, Arbab AS, Yoshikawa T, Ishigame K, Haradome H, Hachiya J (2001) Duct-penetrating sign at

MRCP: usefulness for differentiating inflammatory pancreatic mass from pancreatic carcinomas. Radiology 221: 107–116

Isaji S, Kawarada Y, Uemoto S (2004) Classification of pancreatic cancer: comparison of Japanese and UICC classifications. Pancreas 28:231–234

Johnson PT, Outwater EK (1999). Pancreatic carcinoma versus chronic pancreatitis: dynamic MR imaging. Radiology. 212: 213-8

Jones EC, Chezmar JL, Nelson RC, Bernardino ME (1992) The frequency and significance of small (less than or equal to 15 mm) hepatic lesions detected by CT. AJR Am J Roentgenol 158:535–539

Kanematsu M, Shiratori Y, Hoshi H, Kondo H, Matsuo M, Moriwaki H (2000) Pancreas and peripancreatic vessels: effect of imaging delay on gadolinium enhancement at dynamic gradient-recalled-echo MR Imaging. Radiology 215:95–102

Kartalis N, Lindholm TL, Aspelin P, Permert J, Albiin N (2009) Diffusion-weighted magnetic resonance imaging of pancreas tumours. Eur Radiol 19:1981–1990

Kawaguchi K, Koike M, Tsuruta K, Okamoto A, Tabata I, Fujita N (1991) Lymphoplasmacytic sclerosing pancreatitis with cholangitis: a variant of primary sclerosing cholangitis extensively involving pancreas. Hum Pathol 22:387–395

Kayahara M, Nagakawa T, Ohta T, Kitagawa H, Ueno K, Tajima H, Elnemr A, Miwa K (1999) Analysis of Paraaortic Lymph Node Involvement in Pancreatic Carcinoma. A Significant Indication for Surgery? Cancer 85:583–590

Kim JH, Kim MJ, Chung JJ, Lee WJ, Yoo HS, Lee JT (2002) Differential diagnosis of periampullary carcinomas at MR imaging. Radiographics 22:1335–1352

Klöppel G (2007) Chronic pancreatitis, pseudotumors and other tumor-like lesions. Mod Pathol 20(Suppl 1):S113–S131

Kuroiwa T, Suda T, Takahashi T, Hirono H, Natsui M, Motoyama H, Nomoto M, Aoyagi Y (2002) Bile duct involvement in a case of autoimmune pancreatitis successfully treated with an oral steroid. Dig Dis Sci 47:1810–1816

Lee SS, Byun JH, Park BJ, Park SH, Kim N, Park B, Kim JK, Lee MG (2008). Quantitative analysis of diffusion-weighted magnetic resonance imaging of the pancreas: usefulness in characterizing solid pancreatic masses. J Magn Reson Imaging. 28: 928–36

Lepanto L, Arzoumanian Y, Gianfelice D, Perreault P, Dagenais M, Lapointe R, Létourneau R, Roy A (2002) Helical CT with CT angiography in assessing periampullary neoplasms: identification of vascular invasion. Radiology 222:347–352

Liu RC, Traverso LW (2005) Diagnostic laparoscopy improves staging of pancreatic cancer deemed locally unresectable by computed tomography. Surg Endosc 19:638–642

Lopez Hänninen E, Amthauer H, Hosten N, Ricke J, Böhmig M, Langrehr J, Hintze R, Neuhaus P, Wiedenmann B, Rosewicz S, Felix R (2002) Prospective evaluation of pancreatic tumors: accuracy of MR imaging with MR cholangiopancreatography and MR angiography. Radiology 224:34–41

Lu DS, Reber HA, Krasny RM, Kadell BM, Sayre J (1997) Local staging of pancreatic cancer: criteria for unresectability of major vessels as revealed by pancreatic-phase, thin-section helical CT. AJR Am J Roentgenol 168:1439–1443

Maithel SK, Khalili K, Dixon E, Guindi M, Callery MP, Cattral MS, Taylor BR, Gallinger S, Greig PD, Grant DR, Vollmer CM Jr (2007) Impact of regional lymph node evaluation in staging patients with periampullary tumors. Ann Surg Oncol 14:202–210

Manfredi R, Costamagna G, Brizi MG, Maresca G, Vecchioli A, Colagrande C, Marano P (2000) Severe chronic pancreatitis versus suspected pancreatic disease: dynamic MR cholangiopancreatography after secretin stimulation. Radiology 214:849–855

Matos C, Cappeliez O, Winant C, Coppens E, Devière J, Metens T (2002) MR imaging of the pancreas: a pictorial tour. Radiographics 22:e2

Matsuki M, Inada Y, Nakai G, Tatsugami F, Tanikake M, Narabayashi I, Masuda D, Arisaka Y, Takaori K, Tanigawa N (2007). Diffusion-weighed MR imaging of pancreatic carcinoma. Abdom Imaging. 32: 481–3

Michl P, Pauls S, Gress TM (2006) Evidence-based diagnosis and staging of pancreatic cancer. Best Pract Res Clin Gastroenterol 20:227–251

Miller FH, Rini NJ, Keppke AL (2006) MRI of adenocarcinoma of the pancreas. AJR Am J Roentgenol 187: W365–W374

Morana G, Tapparelli M, Faccioli N, D'Onofrio M, Pozzi Mucelli R (2005) Autoimmune pancreatitis: instrumental diagnosis. JOP 13(6):102–107

Mori H, Miyake H, Aikawa H, Monzen Y, Maeda T, Suzuki K, Matsumoto S, Wakisaka M (1991) Dilated posterior superior pancreaticoduodenal vein: recognition with CT and clinical significance in patients with pancreaticobiliary carcinomas. Radiology 181:793–800

Mueller GC, Hussain HK, Carlos RC, Nghiem HV, Francis IR (2003) Effectiveness of MR imaging in characterizing small hepatic lesions: routine versus expert interpretation. AJR Am J Roentgenol 180:673–680

O'Malley ME, Boland GW, Wood BJ, Fernandez-del Castillo C, Warshaw AL, Mueller PR (1999) Adenocarcinoma of the head of the pancreas: determination of surgical unresectability with thin-section pancreatic-phase helical CT. AJR Am J Roentgenol 173(6):1513–1518

Okazaki K, Chiba T (2002) Autoimmune related pancreatitis. Gut 51:1–4

Oudkerk M, van den Heuvel AG, Wielopolski PA, Schmitz PI, Borel Rinkes IH, Wiggers T (1997) Hepatic lesions: detection with ferumoxide-enhanced T1-weighted MR imaging. Radiology 203:449–456

Pamuklar E, Semelka RC (2005) MR imaging of the pancreas. Magn Reson Imaging Clin N Am 13:313–330

Pancreatic Cancer Registration Committee in Japan Pancreas Society (2003) Pancreatic cancer registration of JPS: the summary for 20 years. J Jpn Pancreas Soc 18:101–169

Pearson RK, Longnecker DS, Chari ST, Smyrk TC, Okazaki K, Frulloni L, Cavallini G (2003) Controversies in clinical pancreatology: autoimmune pancreatitis: does it exist? Pancreas 27:1–13

Petersein J, Spinazzi A, Giovagnoni A, Soyer P, Terrier F, Lencioni R et al (2000) Focal liver lesions: evaluation of the efficacy of gadobenate dimeglumine in MR imaging – a multicenter phase III clinical study. Radiology 215:727–736

Reimer P, Rummeny EJ, Daldrup HE, Hesse T, Balzer T, Tombach B et al (1997) Enhancement characteristics of liver metastases, hepatocellular carcinomas, and hemangiomas with Gd-EOB-DTPA: preliminary results with dynamic MR imaging. Eur Radiol 7:275–280

Robinson PJ, Arnold P, Wilson D (2003) Small "indeterminate" lesions on CT of the liver: a follow-up study of stability. Br J Radiol 76:866–874

Roche CJ, Hughes ML, Garvey CJ, Campbell F, White DA, Jones L, Neoptolemos JP (2003) CT and pathologic assessment of prospective nodal staging in patients with ductal adenocarcinoma of the head of the pancreas. AJR Am J Roentgenol 180:475–480

Sahani DV, Kalva SP, Farrell J, Maher MM, Saini S, Mueller PR, Lauwers GY, Fernandez CD, Warshaw AL, Simeone JF (2004) Autoimmune pancreatitis: imaging features. Radiology 233:345–352

Sahani DV, Shah ZK, Catalano OA, Boland GW, Brugge WR (2008) Radiology of pancreatic adenocarcinoma: current status of imaging. J Gastroenterol Hepatol 23:23–33

Sai M, Mori H, Kiyonaga M, Kosen K, Yamada Y, Matsumoto S (2010). Peripancreatic lymphatic invasion by pancreatic carcinoma: evaluation with multi-detector row CT. Abdom Imaging. 35: 154–62

Schima W, Függer R (2002) Evaluation of focal pancreatic masses: comparison of mangafodipir-enhanced MR imaging and contrast-enhanced helical CT. Eur Radiol 12: 2998–3008

Schima W, Ba-Ssalamah A, Kölblinger C, Kulinna-Cosentini C, Puespoek A, Götzinger P (2007) Pancreatic adenocarcinoma. Eur Radiol 17:638–649

Schneider AR, Adamek HE, Layer G, Riemann JF, Arnold JC (2003) Staging of abdominal metastases in pancreatic carcinoma by diagnostic laparoscopy and magnetic resonance imaging. Z Gastroenterol 41:697–702

Schwartz LH, Gandras EJ, Colangelo SM, Ercolani MC, Panicek DM (1999) Prevalence and importance of small hepatic lesions found at CT in patients with cancer. Radiology 210:71–74

Seiki M, Katsusuke S, Makoto S, Go, Vay Liang WG (2004) Advancements in pancreatic cancer research in Japan and unfolding prospective. Pancreas 28:217–218

Semelka RC, Hussain SM, Marcos HB, Woosley JT (1999) Biliary hamartomas: solitary and multiple lesions shown on current MR techniques including gadolinium enhancement. J Magn Reson Imaging 10(2):196–201

Seneterre E, Taourel P, Bouvier Y, Pradel J, Van Beers B, Daures JP et al (1996) Detection of hepatic metastases: ferumoxides-enhanced MR imaging versus unenhanced MR imaging and CT during arterial portography. Radiology 200:785–792

Sobin LH, Wittekind C (2002) TNM classification of malignant tumors (International Union Against Cancer), 6th edn. Wiley-Liss, New York

Stolte M, Weiss W, Volkholz H, Rösch W (1982) A special form of segmental pancreatitis: "groove pancreatitis". Hepatogastroenterology 29:198–208

Tajima Y, Kuroki T, Tsutsumi R, Isomoto I, Uetani M, Kanematsu T (2007) Pancreatic carcinoma coexisting with chronic pancreatitis versus tumor-forming pancreatitis: diagnostic utility of the time-signal intensity curve from dynamic contrast-enhanced MR imaging. World J Gastroenterol 14(13):858–865

Takahashi S, Kim T, Murakami T, Okada A, Hori M, Narumi Y, Nakamura H (2000). Influence of paramagnetic contrast on single-shot MRCP image quality. Abdom Imaging. 25: 511–3

Takayama M, Hamano H, Ochi Y, Saegusa H, Komatsu K, Muraki T, Arakura N, Imai Y, Hasebe O, Kawa S (2004) Recurrent attacks of autoimmune pancreatitis result in pancreatic stone formation. Am J Gastroenterol 99: 932–937

Takeuchi M, Matsuzaki K, Kubo H, Nishitani H (2008) High-b-value diffusion-weighted magnetic resonance imaging of pancreatic cancer and mass-forming chronic pancreatitis: preliminary results. Acta Radiol 49:383–386

Tamm EP, Silverman PM, Charnsangavej C, Evans DB (2003) Diagnosis, staging, and surveillance of pancreatic cancer. Am J Roentgenol 20(180):1311–1323

Taniguchi T, Kobayashi H, Nishikawa K, Iida E, Michigami Y, Morimoto E, Yamashita R, Miyagi K, Okamoto M (2009) Diffusion-weighted magnetic resonance imaging in autoimmune pancreatitis. Jpn J Radiol 27(3):138–142

Tien YW, Wu YM, Lin WC, Lee HS, Lee PH (2009) Pancreatic carcinoma cells stimulate proliferation and matrix synthesis of hepatic stellate cells. Hepatology 51:307–314

To'o KJ, Raman SS, Yu NC, Kim YJ, Crawford T, Kadell BM, Lu DS (2005) Pancreatic and peripancreatic diseases mimicking primary pancreatic neoplasia. Radiographics 25: 949–965

Tsushima Y, Takano A, Taketomi-Takahashi A, Endo K (2007) Body diffusion-weighted MR imaging using high b-value for malignant tumor screening: usefulness and necessity of referring to T2-weighted images and creating fusion images. Acad Radiol 14:643–650

Wakabayashi T, Kawaura Y, Satomura Y, Watanabe H, Motoo Y, Okai T, Sawabu N (2003) Clinical and imaging features of autoimmune pancreatitis with focal pancreatic swelling or mass formation: comparison with so-called tumor-forming pancreatitis and pancreatic carcinoma. Am J Gastroenterol 98:2679–2687

Ward J, Naik KS, Guthrie JA, Wilson D, Robinson PJ (1999) Hepatic lesion detection: comparison of MR imaging after the administration of superparamagnetic iron oxide with dual-phase CT by using alternative-free response receiver operating characteristic analysis. Radiology 210: 459–466

Wolff RA, Chiao P, Lenzi R, Pisters PW, Lee JE, Janjan NA et al (2000) Current approaches and future strategies for pancreatic carcinoma. Invest New Drugs 18:43–56

Wray CJ, Ahmad SA, Matthews JB, Lowy AM (2005) Surgery for pancreatic cancer: recent controversies and current practice. Gastroenterology 128:1626–1641

Yamada Y, Mori H, Kiyosue H, Matsumoto S, Hori Y, Maeda T (2000) CT assessment of the inferior peripancreatic veins: clinical significance. AJR Am J Roentgenol 174:677–684

Zhang J, Israel GM, Hecht EM, Krinsky GA, Babb JS, Lee VS (2006) Isotropic 3D T2-weighted MR cholangiopancreatography with parallel imaging: feasibility study. AJR Am J Roentgenol 187:1564–1570

Zhong L, Li L, Yao QY (2005) Preoperative evaluation of pancreaticobiliary tumor using MR multi-imaging techniques. World J Gastroenterol 11(24):3756–3761

Zhong L et al (2007) Magnetic resonance imaging in the detection of pancreatic neoplasm. J Dig Dis 8:128–132

Zins M, Petit E, Boulay-Coletta I, Balaton A, Marty O, Berrod JL (2005) Imaging of pancreatic adenocarcinoma. J Radiol 86:759–779

Endoscopic Ultrasonography in Pancreatic Tumors: When and Why?

Angels Ginès, Gloria Fernández-Esparrach, and Carmen Ayuso

Contents

Abstract

> EUS has shown to be superior to other imaging techniques in the diagnosis of pancreatic cancer, especially in tumors < 2cm in diameter. Since the negative predictive value of EUS is 95-100%, EUS should be considered the technique of choice to rule out pancreatic cancer in patients with clinical suspicion and inconclusive previous image techniques. However, there is no agreement on the best technique (EUS or CT) to stage and assess ressectability in pancreatic adenocarcinoma. The most reliable sequential approach consists of a helical CT as the initial test and EUS as a confirmatory technique. EUS FNA is the most accurate and safe modality for tissue diagnosis in patients with suspected pancreatic cancer and is mandatory in unresectable disease. In the case of resectable tumors, the need of EUS FNA is still controversial.

A. Ginès (✉) and G.F.- Esparrach
Endoscopy Unit, Department of Gastroenterology,
Hospital Clínic, ICMDM, IDIBAPS, CIBERehd,
University of Barcelona, Villarroel 170,
08036 Barcelona, Spain
e-mail: magines@clinic.ub.es

C. Ayuso
Department of Radiology, Hospital Clínic,
University of Barcelona, Villarroel 170,
08036 Barcelona, Spain

1 Introduction

Endoscopic ultrasonography (EUS) was first introduced in the mid-1980s in Japan and Germany with the primary aim of better visualization of the pancreas as compared with transabdominal ultrasonography and has quickly gained acceptance.

Two main types of echoendoscopes are used in clinical practice: radial and linear. Radial imaging, either mechanical or electronic, provides a 360° echographic

A. Laghi (ed.), *New Concepts in Diagnosis and Therapy of Pancreatic Adenocarcinoma*,
Medical Radiology, DOI: 10.1007/174_2010_50, © Springer-Verlag Berlin Heidelberg 2011

image in a plane perpendicular to the direction of insertion of the echoendoscope, analogous to the cross-sectional CT. Linear echoendoscope provides sectorial images in a plane parallel to the direction of insertion of the echoendoscope. This physical characteristic allows the visualization of the entire length of the needle, making possible to sample the lesion under real-time EUS guidance, which is directly related to the high performance and safety of this technique. Linear echoendoscopes and the radial electronic as well are equipped with pulse and color Doppler that improves safety.

The widespread use of EUS in the last decade has revolutionized the management of pancreatic diseases since it simultaneously provides primary diagnostic and staging information, as well as enables tissue biopsy.

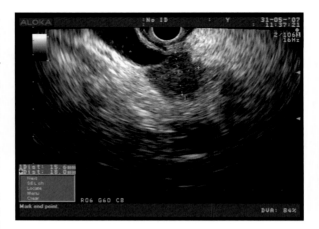

Fig. 1 Small adenocarcinoma of the head of the pancreas (18 × 15.6 mm) causing dilatation of the common bile duct

2 EUS and Diagnosis of Pancreatic Cancer

Pancreatic cancer is one of the main indications of EUS, for either diagnostic or staging purposes. Current indications for EUS in pancreatic masses are shown in Table 1.

The retroperitoneal location of the gland favors EUS beside other imaging techniques especially when FNA is indicated, since the diagnostic yield and safety of EUS-guided FNA (EUS-FNA) are higher than those of the percutaneous approach. Tumors in the body and the tail of the pancreas are visualized via a transgastric window, whereas those located in the head of the pancreas or in the uncinate process are best seen from the duodenum.

Although the echopattern of pancreatic adenocarcinoma is highly variable, the most usual aspect on EUS is a heterogeneous and hypoechoic mass with irregular margins (Fig. 1). Echo-free areas within the tumor are frequent, probably representing areas of necrosis. In

cystic tumors such as mucinous adenocarcinoma, the echo-free or cystic areas may constitute the predominant pattern, whereas the solid part of the tumor consists of an irregular and thickened wall, sometimes with solid papillary projections inside the cyst.

The accuracy of EUS in the diagnosis or detection of pancreatic cancer has been higher than 90% in most series over the years (Rösch and Classen 1992). In most studies published in the early 1990, EUS was proven to be superior to transabdominal ultrasound (US), (CT), endoscopic retrograde colangiopancreatography (ERCP), and angiography in the detection of pancreatic cancer (Rösch 1991; Snady 1992; Yasuda 1988). Later on, other studies comparing EUS with helical CT, magnetic resonance imaging (MRI), and positron-emission tomography (PET) have found that EUS was superior to the other techniques in terms of diagnosis of pancreatic neoplasms (Muller 1994; Gress 1999; Mertz 2000). The advantage of EUS was even greater in tumors <2 cm in diameter, as demonstrated by several investigators (Yasuda 1988; Rösch 1990). For example, in an early study performed in pancreatic tumors of less than 20 mm in diameter, EUS was able to detect them in 100% of cases, while other imaging techniques such as transabdominal US (29%), ERCP (57%), CT scan (29%), and angiography (14%) were significantly less accurate (Yasuda 1988). However, the roles and relative importance of these imaging modalities have changed over the last few decades and continue to change due to the rapid technological advances in medical imaging. Therefore, new investigations are continually required to evaluate and compare new

Table 1 Current indications of EUS in pancreatic masses

Exclusion of pancreatic cancer in doubtful cases

EUS-FNA in nonresectable tumors to confirm malignancy prior to chemotherapy or radiotherapy

EUS-FNA for the differential diagnosis between neoplastic and inflammatory tumor

Aspiration of minimal ascitis or enlarged lymph nodes for tumor staging technology. In this sense, EUS and multidetector spiral CT were first compared for the diagnosis of pancreatic cancer in 2004 (Agarwal 2004; DeWitt 2004). In a first retrospective comparison performed in 81 patients with suspicion of pancreatic cancer, the overall accuracy of spiral CT and EUS was 74 and 94%, respectively. Another prospective study including 80 patients with pancreatic cancer found that EUS was superior to multidetector CT for the detection of the tumor. However, the retrospective approach in the former and the notblinded comparison in the later study limit the value of the conclusions of both investigations.

The debate continues, therefore, on the best diagnostic test in patients with suspicion of pancreatic cancer. In a retrospective study recently published including 693 patients who were suspected of having pancreatic cancer, the negative predictive value (NPV) of EUS in excluding this diagnosis was 100% with a mean follow-up of 25 months (Klapman 2005). In another study including 412 patients, the NPV of EUS was 95%. Therefore, EUS should be considered the technique of choice to rule out pancreatic cancer in patients with clinical suspicion or inconclusive previous image techniques. However, it should be pointed out that most of the studies displaying comparative data between EUS and other cross-sectional imaging techniques are nonblinding, and therefore, an objective assessment of superiority of one test over another is difficult (Wiersema 2001). In everyday clinical practice, the role of CT and EUS in the diagnosis of pancreatic cancer is rather complementary.

A very interesting multicenter study demonstrated that possible factors associated to false-negative EUS for pancreatic cancer are chronic pancreatitis, a diffusely infiltrating carcinoma, a prominent ventral/dorsal split, and a recent episode of acute pancreatitis (Buthani 2004).

When clinical presentation is obstructive jaundice, the likelihood of malignancy is as high as 80–90% whereas jaundice is not present is much lower (around 50%). A very recent study on the diagnostic value of EUS-FNA in the latter subset of patients showed an accuracy of EUS-FNA for diagnosing malignant neoplasm of 97.6% (Krishna 2009) with sensitivity, specificity, positive, and negative predictive values of 96.6, 99, 99.1, and 96.2%, respectively. The authors concluded that EUS-FNA can be used as a definitive diagnostic test in the management of this group of patients.

The differential diagnosis between pancreatic cancer and pseudotumoral chronic pancreatitis or the diagnosis of certainty of pancreatic carcinoma in patients with severe chronic pancreatitis is still a challenge, and, to now, no imaging technique has demonstrated to be superior to the others.

Elastography is a method for real-time evaluation of tissue stiffness, which has been used in organs such as prostate gland and breast. Applying pressure to the tissue, the differences in distortion between hard and soft tissues are used for real-time analysis of the stiffness. Therefore, the obtained images represent tissue elasticity and may reflect histopathological differences. This technique has obtained good results in few recent studies, but because of some methodological problems, at present it is not possible to confirm that elastography is better than the other techniques in the differential diagnosis of pancreatic masses.

When the patient needs a stent because of the obstruction of the biliary tree, EUS should be performed before ERCP and stenting to avoid the interferences of the air and the inflammatory changes in the papilla and periampulary area. These changes due to instrumentation during ERCP can cause hypoechoic changes in the area that may lead to misinterpretation in both senses: overstaging of the lesion or they can be mistaken for a mass lesion by EUS imaging. On the other hand, the inflammation due to the biliary stent also may induce reactive cellular atypia that can mimic the cytologic features of a well-differentiated adenocarcinoma.

3 EUS in the Assessment of Vascular Invasion in Pancreatic Cancer

The most important criterion for the assessment of local resectability in pancreatic cancer is vascular involvement of the vessels that are in close anatomic relationship with the gland: portal vein, confluence with the superior mesenteric vein, superior mesenteric artery, common hepatic artery, and celiac trunk. Invasion of the inferior vena cava is difficult to see by EUS. Criteria for diagnosis of venous involvement are described in Table 2. EUS criteria for vascular involvement that optimize specificity (tumor within the lumen and/or encasement/obstruction) should be used to minimize the possibility of denying the opportunity of a potentially curative surgery. However, when the assessment of vascular involvement is the issue, tumors are usually large. In these cases, EUS may have greater difficulty in

Table 2 Criteria for diagnosis of venous involvement

Loss of tumor-vessel interface
Irregular contours between the tumor and the vessel
Direct visualization of intraluminal tumor growth
Complete obstruction of the vascular lumen
Presence of venous collaterals around or inside the gastrointestinal wall[a]

[a]Indirect sign in absence of portal hypertension

ascertaining the extension of the disease: the decrease in the resolution with the depth of the lesion together with the high frequencies used by EUS results in a limited ability to visualize the region surrounding the portal and the superior mesenteric veins.

In the early 1990, most investigations comparing the accuracy of EUS in the assessment of vascular invasion in pancreatic carcinoma with other imaging techniques showed a clear supremacy of EUS with respect to CT: 81–100% vs. 20–76%, respectively (Rösch and Classen 1992). In fact, a study published by that time (Rösch 1992) showed an accuracy for portal venous involvement of 95, 85, 75, and 55% for EUS, angiography, CT, and transabdominal US, respectively. The results obtained in a coetaneous study (Gress 1999) were very similar. However, the use of nonhelical CT influenced the results in favor of EUS.

After the initial enthusiasm on the performance characteristics of EUS in staging pancreatic cancer, a more moderate approach resulted from further investigations. In this sense, a retrospective study by Ahmad et al. (Ahmad 2000) showed a positive predictive value for resectability of 46%. On the other hand, Rösch et al. performed a very interesting study looking back at the videotapes used in a previous investigation on the ability of EUS to assess mesenteric venous invasion. The review of the videotapes was done in a blinding manner with respect to clinical information and results of other imaging tests. Gold standard used was surgical resection, surgical exploration with biopsy, or unequivocal angiography. Sensitivity and specificity of EUS in predicting mesenteric vascular invasion were 43 and 91%, respectively, as compared with 80 and 91% obtained in the previous nonblinded study (Rösch 2000). Reasons accounting for the inconsistency in data published over the years are methodological (prospective or retrospective design, study population, blinding or not, type of gold standard that lead to different kinds of biases) and

technical (different rates of improvement of the techniques over the years). In a very interesting meta-analysis of the data from 29 studies on the diagnostic accuracy of EUS for vascular invasion in pancreatic and periampullary cancers (Puli 2007), the specificity was 90% whereas the sensitivity was 73%, not as high as suggested in previous studies.

Data from well-designed comparative studies are scarce. In an investigation comparing EUS, helical CT, MRI, and angiography in the preoperative staging and tumor resectability in 62 patients with pancreatic cancer, the decision analysis demonstrated that the best strategy was based on CT or EUS as the initial test, followed by the alternative technique in the potentially respectable cases. A cost minimization analysis suggested that the most reliable sequential approach consists of a helical CT as the initial test and EUS as a confirmatory technique (Soriano 2004). On the other hand, in a recent prospective study that compared EUS and multidetector CT in staging pancreatic cancer, both techniques were similar in terms of nodal staging and assessment of resectability. Other important conclusion of this study was that published investigations are too heterogeneous in terms of design, study populations, and methods to have definitive conclusions on this topic (DeWitt 2004).

4 EUS-Guided FNA in Pancreatic Cancer

The fundamental principle for EUS-FNA is that it should be performed when the information obtained can affect patient's management. Although most patients with pancreatic cancer present with a mass, not every pancreatic mass is a cancer. The differential diagnosis of a solid pancreatic mass includes focal pancreatitis, autoimmune pancreatitis, neuroendocrine tumor, solid pseudopapillary tumor, or metastases among others. Since the image characteristics of these lesions may be similar, a histological or cytological sample is required for establishing a definitive diagnosis.

Sensitivity and accuracy of EUS-FNA of pancreatic tumors lie between 75–92% and 79–95%, respectively, in most series including a variable number of patients (from 43 to 216) (Giovannini 1995; Gress 1997; Wiersema 1997; Chang 1997; Williams 1999; Raut 2003) (Figs. 2 and 3). Failures of EUS-FNA are related

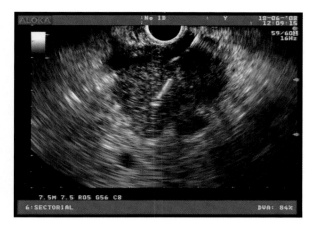

Fig. 2 Adenocarcinoma of the pancreas: hypoechogenic and heterogeneous mass with irregular margins. The needle for cytological assessment is perfectly seen inside the tumor

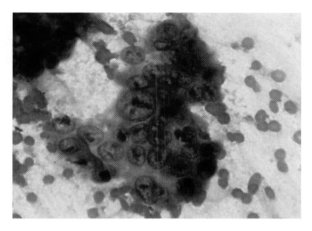

Fig. 3 Cytological smear obtained by EUS-guided FNA (EUS-FNA) consistent with adenocarcinoma

to the interposition of vascular structures, the existence of duodenal stenosis, or the hardness of the tumor itself, especially in cases of chronic pancreatitis. The second limit for sensitivity is the proportion of uninterpretable material because of the presence of blood or the scarce cellularity. The technique of monolayer cytology might improve the interpretability of the material. The size of the tumor seems to be of no effect on sensitivity of EUS-FNA. The opposite happens with cellular differentiation: the more the lesions are well-differentiated, the lower the sensitivity due to the problems in recognizing the tumor among the rest of the parenchyma.

The presence of an on-site cytopathologist or cytotechnician reduces the rate of inadequate specimens as demonstrated in several investigations (Pellisé 2003).

When EUS is available, its use depends on local treatment algorithms, specifically whether neoadjuvant chemotherapy and/or radiation therapy is offered to attempt to downstage patients prior to surgery. If this is the case, EUS-FNA is mandatory for obtaining confirmative cytology before the treatment is administered. When neoadjuvant therapy is not part of the treatment algorithm, the decision of performing or not EUS and EUS-FNA depends on the doctors in charge of the patient.

The pathological confirmation of the diagnosis of pancreatic cancer is one of the well-established indications for EUS-FNA because of the high diagnostic accuracy, low incidence of complications, and the advantages compared with other imaging techniques such as CT scan. One of these advantages is the inclusion of the needle tract in the resection specimen when the head of the pancreas is punctured through the duodenum, thereby minimizing the risk of needle-tract seeding. This would not be the case with pancreatic body and tail neoplasms, which are punctured from the stomach. However, peritoneal carcinomatosis has been reported to have significantly lower association with EUS-FNA than with percutaneous FNA (Micames 2003). Another advantage is the ability of sampling lesions or lymph nodes too small to be identified by other methods.

At present, oncologists have no doubt on the need of having the cytological confirmation of pancreatic cancer before any medical treatment is started in unresectable disease. EUS-FNA has been demonstrated to be the best technique in this setting. In the case of resectable pancreatic cancer, the need of EUS-FNA is still controversial. Reasons against it are the possibility of needle-track dissemination (that is not a problem in the tumors of the head of the pancreas for the reasons explained above) and the fact that the NPV of EUS-FNA in pancreatic masses is not very high; therefore, malignancy cannot be excluded if FNA does not show it. Moreover, although rarely, EUS-FNA may result in complications, which would postpone, interfere, or even exclude surgical treatment. Among arguments in favor of EUS-FNA, it may be argued that the diagnosis of cancer has to be proved before a major surgery, and also those lesions with nonsurgical management such as metastasis, lymphoma, or even infectious diseases have to be excluded. In fact, although the predominant type of pancreatic mass is adenocarcinoma, the differential diagnoses includes squamous cell carcinoma, acinar cell carcinoma, lymphoma, neuroendocrine tumor, solid pseudopapillary tumor, autoimmune pancreatitis, focal pancreatitis and metastases of renal cell carcinoma, melanoma, gastrointestinal stromal tumors, and carcinomas of the breast, ovary, thyroid, lung, prostate, and colon.

Pancreatic metastases seem to be more frequent that it was thought years ago, probably due to the higher accuracy of the current image techniques and the improved survival of patients. They are usually metachronous and characterized by a long period of time between the resection of the primary tumor and their detection. The awareness of the clinical history of the patient, as well as some image characteristics, especially if there are multiple lesions, is crucial for suspicion of this diagnosis (DeWitt 2005).

Autoimmune pancreatitis is a benign inflammatory disease of the pancreas, which may mimic pancreatic carcinoma both clinically and radiologically. EUS-FNA has to be performed if the differential diagnosis is an issue, although it may be difficult to make a definite diagnosis by using cytology alone. However, it has recently been described that EUS-FNA and EUS-guided biopsy with a trucut needle in combination with immunohistochemical staining may be useful for making the specific diagnosis of the disease (Levy 2006).

It has been estimated that approximately 6% of patients undergoing pancreatico-duodenostomy have a benign process. Another 6% of patients may have an "unusual" histological diagnosis. Therefore, some authors strongly recommend a pretreatment tissue.

Finally, not only diagnosis, but also staging of pancreatic cancer may be an indication for EUS-FNA in cases with lymph nodes (especially around the aorta or the celiac axis) and ascites.

It is very important to point out that negative results of EUS-FNA in a pancreatic mass do not rule out malignancy. A large number of studies found an almost 100% specificity with 80–90% sensitivity (Levy 2007), although the pretest likelihood varies among them.

Concerning complications of EUS-FNA, the rate of complications of the technique varies between 0.3 and 2.2% in the larger series of patients (Mortensen 2005; Bournet 2006). The incidence of pancreatitis after EUS-FNA is quite low, although hyperamylasemia occurs in 12% of cases (Eloubeidi 2004; Fernández-Esparrach 2007).

5 Molecular Markers in the Diagnosis of Pancreatic Cancer

After demonstrated that EUS-FNA provides the cytological diagnosis of pancreatic cancer in more than 90% of cases, the interest of some endosonographers turned towards the possibility of performing molecular determinations from the same sample. The rational is that the detection of DNA mutations in the form of point mutations such as K-*ras* and chromosomal losses (loss of heterozygosity) may serve as surrogate markers of malignancy. In this sense, mutations of K-*ras* have been proven to be determined from EUS-FNA material (Pellisé 2003; Tada 2002). Conventional cytology has been compared with K-*ras* mutation analysis in the detection of pancreatic malignancy. Conventional cytology has an overall accuracy of 71–91% compared with 82–84% of K-*ras* mutation analysis, whereas the combination of both methods resulted in an accuracy of 98% (Pellisé 2003). However, limitations exist since up to 20% of pancreatic cancers do not have these mutations, and on the contrary, K-*ras* mutations have been detected in chronic pancreatitis and premalignant conditions such as intraductal papillary mucinous neoplasms. Similar studies have obtained similar results with p53 immunohistochemical analysis (Itoi 2005), telomerase activity (Mishra 2006), and a broad panel of microsatellite allele loss markers (Khalid 2006). Therefore, in cases of inconclusive EUS-FNA cytology, molecular markers could help in establishing the diagnosis of malignancy, and moreover, they open the door to future more individualized treatments, which is the general aim of modern oncology.

References

Ahmad NA (2000) EUS in preoperative staging of pancreatic cancer. Gastrointest Endosc 52:463–468

Agarwal B (2004) Endoscopic ultrasound-guided fine needle aspiration and multidetector spiral CT in the diagnosis of pancreatic cancer. Am J Gastroenterol 99:844–850

Bournet B (2006) Early morbidity of endoscopic ultrasound: 13 years' experience at a referral center. Endoscopy 38:349–354

Buthani MS (2004) The no endosonographic detection of tumor (NEST) study: a case series of pancreatic cancers missed on endoscopic ultrasonography. Endoscopy 36:385–389

Chang KJ (1997) The clinical utility of endoscopic ultrasound-guided fine-needle aspiration in the diagnosis and staging of pancreatic carcinoma. Gastrointest Endosc 45:387–393

DeWitt J (2004) Comparison of endoscopic ultrasonography and multidetector computed tomography for detecting and staging pancreatic cancer. Ann Intern Med 141:753–763

DeWitt J (2005) EUS-guided FNA of pancreatic metastases: a multicenter experience. Gastrointest Endosc 61:689–696

Eloubeidi MA (2004) Acute pancreatitis after EUS-guided FNA of solid pancreatic masses: a pooled analysis from EUS centers in the United States. Gastrointest Endosc 60:385–389

Fernández-Esparrach G (2007) Incidence and clinical significance of hyperamylasemia after endoscopic ultrasound-guided fine-needle aspiration (EUS-FNA) of pancreatic lesions: a prospective and controlled study. Endoscopy 39:720–724

Giovannini M (1995) Fine-needle aspiration cytology guided by endoscopic ultrasonography: results in 141 patients. Endoscopy 27:171–177

Gress FG (1997) Endoscopic ultrasound-guided fine-needle aspiration biopsy using linear array and radial scanning endosonography. Gastrointest Endosc 45:243–250

Gress FG (1999) Role of endoscopic ultrasound in the preoperative staging of pancreatic cancer: a large single-center experience. Gastrointest Endosc 50:786–791

Itoi T (2005) Immunohistochemical analysis of p53 and MIB-1 in tissue specimens obtained from endoscopic ultrasonongraphy-guided fine needle aspiration biopsy for the diagnosis of solid pancreatic masses. Oncol Rep 13:229–234

Khalid A (2006) Endoscopic ultrasound fine needle aspirate DNA analysis to differentiate malignant and benign pancreatic masses. Am J Gastroenterol 101:2493–2500

Klapman JB (2005) Negative predictive value of endoscopic ultrasound in a large series of patients with a clinical suspicion of pancreatic cancer. Am J Gastroenterol 100:1–4

Krishna NB (2009) Diagnostic value of EUS-FNA in patients suspected of having pancreatic cancer with a focal lesion on CT scan/MRI but without obstructive jaundice. Pancreas 38:625–630

Levy MJ (2006) Chronic pancreatitis: focal pancreatitis or cancer. is there a role for FNA/biopsy? Autoimmune pancreatitis. Endoscopy 38(suppl 1):S30–S35

Levy MJ (2007) Endoscopic ultrasound-guided trucut biopsy of the pancreas: prospects and problems. Pancreatology 7:163–166

Mertz HR (2000) EUS, PET, and CT scanning for evaluation of pancreatic adenocarcinoma. Gastrointest Endosc 52:367–371

Micames C (2003) Lower frequency of peritoneal carcinomatosis in patients with pancreatic cancer diagnosed by EUS-FNA vs. percutaneous FNA. Gastrointest Endosc 58:690–695

Mishra G (2006) Determination of qualitative telomerase activity as an adjunct to the diagnosis of pancreatic adenocarcinoma by EUS-guided fine-needle aspiration. Gastrointest Endosc 63:648–654

Mortensen MB (2005) Prospective evaluation of patient tolerability, satisfaction with patient information, and complications in endoscopic ultrasonography. Emdoscopy 37:146–153

Muller MF (1994) Pancreatic tumors: evaluation with endoscopic US, CT and MR imaging. Radiology 190:745–751

Pellisé M (2003) Usefulness of KRAS mutational analysis in the diagnosis of pancreatic adenocarcinoma by means of endosonography-guided fine-needle aspiration biopsy. Aliment Pharmacol Ther 17:1299–1307

Puli SR (2007) Diagnostic accuracy of EUS for vascular invasion in pancreatic and periampullary cancers: a meta-analysis and systematic review. Gastrointest Endosc 65:788–797

Raut C (2003) Diagnostic accuracy of endoscopic-ultrasound guided fine-needle aspiration in patients with presumed pancreatic cancer. J Gastrointest Surg 7:118–128

Rösch T (1990) Preoperative localization of endocrine tumors of the pancreas: endoscopic ultrasound is superior to transabdominal sonography and computed tomography. Gastrointest Endosc 36:199–200

Rösch T (1991) Endoscopic ultrasound in pancreatic tumor diagnosis. Gastrointest Endosc 37:347–352

Rösch T (1992) Staging of pancreatic and ampullary carcinoma by endoscopic ultrasonography. Comparison with conventional sonography, computed tomography and angiography. Gastroenterology 102:188–199

Rösch T (2000) Endoscopic ultrasound criteria of vascular invasion in the staging of pancreatic head cancer: a blinded reevaluation of videotapes. Gastrointest Endosc 52:469–477

Rösch T, Classen M (1992) Gastroenterologic endosonography. Textbook and atlas. Thieme Verlag, New York

Snady H (1992) Endoscopic ultrasonography compared with computed tomography with ERCP in patients with obstructive jaundice or small peri-pancreatic mass. Gastrointest Endosc 38:27–34

Soriano A (2004) Preoperative staging and tumor respectability assessment on pancreatic cancer: prospective study comparing endoscopic ultrasonography, helical computed tomography, magnetic resonance imaging, and angiography. Am J Gastroenterol 99:492–501

Tada M (2002) Quantitative analysis of K-ras gene mutation in pancreatic tissue obtained by endoscopic ultrasonography-guided fine needle aspiration: clinikcal utility for diagnosis of pancreatic tumor. Am J Gastroenterol 97:2263–2270

Wiersema MJ (1997) Endosonography-guided fine-needle aspiration biopsy: diagnostic accuracy and complication assessment. Gastrointest Endosc 112:1087–1095

Wiersema MJ (2001) Accuracy of endoscopic ultrasonography in diagnosis and staging of pancreatic carcinoma. Pancreatology 1:625–632

Williams DB (1999) Endoscopic ultrasound guided fine needle aspiration biopsy: a large centre experience. Gut 44:720–726

Yasuda K (1988) The diagnosis of pancreatic cancer by endoscopic ultrasonography. Gastrointest Endosc 34:1–8

PET/CT in Pancreatic Cancer

Thomas F. Hany and Klaus Strobel

Contents

Abstract

> Hardware- fused positron emission tomography (PET) and computed tomography (CT) to PET/CT as a single-step procedure improves the diagnostic accuracy in many oncological diseases. PET/CT using the most applied tracer F-18 fluorodeoxyglucose (FDG) helps in the differentiation malignant from benign pancreatic mass lesions. In proven exocrine pancreatic cancer, additional use iodinated, intravenous contrast in PET/CT combines the considerable advantages of both imaging modalities in detecting distant metastases as well as local staging regarding vascular invasion. Since FDG-uptake in tumor is correlated with tumor viability, FDG-PET/CT can be used for therapy response assessment in a neo-adjuvant, curative setting as well in monitoring radio-chemotherapy in a palliative setting. Further, FDG-PET/CT is able to detect local as well as distant recurrence rather reliably. For neuroendocrine pancreatic ancer, newly developed tracers like F18-DOPA and 68Ga-DOTA-NOC may revolutionize the diagnostic work-up by combining diagnostic as well as therapy related informations into a single exam.

T.F. Hany (✉) and K. Strobel
Department Medical Radiology, Division of Nuclear Medicine,
University Hospital, Raemistrasse 100, 8091 Zurich,
Switzerland
e-mail: thomas.hany@usz.ch

1 Introduction

Positron emission tomography (PET) using 18F-fluorodeoxyglucose (FDG) for imaging pancreatic ductal adenocarcinoma has been used early after the

A. Laghi (ed.), *New Concepts in Diagnosis and Therapy of Pancreatic Adenocarcinoma*,
Medical Radiology, DOI: 10.1007/174_2010_5, © Springer-Verlag Berlin Heidelberg 2011

introduction of this technology in the late 1990's and the beginning of this decade (Delbeke et al. 1999). Due to missing morphological information, staging by FDG-PET imaging alone was not very successful regarding local disease extension. With the introduction of a combined approach, acquiring PET and CT information in a combined mode on a PET/CT machine, morphological as well as functional information were available. This chapter discusses the current state of PET/CT imaging in staging pancreatic cancer, therapy response, and recurrence.

2 Technique

Since the first proof of the concept PET/CT system devised by Townsend started to operate in 1998 and the first worldwide clinical PET/CT scanner came into operation in March 2001, PET/CT has developed into the fastest growing imaging modality worldwide (Beyer et al. 2000; Hany et al. 2002). Lutetium (LSO, LYSO)-, Germanium (GSO)- as well as Bismutgermanate (BGO)-based crystals are used in different scanner types. PET-emission data are acquired in 2D- as well as in 3D-mode, whereas 3D-mode seems to be the preferential method. Additionally, different new reconstruction algorithms are used to improve image quality (Strobel et al. 2007).

CT data are foremost used for attenuation correction and as anatomic reference frame in PET/CT. Artifacts, which can be generated in PET images due to the use of CT data transformed into μ-maps, are related to the accumulation of highly concentrated CT contrast agents, CT beam-hardening artifacts due to metallic implants and physiologic motion. Additionally, major artifacts occur in the regions adjacent to the heart and the diaphragm including the liver due to mismatch between PET- and CT-data acquisition. An analysis of this problem has shown that with the modern fast CT scanners it is probably best to also acquire the CT data during tidal breathing. Ideally, the CT data are acquired during end expiration, but frequently patient cooperation is problematic to achieve this (von Schulthess et al. 2006). Another approach is to use respiratory gated 4D-PET/CT, which probably has an advantage not only in lungs but also in upper abdominal imaging including the liver (Nehmeh et al. 2004).

Patients have to fast for at least 4 h prior to the FDG injection. Blood glucose measurements are performed

routinely to confirm euglycemia related to fasting and possibly detect patients with a previously undetected diabetes. If patients were truly fasting, blood glucose levels in nondiabetic patients are normally below 6–8 mmol/L. However, in diabetic patients fasting more than 4 h, an elevated blood glucose level above 8 mmol/L can be detected. Nevertheless, routine injection of a standard dose of 370 MBq of FDG can be injected in truly fasting diabetic patients, who did not receive insulin within 4 h prior to FDG injection without decrease in image quality. Therefore, the most important procedure is to ensure that the fasting time has been at least 4 h. In diabetic patients with elevated glucose levels, even though patients have been fasting, injection of fast acting insulin should not be performed since the insulin will move the FDG into the muscles due to insulin-dependent transport. In pancreatic cancer, water as a negative oral contrast agent is given. Bladder voiding just prior to scanning to eliminate the renally excreted FDG is mandatory. The average whole-body patient dose at 40 mAs is approximately 3 mSv and adds up to approximately 8 mSv for a standard dose of 370 MBq FDG. Obviously, the main contraindication is to perform PET/CT in pregnant women.

In pancreatic cancer, dual-phase contrast-enhanced CT (ceCT) of the pancreas/abdomen should be performed. Two different approaches for the use of intravenous contrast have been introduced. In a single-step approach, contrast is given during the acquisition of CT data used for attenuation correction and no further CT scanning is needed. The other approach includes two CT-data acquisitions. One fast, whole-body low-dose CT for AC, and an additional dedicated contrast-enhanced CT in the region of interest after completion of the PET/CT exam if necessary (Strobel et al. 2005, 2008).

Performing a dedicated contrast-enhanced single to multiphase CT-data acquisition after completion of PET/CT in a defined anatomical region has two advantages. First, in cases with extended disease or normal findings, the contrast injection may be unnecessary (Brix et al. 2005). Second, the possibility to acquire a multiphase, contrast-enhanced CT during the arterial, venous, and parenchymal phase is more efficient compared to a single phase acquisition. Therefore, a comprehensive diagnostic workup in a single session can be achieved.

As a general rule for the interval between the end of treatment and PET/CT imaging, PET/CT can be performed 2 weeks after the end of chemotherapy treatment to assess the therapy response. In radiation treatment, a minimum interval of 6 weeks should be used after the end of treatment to reduce FDG-uptake due to inflammatory changes.

3 Characterization of Focal Pancreatic Masses

Differentiation of focal chronic pancreatitis from pancreatic carcinoma remains difficult with all imaging modalities. In an early PET alone study by Zimny et al. (1997), 106 patients were examined due to a suspicious pancreatic mass. In 70% of the cases, adenocarcinoma was histologically confirmed, and 30% were related to chronic pancreatitis. Overall, FDG-PET detected 63 of 74 malignant tumors and 27 of 32 cases of nonmalignant origin. Overall, sensitivity and specificity in the detection of pancreatic cancer were 85% and 84%, respectively. Other studies reported similar results, in a fair amount of cases better than morphological imaging studies. In a study by Heinrich et al. (2005), 59 patients with suspected pancreatic cancer were staged by abdominal CT, chest X-ray and CA 19-9 measurement, and FDG-PET/CT, and findings were confirmed by histology. Cost benefit analysis was performed based on charged cost of PET/CT and pancreatic resection. The positive and negative predictive values for pancreatic cancer were 91% and 64%, respectively. False-positive results were due to inflammatory pseudotumor, pancreatic tuberculosis, chronic pancreatitis, and focal high-grade dysplasia, which was suspicious for malignancy by brush cytology. PET/CT detected additional distant metastases in five and a synchronous rectal cancer in two patients. PET/CT findings changed the management in 16% of patients with pancreatic cancer deemed resectable after routine staging ($p=0.031$). In total, PET/CT reduced cost by $74,925 ($1,270 per patient).

In a study by Schick et al. (2008), 46 patients with a solid pancreatic lesion >10 mm and suspicion of a pancreatic neoplasm underwent dual-phase, contrast-enhanced FDG-PET/CT. Results were compared to endoscopic ultrasound (EUS), endocopic retrograde cholangio-pancreatography (ERCP), intraductal ultrasound (IUDS), abdominal ultrasound, and histopathology. In 27 patients, a pancreatic malignancy was proven by histopathology, whereas the sensitivity of

PET/CT in the detection of malignant disease was 89% with a specificity of 74%. There were no significant differences between sensitivity, specificity, and positive and negative predictive values compared to the other imaging modalities. The increased specificity was attributed to the contrast-enhanced CT of the integrated PET/CT; however, local invasion of the local vasculature was not assessed in this study.

4 Staging of Pancreatic Ductal Adenocarcinoma

The most important information from any imaging modality is arterial vascular involvement of the primary tumor, the presence of peritoneal carcinomatosis, and the detection of distant metastases (Fig. 1). Regarding the performance of PET/CT now, available data are rather sparse. In a study by Farma et al. (2008), 82 patients with assumed resectable pancreatic cancer underwent staging with noncontrast-enhanced PET/CT and ceCT of the chest and abdomen. The sensitivity and specificity of PET/CT in diagnosing pancreatic cancer were 89% and 88%, respectively. Sensitivity of detecting metastases for PET/CT, ceCT, and the combination of both were 61, 57, and 87%, respectively. PET/CT findings influenced the clinical management in seven patients (11%), essentially all due to distant metastases. As a major drawback of this study, the CT component of the PET/CT was not performed using a contrast-enhanced triple-phase CT. In a study by Strobel et al. (2008), 50 patients with biopsy-proven pancreatic cancer (adenocarcinoma) were evaluated by integrated three-phase contrast-enhanced PET/CT regarding resectability and overall staging. Criteria for unresectability were distant metastases, peritoneal carcinomatosis, arterial infiltration, or infiltration of neighboring organs other than the duodenum. Histology, intraoperative findings, and follow-up CT with clinical findings were used as standard of reference. According to standard, 27 patients had unresectable disease because of distant metastases ($n=17$), peritoneal carcinomatosis ($n=5$), or local infiltration ($n=5$) (Fig. 2). In the assessment of resectability, PET alone had a sensitivity of 100%, specificity of 44%, accuracy of 70%, positive predictive value of 61%, and negative predictive value of 100%; unenhanced PET/CT had respective values of 100, 56, 76, 66, and 100%; and

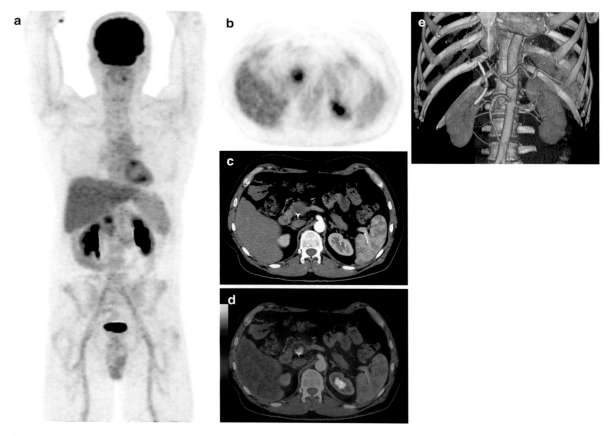

Fig. 1 43-year-old male patient with a proven adenocarcinoma of the pancreas, stenting of the choeldochus due symptomatic cholostasis, patient referred for staging. Maximum intensity projection image (MIP, **a**) demonstrates focal FDG-uptake in the right mid-abdomen, no evidence of further pathological uptake. In the axial PET (**b**), ceCT (**c**) and fused image (**d**), the focal uptake is clearly localized to the pancreatic head lesion without evidence of local arterial invasion. Volume rendered, fused PET/CT image (**e**) delineates the proximity to the stent and clear delineation for arterial vasculature of the celiac trunk

enhanced PET/CT, 96, 82, 88, 82, and 96%. In five patients, unresectability was missed by all imaging methods and was diagnosed intraoperatively. Enhanced PET/CT was significantly superior to PET alone ($p = 0.035$), and there was a trend for enhanced PET/CT to be superior to unenhanced PET/CT ($p = 0.070$). From the above mentioned data, it is clear that noncontrast-enhanced PET/CT is able to detect distant metastases in a large proportion of cases; however, local extent is not possible. Furthermore, in a rather considerable proportion of patients, only intraoperative findings do reveal surgery-precluding factors such as deep retroperitoneal infiltration, small liver metastases, or peritoneal involvement. It seems that an approach including an intravenous contrast-enhanced CT into the PET/CT protocol seems to be most favorable, but does not reflect clinical practice, since most patients with a suspicion of a pancreatic lesion rapidly undergo contrast-enhanced CT or MRI.

5 Therapy Response Evaluation

Standard treatment for advanced adenocarcinoma of the pancreas (stage III and higher) includes chemotherapy with or without radiation treatment. In general, assessment of treatment response has an impact on treatment strategies and obviously outcome. In FDG-PET imaging, FDG-uptake is rather strongly correlated to a number of tumor cells as well as tumor cell viability. Probably, the best-studied group of malignant disease regarding tumor response assessment is lymphomas, including Hodgkin's as well as Non-Hodgkin's

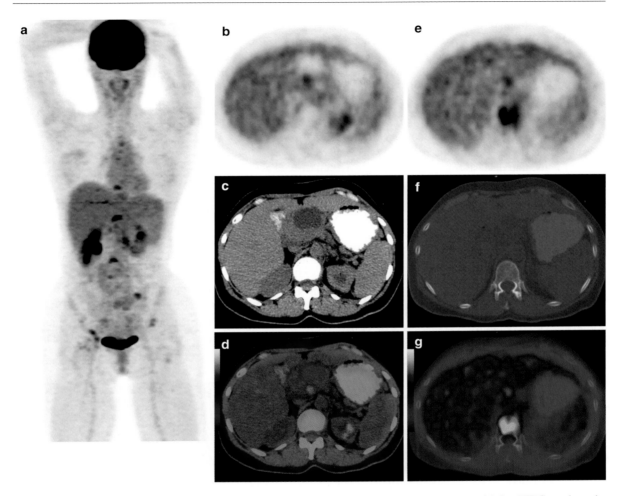

Fig. 2 46-year-old female patient with proven cystadenocarcinoma of the pancreas. Maximum intensity projection image (MIP, **a**) with faint uptake in the region of the mid-abdomen but multiple focal FDG-uptake in projection of the midline. In the axial PET (**b**), non-enhanced CT (**c**) and fused image (**d**), the cystic lesion of the pancreas is seen with focal FDG-uptake at the rim. Axial PET (**e**), CT (**f**) and fused image (**g**) at he the level of the 12th thoracic spine demonstrates high FDG-uptake in the vertebral body without considerable osseous destruction, corresponding to an osseous metastases, previously not detected in CT

lymphoma. Reduction FDG-uptake to so-called normal values in the affected regions is related strongly to successful treatment as well as progression-free survival (Jerusalem et al. 2001). Standard treatment options for patients with stage I and II pancreatic cancer include pancreaticoduodenectomy with adjuvant treatment including chemo- and/or radiation therapy. Here, obviously no data regarding the use of PET/CT in this setting are available. For patients with advanced nonresectable cancer, a combination of chemo-radiation treatment is given in a palliative intent. Only small studies are available, using PET stand-alone as well as separate CT scans for therapy evaluation. In studies by Maisey et al. (2000) as well as Yoshioka et al. 2003), a decrease of FDG was seen before any changes in CT were visible. In a study by Bang et al. (2006), a small patient population of 15 patients receiving radio-chemotherapy was followed up. FDG-PET detected treatment response in 5 out of 15 cases, whereas CT was not able to see any differences due to similar tumor size before and after treatment. Furthermore, time-to-tumor progression was significantly longer in PET-responders. It seems that, overall, regarding therapy response assessment in this clinical setting of palliative treatment, PET has a certain value; however, data regarding the appropriate use of costly PET/CT exams are missing.

Heinrich et al. (2008) evaluated a somehow novel approach, using gemcitabine-based chemotherapy in a neoadjuvant setting for potentially resectable pancreatic cancer. FDG-PET/CT was used pre and postchemotherapy for tumor response assessment in 28 patients before pancreaticoduodenectomy. A significant decrease in FDG-uptake occurred during chemotherapy ($p=0.031$), which correlated with the baseline FDG-uptake ($p=0.001$), Ki-67 expression ($p=0.016$), and histologic response ($p=0.01$). Regarding patient outcome, neither the metabolic nor the histologic response was predictive of the median disease-free (9.2 months) or overall survival (26.5 months).

6 Recurrent Disease

Serial measurements of tumor marker levels (CA 19-9) are a sensitive indicator of disease recurrence. However, differentiation of local scar from tumor is difficult. Ruf et al. (2005) demonstrated in a study of 31 patients

with suspected recurrent disease a sensitivity of 96% in the detection of local recurrences by FDG-PET compared to 23% by CT or MRI. In detecting metastatic disease in the liver, CT and MRI were more sensitive, particularly in identifying small lesions, but FDG-PET additionally helped to detect occult nonregional and extraabdominal disease (Fig. 3).

7. Endocrine pancreatic cancer

Neuroendocrine tumors of the pancreas account for less than 5% of all malignant tumors of the pancreas. PET imaging using FDG has limited value, since this tumor entity has often a slow tumor growth and according low metabolism (Pasquali et al. 1998). Beside morphological imaging modalities including ceCT and MRI, Somatostatin receptor scintigraphy (SRS) is generally used to localize and characterize neuroendocrine tumors in general and specially of the pancreas.

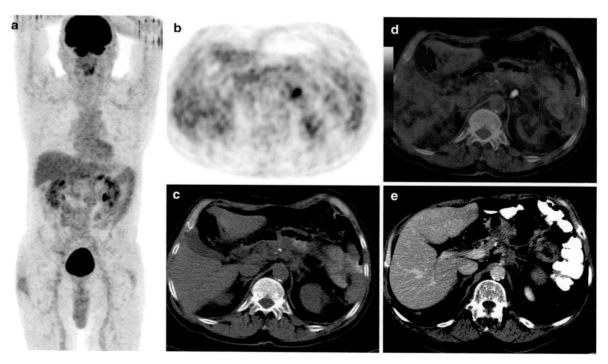

Fig. 3 63-year-old male patient with suspicion of recurrent pancreatic carcinoma of the pancreatic tail after left pancreatic resection. Maximum intensity projection image (MIP, **a**) demonstrates focal FDG-uptake left upper abdomen. In the axial PET (**b**), non-enhanced CT (**c**) and fused image (**d**), the focal uptake is localized to a soft tissue mass in the former region of the pancreatic tail, corresponding to a local recurrence, which was regarded a focal scar in the previously performed ceCT (**e**)

Interpretation of SRS can be challenging due to the difficulty of distinguishing tumors from intestinal structures, and due to the variable density of somatostatin receptors on the different tumors. Overall, a significant rate of false negative results with sensitivities ranging between 50% and 78% in detection of NET depending on the localisation, have been reported (Gibril et al. 1996). Positron emission tomography (PET) using the catecholamine precursor 6-(fluoride-18) fluoro-dopa (F18-DOPA) has been proposed as a valuable imaging option for NET (Koopmans et al. 2006). It highlights the intracellular decarboxylase activity and provides, being a PET-tracer, a higher spatial resolution than SRS-imaging (Fig.4). A major drawback of this tracers is the essential physiological uptake of this tracer into the pancreas, obscuring in certain cases the detection of the primary tumor. Another rather newly developed PET-tracer uses the same basic principle of SRS by labeling somtostatin to Ga-68. In a study by Ambrosini et al. both tracers were

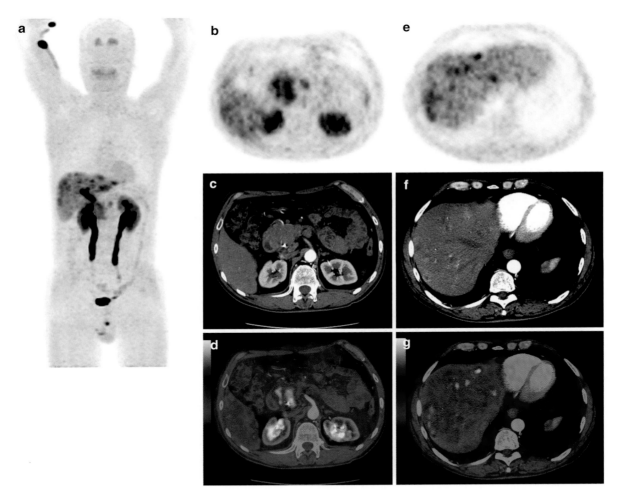

Fig. 4 56-year-old male patient with a proven neuroendocrine tumor of the pancreas with a high proliferation rate referred for a DOPA-PET/CT. Maximum intensity projection image (MIP, a) demonstrates multiple focal DOPA-uptake in both liver lobes, uptake in the large primary tumor and physiological uptake in the basal ganglia as well as excretion into the bile duct. In the axial PET (b), arterial phase ceCT (c) and fused images (d), the DOPA-uptake in the primary tumor of the pancreatic head as well as an adjacent lymph node metastasis left to the mesenteric artery is seen. Further, typical focal DOPA-uptake in multiple, early arterial enhancing liver metastasis can be demonstrated (PET (e), arterial phase ceCT (f) and fused image (g))

compared in a rather small group of 13 patients (Ambrosini et al. 2008). 68Ga-DOTA-NOC demonstrated to be an accurate tracer for the assessment of NET cases; 68Ga- DOTA-NOC was found to be more accurate than 18-F-DOPA for the detection of NET primary tumour and metastatic sites of disease. Especially for pancreatic primary tumours, the accuracy was better for 68Ga-DOTA-NOC. The authors concluded, that since pancreas is the most frequent site of NET the routine use of 68Ga-DOTA-NOC seems to be more appropriate. Here, obviously, larger, comparative studies including morphological imaging modalities have to be performed to determine the role of PET/CT in neuroendocrine tumors of the pancreas.

References

Ambrosini V, Tomassetti P, Castellucci P, Campana D, Montini G, Rubello D, Nanni C, Rizzello A, Franchi R, Fanti S (2008) Comparison between 68Ga-DOTA-NOC and 18F-DOPA PET for the detection of gastro-entero-pancreatic and lung neuro-endocrine tumours. Eur J Nucl Med Mol Imaging 35(8): 1431-1438

Bang S, Chung HW, Park SW, Chung JB, Yun M, Lee JD, Song SY (2006) The clinical usefulness of 18-fluorodeoxyglucose positron emission tomography in the differential diagnosis, staging, and response evaluation after concurrent chemoradiotherapy for pancreatic cancer. J Clin Gastroenterol 40(10):923–929

Beyer T, Townsend DW, Brun T, Kinahan PE, Charron M, Roddy R, Jerin J, Young J, Byars L, Nutt R (2000) A combined PET/CT scanner for clinical oncology. J Nucl Med 41(8):1369–1379

Brix G, Lechel U, Glatting G, Ziegler SI, Munzing W, Muller SP, Beyer T (2005) Radiation exposure of patients undergoing whole-body dual-modality 18F-FDG PET/CT examinations. J Nucl Med 46(4):608–613

Chang L, Stefanidis D, Richardson WS, Earle DB, Fanelli RD (2009) The role of staging laparoscopy for intraabdominal cancers: an evidence-based review. Surg Endosc 23(2): 231-241

Delbeke D, Rose DM, Chapman WC, Pinson CW, Wright JK, Beauchamp RD, Shyr Y, Leach SD (1999) Optimal interpretation of FDG PET in the diagnosis, staging and management of pancreatic carcinoma. J Nucl Med 40(11):1784–1791

Farma JM, Santillan AA, Melis M, Walters J, Belinc D, Chen DT, Eikman EA, Malafa M (2008) PET/CT fusion scan enhances CT staging in patients with pancreatic neoplasms. Ann Surg Oncol 15(9):2465–2471

Gibril F, Reynolds JC, Doppman JL, Chen CC, Venzon DJ, Termanini B, Weber HC, Stewart CA, Jensen RT (1996) Somatostatin receptor scintigraphy: its sensitivity compared with that of other imaging methods in detecting primary and metastatic gastrinomas. A prospective study. Ann Intern Med 125(1): 26-34

Hany TF, Steinert HC, Goerres GW, Buck A, von Schulthess GK (2002) PET diagnostic accuracy: improvement with in-line PET-CT system: initial results. Radiology 225(2):575–581

Heinrich S, Goerres GW, Schafer M, Sagmeister M, Bauerfeind P, Pestalozzi BC, Hany TF, von Schulthess GK, Clavien PA (2005) Positron emission tomography/computed tomography influences on the management of resectable pancreatic cancer and its cost-effectiveness. Ann Surg 242(2): 235–243

Heinrich S, Schafer M, Weber A, Hany TF, Bhure U, Pestalozzi BC, Clavien PA (2008) Neoadjuvant chemotherapy generates a significant tumor response in resectable pancreatic cancer without increasing morbidity: results of a prospective phase II trial. Ann Surg 248(6):1014–1022

Jerusalem G, Beguin Y, Najjar F, Hustinx R, Fassotte MF, Rigo P, Fillet G (2001) Positron emission tomography (PET) with 18F-fluorodeoxyglucose (18F-FDG) for the staging of low-grade non-Hodgkin's lymphoma (NHL). Ann Oncol 12(6): 825–830

Koopmans KP, de Vries EG, Kema IP, Elsinga PH, Neels OC, Sluiter WJ, van der Horst-Schrivers AN, Jager PL (2006) Staging of carcinoid tumours with 18F-DOPA PET: a prospective, diagnostic accuracy study. Lancet Oncol 7(9): 728-734

Long EE, Van Dam J, Weinstein S, Jeffrey B, Desser T, Norton JA (2005) Computed tomography, endoscopic, laparoscopic, and intra-operative sonography for assessing resectability of pancreatic cancer. Surg Oncol 14(2): 105-113

Maisey NR, Webb A, Flux GD, Padhani A, Cunningham DC, Ott RJ, Norman A (2000) FDG-PET in the prediction of survival of patients with cancer of the pancreas: a pilot study. Br J Cancer 83(3):287–293

Nehmeh SA, Erdi YE, Pan T, Yorke E, Mageras GS, Rosenzweig KE, Schoder H, Mostafavi H, Squire O, Pevsner A, Larson SM, Humm JL (2004) Quantitation of respiratory motion during 4D-PET/CT acquisition. Med Phys 31(6):1333–1338

Palazzo L, Roseau G, Gayet B, Vilgrain V, Belghiti J, Fekete F, Paolaggi JA (1993) Endoscopic ultrasonography in the diagnosis and staging of pancreatic adenocarcinoma. Results of a prospective study with comparison to ultrasonography and CT scan. Endoscopy 25(2): 143-150

Pasquali C, Rubello D, Sperti C, Gasparoni P, Liessi G, Chierichetti F, Ferlin G, Pedrazzoli S (1998) Neuroendocrine tumor imaging: can 18F-fluorodeoxyglucose positron emission tomography detect tumors with poor prognosis and aggressive behavior? World J Surg 22(6): 588-592

Ruf J, Lopez Hanninen E, Oettle H, Plotkin M, Pelzer U, Stroszczynski C, Felix R, Amthauer H (2005) Detection of recurrent pancreatic cancer: comparison of FDG-PET with CT/MRI. Pancreatology 5(2–3):266–272

Schick V, Franzius C, Beyna T, Oei ML, Schnekenburger J, Weckesser M, Domschke W, Schober O, Heindel W, Pohle T, Juergens KU (2008) Diagnostic impact of 18F-FDG PET-CT evaluating solid pancreatic lesions versus endosonography, endoscopic retrograde cholangio-pancreatography with intraductal ultrasonography and abdominal ultrasound. Eur J Nucl Med Mol Imaging 35(10):1775–1785

Smith SL, Rajan PS (2004) Imaging of pancreatic adenocarcinoma with emphasis on multidetector CT. Clin Radiol 59(1): 26-38

Soriano A, Castells A, Ayuso C, Ayuso JR, de Caralt MT, Gines MA, Real MI, Gilabert R, Quinto L, Trilla A, Feu F,

Montanya X, Fernandez-Cruz L, Navarro S (2004) Preoperative staging and tumor resectability assessment of pancreatic cancer: prospective study comparing endoscopic ultrasonography, helical computed tomography, magnetic resonance imaging, and angiography. Am J Gastroenterol 99(3): 492-501

Strobel K, Heinrich S, Bhure U, Soyka J, Veit-Haibach P, Pestalozzi BC, Clavien PA, Hany TF (2008) Contrast-enhanced 18F-FDG PET/CT: 1-stop-shop imaging for assessing the resectability of pancreatic cancer. J Nucl Med 49(9):1408–1413

Strobel K, Rudy M, Treyer V, Veit-Haibach P, Burger C, Hany TF (2007) Objective and subjective comparison of standard 2-D and fully 3-D reconstructed data on a PET/CT system. Nucl Med Commun 28(7):555–559

Strobel K, Thuerl CM, Hany TF (2005) How much intravenous contrast is needed in FDG-PET/CT? Nuklearmedizin 44(suppl 1):S32–S37

von Schulthess GK, Steinert HC, Hany TF (2006) Integrated PET/CT: current applications and future directions. Radiology 238(2):405–422

Wray CJ, Ahmad SA, Matthews JB, Lowy AM (2005) Surgery for pancreatic cancer: recent controversies and current practice. Gastroenterology 128(6): 1626-1641

Yeo CJ, Abrams RA, Grochow LB, Sohn TA, Ord SE, Hruban RH, Zahurak ML, Dooley WC, Coleman J, Sauter PK, Pitt HA, Lillemoe KD, Cameron JL (1997) Pancreaticoduodenectomy for pancreatic adenocarcinoma: postoperative adjuvant chemoradiation improves survival. A prospective, single-institution experience. Ann Surg 225(5): 621-633; discussion 633-636

Yoshioka M, Sato T, Furuya T, Shibata S, Andoh H, Asanuma Y, Hatazawa J, Koyama K (2003) Positron emission tomography with 2-deoxy-2-[(18)F] fluoro- d-glucose for diagnosis of intraductal papillary mucinous tumor of the pancreas with parenchymal invasion. J Gastroenterol 38(12):1189–1193

Zimny M, Bares R, Fass J, Adam G, Cremerius U, Dohmen B, Klever P, Sabri O, Schumpelick V, Buell U (1997) Fluorine-18 fluorodeoxyglucose positron emission tomography in the differential diagnosis of pancreatic carcinoma: a report of 106 cases. Eur J Nucl Med 24(6):678–682

A Cost Decision Analysis for Diagnosing and Staging

Stephan L. Haas, Konstantin von Heydwolff, and J.-Matthias Löhr

Contents

S.L. Haas (✉)
Department of Medicine II, Gastroenterology and Oncology,
Klinikum Aschaffenburg, Teaching Hospital of the University
of Würzburg, Am Hasenkopf 1, D-63739 Aschaffenburg,
Germany
e-mail: stephan.haas@klinikum-aschaffenburg.de

K. von Heydwolff
Financial Controlling Unit, Teaching Hospital of the University
of Würzburg, Am Hasenkopf 1, D-63739 Aschaffenburg,
Germany
e-mail: konstantin.vonheydwolff@klinikum-aschaffenburg.de

J.-M. Löhr
CLINTEC, K53; Department of Surgical Gastroenterology,
Karolinska University Hospital Huddinge, SE-141 86,
Stockholm, Sweden
e-mail: matthias.lohr@ki.se

Abstract

> Diagnostic technologies have no major contributory role in the observed continuous increase in health care spendings of Western societies. Although cost-benefit analyses were mainly performed to evaluate therapeutic interventions, the evaluation of different diagnostic procedures became the focus of health technology assessments in recent years. So-called decision trees proved to be a valuable tool for studying cost-effectiveness.

> On average 4,000 € have to be spent each month for a patient with pancreatic cancer (PC) when indirect costs are included. Diagnostic imaging accounts for 9% of all costs during hospitalisation.

> In more than 80% of PC patients a combination of abdominal US and CT clearly defines the locally progressed or even metastasized state and is associated with limited costs. According to cost-effectiveness models, the combination of CT with EUS, EUS-FNA or laparoscopy was associated with higher costs for diagnosis and staging but reduced total costs by avoiding unnecessary laparotomies in patients with peritoneal carcinomatosis or non-locoregional lymph node metastases. Further studies have to prove cost-effectiveness when state of the art multidetector row CT scanners with very high accuracy rates are combined with complimentary diagnostic modalities.

A. Laghi (ed.), *New Concepts in Diagnosis and Therapy of Pancreatic Adenocarcinoma*,
Medical Radiology, DOI: 10.1007/174_2010_69, © Springer-Verlag Berlin Heidelberg 2011

> ❯ Screening for pancreatic cancer in high risk populations (familial pancreatic cancer families, hereditary pancreatitis, Peutz-Jeghers syndrome) offers the possibility to detect (pre)malignant pancreatic lesions at an early stage when a curative resection is still possible. Studies demonstrated that screening might be cost-effective only in subgroups of patients with the highest cancer risk. EUS-based screening programmes are hampered by a significant number of false-positive results leading to unnecessary diagnostic and therapeutic procedures contributing to high expenditures.

Abbreviations

CT   Computed tomography
MDCT   Multidetector-row computed tomography
EUS   Endoscopic ultrasound
FN   Fine needle
FNA   Fine needle aspiration
ICER   Incremental cost effectiveness ratio
MRI   Magnetic resonance imaging
PC   Pancreatic cancer
US   Ultrasound

1 Cancer and Health Economics

Cancer represents a leading cause of death in Western civilization and poses a major burden on society. Due to the demographic changes an increase of 2% in the cancer incidence is predicted (Bosanquet and Sikora 2004). More than 1,300,000 new cancers are diagnosed in the European Union annually (van der Schueren et al. 2000).

The continuing rise of the expenses for the health care system in conjunction with constrained budgets can be regarded as the major stimulus for applying economic decision analyses in the field of health care.

The USA spends approximately 16% (more than $2 trillion) of its gross domestic product on health care (Keehan et al. 2008). Alarmingly, the growth in health care spending exceeds that of the overall economy (approximately 6–8% versus 4–6%). Growth figures in

European countries are similar (van der Schueren et al. 2000). According to the National Institute of Health (NIH), direct health care spendings were totaling $89 billion in 2007 and were even higher ($219.2 billion) when indirect costs as lost productivity due to premature death and morbidity were included.

Cancer care accounts for 5% of all health care spending and is supposed to increase significantly. Besides new technologies, novel antineoplastic substance groups (biologicals like antibodies and "small molecules") represent a relevant driving force for the observed cost increase in the previous years. In 2005–2006, a 20.8% increase in clinic drug expenditures was noted in the USA (Meropol et al. 2009).

In contrast, cost for new diagnostic technologies do not appear to play a major role for the cost increase (Beinfeld and Gazelle 2005).

The economic evaluation of health care interventions date back to the early 1960s. The later Nobel Prize laureate Kenneth Arrow discussed in his seminal article the similarities and distinctions between health care services and other economic goods and services (Arrow 1963).

Nowadays, the assessment of health technology is performed primarily by agencies and institutes for health technology assessment (HTA). In 1993, the International Network of Agencies for Health Technology Assessment (INAHTA) was established and consists of 50 member agencies (http://www.inahta.org/) with the secretariat located in Stockholm.

HTA may be defined as "… a comprehensive evaluation of the medical, economic and social consequences of a given technology. It is a form of policy analysis that examines the short and long-term consequences of the application of technology. The goal of technology assessment is to provide policy-makers with information on alternatives."

It has to be taken into account that the term technology covers diagnostics, medical treatments, screening, and all forms of medical interventions (Abelson et al. 2007; Waugh 2006).

Further examples of institutions which perform HTA are governmental organizations like the National Institute for Health and Clinical Excellence (NICE) in Britain (http://www.nice.org.uk/) or university-affiliated departments of public health or health economics.

Traditionally, therapeutic interventions were the main focus for health economic analyses (Eddama and Coast 2008). During the last decade, oncology proved to be an intensively studied area of research (Neymark

1999a, b; Tappenden et al. 2007). In recent years more and more decision analyses were performed in the field of diagnostics (Plevritis 2005).

2 Pancreatic Cancer: Costs We Have to Encounter

In a US study by Elixhauser and Halpern costs for pancreatic cancer accounted for 1.8% of the total costs of cancer care ($2.6 billion of $146 billion) (Elixhauser and Halpern 1999). In another study, which applied a prevalence-based human capital approach to estimate direct and indirect costs of pancreatic cancer, total annual costs were $4.6 billion (Wilson and Lightwood 1999). This appears to be only a rather limited fraction of the total expenses for cancer care and is explained by the relatively low incidence rate of pancreatic cancer and a short survival time. Due to the differing health care systems the average costs can vary substantially when comparing the expenses in different countries (Table 1). Higher costs in patients with resectable disease result from surgical resections which are associated with higher expenses, whereas palliative treatment in metastatic patients is less costly.

In a German prospective study all direct and indirect costs were calculated in 45 patients with pancreatic cancer (Müller-Nordhorn et al. 2005). Total costs were 4,078 € per patient and month when indirect costs were added which represent costs from a societal perspective. Interestingly costs for hospitalization accounted for 75% of total costs. During hospitalization major diagnostic procedures including all imaging modalities represented 9.4% of the costs (Fig. 1). Very similar, diagnostics represented 9% of all costs in a study from the Swedish Institute for Health Economics (IHE) (Hjelmgren et al. 2003). Of note, costs are U-shaped with a large fraction spent in the first months for hospitalization, diagnostics, and therapy (e.g. surgery). Following the initial phase there is a

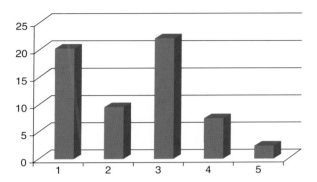

Fig. 1 Hospitalization costs for pancreatic cancer patients in percent of total costs (Müller-Nordhorn et al. 2005). Percent of total hospitalization costs (%). *1.* All diagnostic procedures (3,271 €), *2.* Major diagnostic procedures including imaging (1,531 €), *3.* Chemotherapy (3,569 €), *4.* Medication other than chemotherapy (1,181 €), and *5.* Surgery (360 €). Total costs: 16,264 €

period where the average monthly costs diminish followed by a costly terminal phase prior to death.

3 Decision Making for Diagnosing and Staging Pancreatic Cancer

Economic considerations are increasingly relevant for diagnostic decisions. At the same time, the clinician is confronted with a growing number of diagnostic and therapeutic modalities (Table 2). In contrast to the growing pressure to consider economic factors there is a clear paucity of studies that have performed a systematic economic decision analysis regarding the best approach in the diagnosis and staging of pancreatic cancer.

In the previous chapters a comprehensive analysis of key imaging modalities has been performed. In this chapter a diagnostic algorithm will be discussed with the goal of integrating the different imaging techniques with a focus on cost-minimization (Fig. 2).

In the majority of patients the initial diagnostic steps are triggered by unspecific signs and symptoms

Table 1 Cost comparison of pancreatic cancer treatment by country

Average	Resectable disease	Locally advanced disease	Metastatic disease	Country	Citation
$19,499	$27,161	$22,671	$14,277	Sweden	Hjelmgren et al. (2003)
$35,892	$46,250	$34,626	$29,658	Japan	Ishii et al. (2005)
$48,803	$65,335	$54,717	$35,809	United States	Du et al. (2000)

Table 2 Methods to diagnose and stage pancreatic cancer

A. Imaging
  I. Noninvasive imaging
    1. Transabdominal ultrasound (US) (+/– contrast-enhanced, +/– color-Doppler mode)
    2. Contrast-enhanced multidetector-row computed tomography (MDCT)
    3. Contrast-enhanced magnetic-resonance imaging (+/– MRCP, +/– MR-angiography)
    4. Positron emission tomography (PET)
    5. PET/CT
  II. Invasive imaging
    1. Endoscopic ultrasound (EUS) (+/– contrast-enhanced, +/– elastography)
    2. Laparoscopic ultrasound (LPUS)
    3. Intraoperative ultrasound (IOUS)
    4. Intraductal ultrasound (IDUS)
    5. Endoscopic-retrograde cholangiopancreaticography (ERCP)
    6. Pancreatoscopy
    7. Percutaneous transhepatic cholangiography (PTC)

B. Biomarkers from: serum, bile, cyst fluid

C. Cytology/histology: bile fluid, brush cytology from bile duct or pancreatic duct, biopsies (US-guided, CT-guided, EUS-guided), fine-needle aspiration cytology (FN-aspiration cytology), cytology from peritoneal "washing"

D. Surgery: laparoscopy (+/– biopsies, +/– ultrasound, +/– washings for cytology), surgical exploration

like jaundice, abdominal pain, anorexia, and weight loss. Thorough clinical examination is of importance offering the possibility to detect signs of metastases (e.g., ascites) and enabling a first assessment of the general performance status. Patients with a low performance status are no candidates for surgical treatment. Thus a meticulous diagnostic workup to confirm resectability and to rule out metastases can be omitted.

In most countries abdominal ultrasound (US) is the first screening technique. Abdominal US is readily available and inexpensive (Table 3). In addition, the sensitivity is high for ruling out gallstone disease with subsequent biliary obstruction and to detect even very small amounts of ascites which might be indicative for peritoneal carcinosis. Disadvantages are operator-dependency and the limited sensitivity to detect lesions in the pancreatic tail. Visualization of the pancreas is frequently hampered by bowel gas or by obesity.

In a considerable number of cases a typical hypoechoic cancer of the pancreatic head with liver metastases can be demonstrated. In the multimorbid patient of older age who is unfit for chemotherapy, no further diagnostics have to be performed and best supportive care remains the only option (Fig. 2).

In the presence of a pancreatic tumor in conjunction with biliary obstruction and cholangitis, an ERCP is mandatory to alleviate biliary obstruction by papillotomy and stent placement to prevent biliary sepsis. Beside this therapeutic maneuver ERCP can exhibit characteristic features of pancreatic cancer like a

double-duct sign or an isolated irregular stenosis of the pancreatic duct with prestenotic dilatation.

In a cost-benefit analysis including 126 patients with pancreatic cancer Alvarez and coworkers compared the benefit of CT, ERCP, and fine-needle aspiration (FNA) and found that ERCP did not change the management of a single patient with a mass in the pancreatic head but had a benefit in patients with atypical CT findings (Alvarez et al. 1993). Nowadays, ERCP does not play a role as a mere diagnostic tool. Formerly, some institutions had performed ERCP if a clinical suspicion for pancreatic cancer was present, although CT was unable to demonstrate a pancreatic tumor (Böttger et al. 1998). Instead of ERCP, most centers would currently favor EUS for further clarification in those cases.

For assessing loco-regional extension, vascular invasion, and metastatic spread of pancreatic cancer contrast-enhanced dual-phase multidetector-row computed tomography (MDCT) has the unchallenged leading role and provides the clinician with answers to the following pivotal questions: Is there a mass in the pancreas (anatomy), is it cancer (predict pathology), and is it resectable ("dictate" management). In comparison to CT, magnetic-resonance imaging has a comparable accuracy for diagnosing and staging but is significantly more expensive (401 € vs. 182 €, see Table 4), which is one of the main reasons why MRI is not used as the primary diagnostic method but proved to be a powerful tool as a "problem-solver" when results of CT scans are ambiguous.

Fig. 2 Algorithm for the diagnosis, staging, and management of pancreatic cancer. ECOG, Eastern Cooperative Oncology Group performance status; risk factors: large primary tumor, markedly elevated CA 19–9, tumors in the body and tail

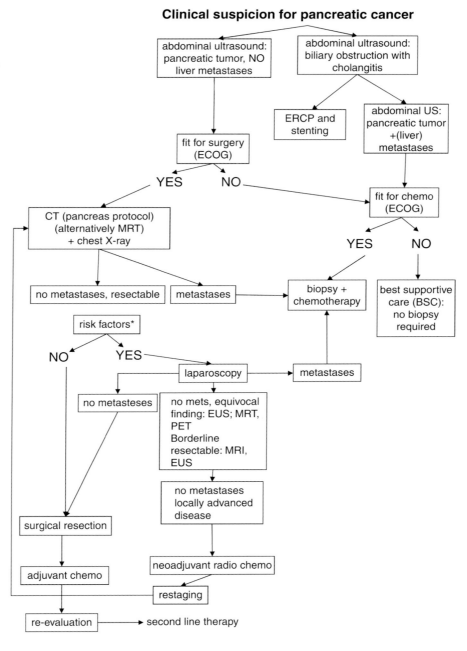

Bearing in mind that more than 80% of patients with pancreatic cancer are diagnosed at a late stage with unresectable cancer and/or distant metastases, MDCT will clearly define this patient group in the vast majority of cases – not necessitating further diagnostics. Böttger and coworkers conducted a prospective observational study with the inclusion of 307 patients with histologically proven pancreatic cancer in a German tertiary-referral center. In 95% of all cases abdominal US and CT were sufficient for diagnosing and staging with a sensitivity rate of 89.4% for US and a sensitivity rate of 97.8% for CT, respectively (Böttger et al. 1998).

Due to the high accuracy of CT and the comparably low negative predictive value of biopsies a histologic confirmation of pancreatic cancer is confined to few scenarios. Prior to initiation of chemotherapy a histologic confirmation of pancreatic cancer is mandatory.

Table 3 Costs for key imaging modalities and the Whipple procedure

Imaging modality	Costs (€)[a]
Transabdominal US	46.5
CT	182
MRI	401
EUS	155
EUS + fine-needle biopsy	180
Laparoscopy	395
ERCP – diagnostic	382
ERCP – therapeutic	523
PET	540
Surgery	
Whipple procedure	13,000–18,800

US ultrasound, *CT* contrast-enhanced computed tomography, *MRI* magnetic resonance tomography, *EUS* endoscopic ultrasound, *ERCP* endoscopic retrograde cholangiopancreaticography
[a] Calculated by personnel and material costs in Germany

Table 4 Risk factors for the development of pancreatic cancer

- Older age
- Smoking
- Idiopathic acute pancreatitis (>50 years)
- Chronic pancreatitis
- Long-standing type II diabetes
- New-onset diabetes
- Cystic fibrosis
- Familial pancreatic cancer
- Hereditary pancreatitis (HP)
- Peutz–Jeghers syndrome (PJS)
- Hereditary nonpolyposis colorectal cancer (HNPCC)
- Familial atypical multiple mole melanoma syndrome (FAMMM)

The general rule is that the primary tumor or a metastasis is biopsied which is accessible with the lowest risk. Frequently, a simple transabdominal US-guided biopsy of a liver metastasis is the best and least expensive option. In contrast, EUS-guided fine-needle aspiration (EUS-FNA) of the pancreatic mass is the standard procedure in those patients planned for neoadjuvant radiochemotherapy – and is associated with higher costs (EUS-FNA: 180 €, Table 3). Although the risk for tumor seeding as a result of a transabdominal biopsy is extremely low, biopsy by EUS guidance is generally preferred and recommended by current guidelines (http://www.nccn.org/professionals/physician_gls/f_guidelines.asp).

Histologic or cytologic confirmation in patients with a high suspicion for resectable pancreatic cancer without metastases is not needed. The negative predictive value of an EUS-FNA is too low – in other words, the number of false-negative findings would be unacceptably high excluding patients from the only potentially curative treatment. On the other hand, in up to 13% of patients with presumed pancreatic cancer the diagnosis is incorrect (Barone 2008).

For two reasons correct staging to assess local progression and distant metastases is of utmost importance. Overstaging would exclude a patient from resection which is currently the treatment option that is associated with the highest survival rate. Contrary, understaging would lead to an unnecessary laparotomy in a patient with few months to live.

A Spanish study performed a cost-minimization analysis in 62 patients who were assessed for resectability of pancreatic cancer by CT, MRI, EUS, and angiography. Analyzing different combinations a sequential imaging of CT and EUS proved to be the best strategy. EUS was used as a confirmatory technique in those patients in whom helical CT suggested resectability (Soriano et al. 2004). Although the combination of EUS and CT leads to higher expenses costs were eventually saved as unnecessary exploratory laparotomies were avoided.

A similar study from the Decision Analysis and Technology Assessment Group of the Massachusetts General Hospital in Boston addressed the same topic (McMahon et al. 2001). Different imaging technologies and their combinations were analyzed for cost-effectiveness to evaluate resectability. Costs for CT, MRI, laparoscopy, laparoscopic ultrasound (LPUS), and EUS were calculated and compared with costs of best supportive care and surgery. Interestingly, the main outcome parameter was life-years gained. This is an outcome parameter widely used in decision analyses of therapeutic technologies (e.g., surgery, chemotherapy) but less frequently applied to assess the effectiveness of diagnostic strategies. Interestingly, few statistically significant differences in effectiveness between the analyzed diagnostic options to assess resectability were found. But costs differed significantly. The least expensive strategy proved to be CT in combination with laparoscopy or LPUS, respectively. This strategy had an incremental cost-effectiveness ratio (ICER) of $87,502 per life-year saved. Due to the detrimental prognosis of pancreatic cancer, high amounts of money have to be spent per each additional year saved. The second most cost-effective strategy was the combination of CT with EUS. The combination of CT with laparoscopy or EUS was more expensive than a single imaging modality, but cost savings by reducing the number of unnecessary laparotomies outweighed those additional costs by far.

Other authors addressed the question whether the addition of a more extended diagnostic work-up will detect metastases in a higher number of patients which would reduce the number of unnecessary surgical procedures in metastasized patients.

For a cost-minimization analysis from the Mayo Clinic a decision-tree model was applied (Harewood and Wiersema 2001, Fig. 3). Three different approaches were investigated in a hypothetical group of patients with local resectability and no obvious metastases but suspicious distant (non-peripancreatic) lymphnodes: (a) proceed directly to surgery, (b) EUS-fine needle aspiration (EUS-FNA) of the suspicious lymphnode, and (c) CT-guided fine-needle aspiration (CT-FNA) of the suspicious lymphnode. Costs, sensitivities, and probabilities were derived from the literature. A sensitivity rate of 80% for EUS-guided FNA and a sensitivity rate of only 40% for CT-FNA were used as a basis for further calculations.

The EUS-FNA approach was the least costly with $15,938 and avoided 16 unnecessary surgeries

in 100 patients. Costs for CT-FNA were slightly higher ($16,378) and avoided laparotomies in 8 of 100 patients.

Heinrich and coworkers from Switzerland sought to elucidate whether PET/CT would be cost-effective in 59 patients with presumed resectable pancreatic cancer (Heinrich et al. 2005). PET/CT detected additional distant metastases in five and synchronous rectal cancer in two patients thus changing the management in 16% of all included patients. Following their calculation $62,912 were finally saved. Expenses for 59 PET/CTs were calculated to be $125,588. Avoiding five pancreatic resections resulted in cost savings of $188,500. This cost calculation appeared to be too optimistic in favor of PET/CT, as the two rectal cancers and one abdominal wall metastasis were visible on the initial CT. Consequently, those patients did not fulfill the entry criteria for this study and biased the result (Goh 2006).

3.1 Summary

In conclusion, it can be summarized that various studies could demonstrate that increasing the accuracy of staging strategies – in terms of assessing resectability and the presence of metastases – offers a potential to reduce costs by preventing laparotomies. This refers to the rather small group of patients with presumed resectability.

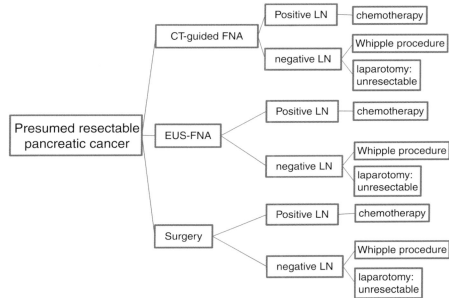

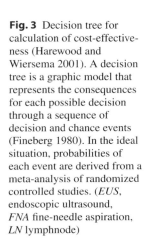

Fig. 3 Decision tree for calculation of cost-effectiveness (Harewood and Wiersema 2001). A decision tree is a graphic model that represents the consequences for each possible decision through a sequence of decision and chance events (Fineberg 1980). In the ideal situation, probabilities of each event are derived from a meta-analysis of randomized controlled studies. (*EUS*, endoscopic ultrasound, *FNA* fine-needle aspiration, *LN* lymphnode)

Results of published cost-effectiveness studies have to be interpreted with caution, as the assumptions for costs in US studies do not frequently mirror costs in European or other non-US countries. In addition, imaging technology has experienced a dramatic progress in the last decade, so that cost-effectiveness studies have to be conducted with the state-of-the-art technology. Based on the excellent accuracy rates of current MDCT scanners for diagnosing and staging pancreatic cancer it can be anticipated that the addition of further diagnostic methods would prove to be cost-effective only in a very selected group of patients. As the detection of metastases to the peritoneum is still problematic, new cost-effectiveness analyses with the inclusion of laparoscopy for high-risk patients appear to be most urgently needed. Additionally, further studies are needed to demonstrate cost-effectiveness of EUS and PET/CT.

4 Screening for Pancreatic Cancer

Typically the patient is diagnosed with pancreatic cancer when a curative resection is impossible as the tumor has locally progressed or even metastasized. Screening for pancreatic cancer appeared to be an attractive strategy to detect pancreatic cancer at an early stage thus enabling curative resection. Complete resection of small pancreatic cancers (T1, ≤2 cm) leads to 5-year survival rates ranging from 30% to 60% (Furukawa et al. 1996; Ishikawa et al. 1999; Shimizu et al. 2005). Stage 1 tumors with a size ≤1 cm ("minute" pancreatic cancer) have even higher 5-year survival rates, exceeding 75% (Tsuchiya et al. 1986; Ishikawa et al. 1999). Concurrently, early diagnosis has the potential to detect the tumor prior to metastatic spread. In one series, even in ≤2 cm cancers only 44% were confined to the pancreas (Tsuchiya et al. 1986). Frequently duct dilation and the cut-off sign represented the earliest CT findings and were the only morphological changes when the tumor was still invisible (Shimizu et al. 2005; Gangi et al. 2004), keeping in mind that in those studies current state-of-the-art MDCT scanners were not used.

In the general population the life-time risk for developing cancer is 1.27% or one in every 80 men or women (http://seer.cancer.gov/statfacts/html/pancreas. html?statfacts_page=pancreas.html&x=9&y=20). A general screening program would never be cost-

effective and would result in a high absolute number of false-positive results. This can be exemplified by a simple calculation: the age-adjusted incidence of pancreatic cancer in individuals 50 years of age or older is 38 per 100,000. If we had a test with 99% sensitivity and 99% specificity for pancreatic cancer and would screen 100,000 individuals aged >50 years, nearly all 37 patients with pancreatic cancer would be identified. At the same time, the test would falsely identify nearly 1,000 individuals as having cancer.

In a recent study effectiveness and costs of a whole-body CT scan as a general screening tool in asymptomatic 50-year-old men were calculated (Beinfeld et al. 2005). Eight different cancer entities were included in the model. Most subjects (95.8%) had at least one positive finding, but only 2% had disease. The work-up of false-positive results would account for 32% of total costs. Altogether, this would cost 151,000 per life-year saved. In general, $55,000–$80,000 – which reflect costs per life-year gained of patients treated with hemodialysis – represent the upper limit society is willing to pay when assessing health technologies.

Several factors and cancer syndromes were characterized to be associated with a significantly enhanced risk for developing pancreatic cancer (Vitone et al. 2006; Table 4).

Familial pancreatic cancer (≥3 affected first-degree relatives, relative risk for pancreatic cancer: 32), Peutz–Jeghers syndrome (relative risk for pancreatic cancer: 132), and hereditary pancreatitis (cumulative life time risk for pancreatic cancer: 40%) have the highest inherent risk for pancreatic cancer, and screening programs were proposed for subjects referring to this high-risk groups. An expert panel at the Fourth International Symposium of Inherited Diseases of the Pancreas stated that a surveillance program should be recommended for patients who have a more than tenfold greater risk for the development of pancreatic cancer (Brand et al. 2007).

All currently used screening protocols apply EUS for regular screening (Del Chiaro et al. 2010) which reflects the very high sensitivity to detect pancreatic abnormalities compared to all other imaging modalities. In addition EUS is safe with a very low complication rate and involves no radiation. In contrast, ERCP poses a low but significant risk for complications like pancreatitis, bleeding, and perforation excluding this method for a general use in screening programs. According to the majority of screening protocols, only pancreatic lesions that were identified by EUS have to be confirmed by ERCP before therapeutic decisions are made. In high-risk populations chronic-pancreatitis-like abnormalities and (pre)malignant lesions like pancreatic intraepithelial neoplasias (PanIn I-III) or intraductal papillary mucinous neoplasms (IPMN) are detected in significant numbers (Larghi et al. 2009). These pathologies are reflected by nodules, cysts, or echogenic foci, strands, and hyperechoic pancreatic duct walls. The relatively low specificity of these changes represent a problem, and in all screening centers cases are well-known where a pancreatectomy was performed and no relevant (pre)malignant lesions were found by the pathologists. Based on the low specificity of EUS, patients with hereditary pancreatitis are the least suitable high-risk group for regular EUS examination as all pancreata exhibit abnormalities.

Cost-effectiveness of screening programs is still a matter of debate and a number of cost-effectiveness studies were conducted. In a decision analysis Rulyak and coworkers from the University of Washington compared one-time screening for pancreatic dysplasia with EUS to no screening in a hypothetical cohort of 100 members of familial pancreatic cancer (Rulyak et al. 2003). Pathologic EUS findings were confirmed by ERCP prior to total pancreatectomy. Calculations were based on a prevalence rate of 20% for pancreatic dysplasias and a sensitivity rate of 90% for EUS and ERCP. Endoscopic screening was cost-effective and following this model $16,885 had to be paid for one life-year saved (incremental cost-effectiveness ratio: $16,885/life-year saved). A sensitivity analysis proved that screening remained cost-effective if the prevalence of dysplasia was greater than 16% or if the sensitivity of EUS was greater than 84%. The authors deduced that screening of high-risk family members is cost-effective and justified. This study was criticized as one-time screening is not the approach of current screening programs where regular controls are required to detect newly formed dysplasias or malignancies. Consequently, it is unproven if a screening interval of 1 or 3 years would be still cost-effective.

In a similar study, costs were calculated when patients with hereditary pancreatitis were screened annually with EUS from 40 to 55 years of age with the expectation to identify seven pancreatic cancers. This model led to a total cost of $164,285 per newly detected pancreatic cancer – which is a substantial amount of money.

In a third analysis from Liverpool, cost-effectiveness of a screening program – according to US und EU

protocols – for patients with Peutz–Jeghers was assessed (Latchford et al. 2006). A screening would cost $350,000 per life saved – which is far from cost-effective. Of note, further risk stratification could reduce costs so that ultimately only $50,000 would be required to save one life. This exemplifies that a screening might be only cost-effective if highly selected subjects are included in the screening program.

References

Abelson J, Giacomini M, Lehoux P, Gauvin FP (2007) Bringing 'the public' into health technology assessment and coverage policy decisions: from principles to practice. Health Policy 82:37–50

Alvarez C, Livingston EH, Ashley SW, Schwarz M, Reber HA (1993) Cost-benefit analysis of the work-up for pancreatic cancer. Am J Surg 165:53–58

Arrow K (1963) Uncertainty and the welfare economics of medical care. Am Econ Rev 53:941–973

Barone JE (2008) Pancreaticoduodenectomy for presumed pancreatic cancer. Surg Oncol 17:139–144

Beinfeld MT, Gazelle GS (2005) Diagnostic imaging costs: are they driving up the costs of hospital care? Radiology 235:934–939

Beinfeld MT, Wittenberg E, Gazelle GS (2005) Cost-effectiveness of whole-body CT screening. Radiology 234:415–422

Bosanquet N, Sikora K (2004) The economics of cancer care in the UK. Lancet Oncol 5:568–574

Böttger TC, Boddin J, Düber C, Heintz A, Küchle R, Junginger T (1998) Diagnosing and staging of pancreatic carcinoma – what is necessary? Oncology 55:122–129

Brand RE, Lerch MM, Rubinstein WS, Neoptolemos JP, Whitcomb DC, Hruban RH, Brentnall TA, Lynch HT, Canto MI, Participants of the Fourth International Symposium of Inherited Diseases of the Pancreas (2007) Advances in counselling and surveillance of patients at risk for pancreatic cancer. Gut 56:1460–1469

Del Chiaro M, Zerbi A, Capurso G, Zamboni G, Maisonneuve P, Presciuttini S, Arcidiacono PG, Calculli L, Falconi M (2010) Familial pancreatic cancer in Italy. Risk assessment, screening programs and clinical approach: a position paper from the Italian Registry. Dig Liver Dis 42:597–605

Du W, Touchette D, Vaitkevicius VK, Peters WP, Shields AF (2000) Cost analysis of pancreatic carcinoma treatment. Cancer 89:1917–1924

Eddama O, Coast J (2008) A systematic review of the use of economic evaluation in local decision-making. Health Policy 86:129–141

Elixhauser A, Halpern MT (1999) Economic evaluations of gastric and pancreatic cancer. Hepatogastroenterology 46:1206–1213

Fineberg HV (1980) Decision trees. Construction, uses, and limits. Bull Cancer 67:395–404

Furukawa H, Okada S, Saisho H, Ariyama J, Karasawa E, Nakaizumi A, Nakazawa S, Murakami K, Kakizoe T (1996)

Clinicopathologic features of small pancreatic adenocarcinoma. A collective study. Cancer 78:986–990

Gangi S, Fletcher JG, Nathan MA, Christensen JA, Harmsen WS, Crownhart BS, Chari ST (2004) Time interval between abnormalities seen on CT and the clinical diagnosis of pancreatic cancer: retrospective review of CT scans obtained before diagnosis. AJR Am J Roentgenol 182:897–903

Goh BK (2006) Positron emission tomography/computed tomography influences on the management of resectable pancreatic cancer and its cost-effectiveness. Ann Surg 243:709–710

Harewood GC, Wiersema MJ (2001) A cost analysis of endoscopic ultrasound in the evaluation of pancreatic head adenocarcinoma. Am J Gastroenterol 96:2651–2656

Heinrich S, Goerres GW, Schäfer M, Sagmeister M, Bauerfeind P, Pestalozzi BC, Hany TF, von Schulthess GK, Clavien PA (2005) Positron emission tomography/computed tomography influences on the management of resectable pancreatic cancer and its cost-effectiveness. Ann Surg 242:235–243

Hjelmgren J, Ceberg J, Persson U, Alvegård TA (2003) The cost of treating pancreatic cancer – a cohort study based on patients' records from four hospitals in Sweden. Acta Oncol 42:218–226

Ishii H, Furuse J, Kinoshita T, Konishi M, Nakagohri T, Takahashi S, Gotohda N, Nakachi K, Suzuki E, Yoshino M (2005) Treatment cost of pancreatic cancer in Japan: analysis of the difference after the introduction of gemcitabine. Jpn J Clin Oncol 35:526–530

Ishikawa O, Ohigashi H, Imaoka S, Nakaizumi A, Uehara H, Kitamura T, Kuroda C (1999) Minute carcinoma of the pancreas measuring 1 cm or less in diameter – collective review of Japanese case reports. Hepatogastroenterology 46:8–15

Keehan S, Sisko A, Truffer C, Smith S, Cowan C, Poisal J, Clemens MK, National Health Expenditure Accounts Projections Team (2008) Health spending projections through 2017: the baby-boom generation is coming to Medicare. Health Aff (Millwood) 27:w145–55

Larghi A, Verna EC, Lecca PG, Costamagna G (2009) Screening for pancreatic cancer in high-risk individuals: a call for endoscopic ultrasound. Clin Cancer Res 15:1907–1914

Latchford A, Greenhalf W, Vitone LJ, Neoptolemos JP, Lancaster GA, Phillips RK (2006) Peutz-Jeghers syndrome and screening for pancreatic cancer. Br J Surg 93:1446–1455

McMahon PM, Halpern EF, Fernandez-del Castillo C, Clark JW, Gazelle GS (2001) Pancreatic cancer: cost-effectiveness of imaging technologies for assessing resectability. Radiology 221:93–106

Meropol NJ, Schrag D, Smith TJ, Mulvey TM, Langdon RM Jr, Blum D, Ubel PA, Schnipper LE, American Society of Clinical Oncology (2009) American Society of Clinical

Oncology guidance statement: the cost of cancer care. J Clin Oncol 27:3868–3874

Müller-Nordhorn J, Brüggenjürgen B, Böhmig M, Selim D, Reich A, Noesselt L, Roll S, Wiedenmann B, Willich SN (2005) Direct and indirect costs in a prospective cohort of patients with pancreatic cancer. Aliment Pharmacol Ther 22:405–415

Neymark N (1999a) Techniques for health economics analysis in oncology: Part 1. Crit Rev Oncol Hematol 30:1–11

Neymark N (1999b) Techniques for health economics analysis in oncology: part 2. Crit Rev Oncol Hematol 30:13–24

Plevritis SK (2005) Decision analysis and simulation modeling for evaluating diagnostic tests on the basis of patient outcomes. AJR Am J Roentgenol 185:581–590

Rulyak SJ, Kimmey MB, Veenstra DL, Brentnall TA (2003) Cost-effectiveness of pancreatic cancer screening in familial pancreatic cancer kindreds. Gastrointest Endosc 57:23–29

Shimizu Y, Yasui K, Matsueda K, Yanagisawa A, Yamao K (2005) Small carcinoma of the pancreas is curable: new computed tomography finding, pathological study and postoperative results from a single institute. J Gastroenterol Hepatol 20:1591–1594

Soriano A, Castells A, Ayuso C, Ayuso JR, de Caralt MT, Ginès MA, Real MI, Gilabert R, Quintó L, Trilla A, Feu F, Montanyà X, Fernández-Cruz L, Navarro S (2004) Preoperative staging and tumor resectability assessment of pancreatic cancer: prospective study comparing endoscopic ultrasonography, helical computed tomography, magnetic resonance imaging, and angiography. Am J Gastroenterol 99:492–501

Tappenden P, Jones R, Paisley S, Carroll C (2007) The cost-effectiveness of bevacizumab in the first-line treatment of metastatic colorectal cancer in England and Wales. Eur J Cancer 43:2487–2494

Tsuchiya R, Noda T, Harada N, Miyamoto T, Tomioka T, Yamamoto K, Yamaguchi T, Izawa K, Tsunoda T, Yoshino R et al (1986) Collective review of small carcinomas of the pancreas. Ann Surg 203:77–81

van der Schueren E, Kesteloot K, Cleemput I (2000) Economic evaluation in cancer care: questions and answers on how to alleviate conflicts between rising needs and expectations and tightening budgets. Eur J Cancer 36:13–36, Federation of European Cancer Societies. Full report

Vitone LJ, Greenhalf W, McFaul CD, Ghaneh P, Neoptolemos JP (2006) The inherited genetics of pancreatic cancer and prospects for secondary screening. Best Pract Res Clin Gastroenterol 20:253–283

Waugh N (2006) Health technology assessment in cancer: a personal view from public health. Eur J Cancer 42:2876–2880

Wilson LS, Lightwood JM (1999) Pancreatic cancer: total costs and utilization of health services. J Surg Oncol 71:171–181

Part III

Therapy

The Case for Surgery

Claudio Bassi, Matilde Bacchion, and Giovanni Marchegiani

Contents

Abstract

> The treatment of choice for ductal adenocarcinoma of the pancreas has to deal with the symptoms and general clinic conditions of the patients, eventual comorbidities, prognostic factors, and survival expectancy. It is nowadays assumed that radical surgery, once a correct indication for a demolitive intervention is given, is the first therapeutical step to positively influence patient's long survival, even though a complete recovery can seldom be reached (Sener et al. (1999) J Am Coll Surg 189:1–7).

1 Radical Surgery

Curative resection of pancreatic cancer can be performed only in 20% of patients because of advanced stage. After radical surgery, when associated with adjuvant treatments, an overall 5-year survival rate of around 20% is expected (Sener et al. 1999; Sohn et al. 2000; Wagner et al. 2004). Improvements in technique and perioperative management have led to a significant reduction of postoperative mortality in experienced centers (Sohn et al. 2000; Wagner et al. 2004; Geer and Brennan 1993).

1.1 Duodenopancreatectomy

Duodenopancreatectomy (DP) represents the treatment of choice for neoplastic processes of pancreatic head and consists of three operative phases: the explorative,

C. Bassi (✉), M. Bacchion, and G. Marchegiani
Department of Radiology, Policlinico "GB Rossi", University of Verona, Piazzale LA Scuro, 10, 37134 Verona, Italy
email: claudio.bassi@univr.it

A. Laghi (ed.), *New Concepts in Diagnosis and Therapy of Pancreatic Adenocarcinoma*,
Medical Radiology, DOI: 10.1007/174_2010_1, © Springer-Verlag Berlin Heidelberg 2011

the resective, and the reconstructive ones (Jaeck et al. 1998a).

Since both peritoneal and liver metastases are considered absolute contraindications for the execution of a DP, the first step of the surgery consists in an accurate analysis of their presence through direct vision, manual exploration, and intraoperative ultrasounds. Moreover, a closer examination of the pancreas allows a thorough evaluation of neoplastic resectability.

This exploration phase requires three fundamental moments: the complete dissection of gastrocolic ligament extended to the hepatic colic flexure; the Kocher maneuver extended to the right margin of the aorta and finally the cleavage between the posterior surface of the pancreas and the portal-mesenteric trunk.

If the lesion is limited to the pancreatic parenchyma and there is no evidence of extrapancreatic disease, the operation can proceed to the next phase.

The exeresis consists of four steps: first the gallbladder and the cystic duct are mobilized, then the common bile duct and the gastroduodenal artery are carefully sectioned under direct vision. This phase is followed by the removal of the distal portion of the stomach in case of a nonpylorus-preserving Whipple DP (whereas the whole organ is preserved if a Traverso-Longmire DP is performed). Finally, the resection of the pancreas together with the duodenum and the retroportal pancreatic lamina is completed.

The last phase, the reconstructive one, consists of the restoring of pancreatic, biliary, and gastric continuity, through the anastomosis of the common bile duct, the pancreatic stump, and the stomach with a proximal jejunal loop. This method guarantees an efficient drainage of both pancreatic and biliary secretions. The jejunal proximal extremity could eventually be passed through the retroperitoneal transmesocolic breach created with the previous dissecting maneuver. It is, nevertheless, preferable to close this pathway and let the loop pass anterior to the mesenteric vessels and then through an intraperitoneal transmesocolic breach in order to avoid any risk of compression on the loop.

At this point, everything is properly set up for the execution of the following anastomosis:

• Pancreatic-jeunal: it is the most delicate. The pancreatic anastomosis "risk" depends on severe factors. In the ductal cancer cases the remaining tissue can be characterized by different texture. The more tender the pancreatic stump is, the easier it is torn by surgical threads and predisposed to arouse an inflammatory reaction resulting in necrosis, anastomotic leakage, and postoperative fistulas. The end-to-end pancreatic-jejunal anastomosis has been now quite completely replaced by the end-to-side pancreatic-jejunal one. The previously closed jejunal loop and the pancreatic stump are brought close by, thereby permitting the execution of the anastomosis at the level of the antimesenteric margin 2–3 cm below the loop proximal extremity.

• Hepatic-jejunal: performed distally about 20 cm below the previous one, in order to avoid a possible involvement of this latter anastomosis, whereas an undesired pancreatic fistula should occur. This would lead to a more perilous pancreatic-biliary one.

• Gastric-jejunal: a sufficiently wide, left transmesocolic breach is performed through which the gastric stump is lowered. The anastomosis is thus performed at least 40 cm distally to the bilio-jejunal one in order to prevent any risk of tension on it. If the transmesocolic breach cannot be executed, the anastomosis can be anyway performed in an antecolic position. It is also advisable to add, when possible, a side-to-side 4–5 cm long anastomosis between the afferent and efferent loops to the stomach (Brown procedure). This expedient can ease the efferent loop's emptying.

It is, moreover, mandatory to underline how the classic DP procedure (the so-called Whipple one) has now been replaced, when possible, by the one proposed by Traverso and Longmire. This pylorus-preserving technique, thanks to the consequent sparing of the Letarjet plexus, seems to result in a more physiologic gastric emptying with a consequent reduced gastro-jejunal reflux and "dumping syndrome" presentation. Long-term results testify a lower incidence of postoperative malnutrition connected to the pylorus sparing procedure.

The section of the duodenum is classically executed 3–4 cm distally from the pylorus sphincter and is followed by one of the gastroduodenal arteries. Restoring of gastrointestinal continuity is realized as previously described (Fig. 1).

When the pylorus cannot be technically preserved, two different reconstructive strategies have been proposed in order to avoid biliary and pancreatic reflux on the gastric stump. Besides the previously described side-to-side 4–5 cm long anastomosis between the afferent and efferent loops to the stomach (Brown

Fig. 1 Reconstruction after DP

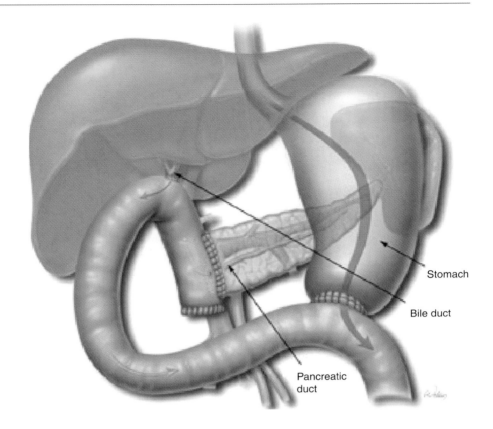

Stomach

Bile duct

Pancreatic duct

procedure), an "en-Y" gastro-jejunal anastomosis can be successfully performed with good results in terms of a more physiologic gastric emptying.

1.2 Distal Pancreatectomy

Distal pancreatectomy (DPa) is considered the standard technique for the management of malignant disorders of the body-tail of the pancreas (Jaeck et al. 1998b). In general, the operation is performed en bloc along with resection of the spleen; however, splenic preservation has recently been advocated whenever technically feasible and safe. Indications for spleen preserving DPa are represented by benign-borderline disorders of the gland, such as chronic pancreatitis, pseudocysts, cystic tumors, pancreatic traumas, and fistulas related to previous pancreatic surgeries. By the way, once a correct diagnosis of malignant neoplasm of the body-tail of the pancreas is given, the treatment of choice is represented by a standard distal splenopancreatectomy

(Aldridge and Williamson 1991; Richardson and Scott-Conner 1989; Fernandez-Cruz et al. 2005).

The patient is placed in the supine position. Axifoid-umbilical midline incision is performed. After the division of the gastrocolic ligament, the body-tail of the pancreas is best exposed by displacing the omentum and the colon with its mesocolon inferiorly away from the pancreas. The dissection is continued up to the uppermost short gastric vessels, which are legated and divided thus freeing the spleen from the greater curvature of the stomach. Division of adhesions between the posterior wall of the stomach and pancreas allows the stomach to be retracted superiorly. The celiac axis is then visualized at the upper border of the body of the pancreas; the hepatic artery is identified and freed from the superior margin of the pancreas; this artery is then followed to the left until it merges with the splenic artery at its origin from the celiac trunk. The splenic artery is consequently ligated and divided.

The posterior aspect of the body of the pancreas is mobilized out of the retroperitoneum until the superior

Fig. 2 Distal pancreatectomy

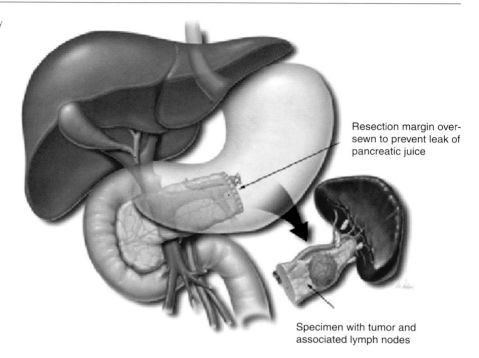

Resection margin over-
sewn to prevent leak of
pancreatic juice

Specimen with tumor and
associated lymph nodes

mesenteric vein is clearly identified. Once the lienore-nal and lienophrenic ligaments are divided, the spleno-pancreatic-block can be fully mobilized and brought over the right side of the patient; the splenic vein and the pancreas are, therefore, dissected via linear stapling device. The pancreatic stump is properly sutured and a single drainage is placed (Fernandez-Cruz 2006).

In general, the DPa procedure is nowadays becom-ing more and more popular by laparoscopic-mini inva-sive approach, even if it is not yet indicated for adenocarcinoma (Fig. 2).

1.3 Total Pancreatectomy

The role of total pancreatectomy (TP) for the man-agement of pancreatic adenocarcinoma is nowadays confined: (a) in case of a soft and corrupted pancre-atic stump resulting from a previous partial resection not allowing a safe anastomosis and (b) for recurring positivity for neoplasm of the pancreatic margin dur-ing intraoperative examination after a partial pancre-atic resection (Butturini et al. 2008; Muller et al. 2007; Schmidt et al. 2007).

The operative technique utilized for TP depends upon whether the patient has undergone previous

pancreatic resection. Distal pancreatectomy can be performed in patients who had a previous pancreatodu-odenectomy. Patients with a previous distal pancreate-ctomy are candidates for either duodenum-preserving pancreatectomy or completion pancreaticoduodenec-tomy (Heidt et al. 2007).

The operative procedure begins with a thorough exploration to evaluate the presence of extrapancre-atic disease. The right colon and hepatic flexure of the colon are mobilized to provide access to the second part of the duodenum. A wide Kocher maneuver is per-formed and the duodenum and pancreas are elevated off the inferior vena cava until the left border of the abdominal aorta can be palpated. The Kocher maneu-ver is extended by continuing mobilization of the third portion of the duodenum until the superior mesenteric vein is encountered. The gastrocolic ligament is widely divided to allow access to the body of the pancreas. The anterior surface of the superior mesenteric vein is identified and dissected under direct vision. Using a proper retractor, the neck of the pancreas is lifted, and entering this avascular plane, the superior mesen-teric vein is traced proximally to its confluence with the portal vein. Following cholecystectomy, the peritoneal reflection over the hepatoduodenal ligament is care-fully opened and the common bile duct and common hepatic artery are carefully dissected, and vessel loops are placed around them. The gastroduodenal artery is identified and ligated in continuity to facilitate access to the portal vein at the superior aspect of the pancreas. The splenorenal ligament is divided, and the spleen is drawn medially together with the tail of the pancreas, thus opening the retropancreatic plane. The splenic vein and artery are ligated. Next, the distal part of the stomach is mobilized and transected in case of a non-pylorus preserving procedure, while if the sphincter can be spared, the transaction is performed 2–3 cm distally to it, at the level of the first duodenal portion. The duodenojejunal flexure is located and dissected free from the retroperitoneum by dividing the ligament of Treitz. Approximately 10–15 cm distal to the duodenojejunal flexure, the vessels within the mesentery and subsequently the small bowel are divided. The pancreas, distal stomach, duodenum, and spleen are removed en bloc. To restore gastrointestinal continuity, an end-to-side choledochojejunal anastomosis is performed. The stomach is then anastomosed to the jejunum in two layers (Lillemoe et al. 1999; Sohn et al. 1999).

Recent international literature data and our experience attest that TP can nowadays be performed safely in high-volume centers (Billings et al. 2005). The overall quality of life after the intervention is now considered to be acceptable thanks to the newest techniques of management of the apancreatic status. Moreover, the limitations due to this condition do not justify avoiding the procedure in patients in whom the complete removal of the pancreas is required for oncologic, technical, prophylactic, or complication-related reasons. Therefore, TP should no longer be generally avoided, because it is a viable option in selected patients.

2 Palliative Surgery

As already stressed, adenocarcinoma remains a disease associated with a poor prognosis. The majority of patients are not candidates for resection at the time of diagnosis (Trede 1985), and between 25 and 75% of patients who undergo exploratory surgery are found to have unresectable disease (Lillemoe et al. 1999).

Surgical palliation continues to play an important role in the management of periampullary carcinoma, and it can be performed with minimal perioperative mortality, acceptable morbidity, and good long-term palliation, being the treatment of choice for selected patients with unresectable tumors (Sohn et al. 1999; Lillemoe et al. 1993).

Palliation from obstructive jaundice is associated with important physiological benefits (improved hepatocyte metabolism, protein synthesis, absorption and digestion of fats, bacterial clearance) as well as with the relief of disturbing clinical symptoms (maldigestion, itching, peripheral edema).

The results of controlled clinical trials and large multicentre studies comparing operative biliary bypass and biliary stent insertion in unresectable pancreatic tumors have shown how the initial success rate in palliation of jaundice is similar after endoscopic stent insertion and biliary bypass operation (Schwarz and Beger 2000). Other studies have demonstrated how morbidity and 30-day mortality are higher after bypass operation, whereas stent insertion is accompanied by a higher rate of hospital readmission and reintervention because of infections and recurrent jaundice (Smith et al. 1994; Luque-de Leon et al. 1999).

Debate still exists in literature in the case of intraoperative evidence of systemic diffusion of cancer (peritoneal or liver metastasis): in some high-volume centers, such as in the John Hopkins Group, intraoperative diagnosis of metastasis does not contraindicate surgical palliation (Butturini et al. 2008), while on the other hand – according to other authors (Luque-de Leon et al. 1999; Falconi et al. 2004; Potts et al. 1990) – in patients in stage IV there is no indication to proceed with a surgical biliary bypass considering the short expectancy of life (<6 months). In case of intraoperative diagnosis of unresectability for the local extension of the tumor with local nodal or vascular involvement, in the presence of jaundice or main biliary duct dilation, biliary bypass should be performed (Luque-de Leon et al. 1999; Potts et al. 1990), particularly for younger patients without comorbid conditions (Luque-de Leon et al. 1999).

For tumors located in the head of the pancreas, combined biliary and gastric bypass would be the elected procedure, due to the high risk of developing obstructive jaundice.

Surgical palliation could include different options such as cholecystojujenostomy, choledochoduodenostomy, or hepatico-(choledocho)-jejunostomy. In several authors' opinion, the overall outcomes of these three techniques are similar (Deziel et al. 1996).

Cholecystojujenostomy is a quick and safe method of drainage and minimal expertise is required as the dissection of the biliary tree is not necessary.

More recently, Falconi et al. (2004) proposed with good results a pylorus-preserving gastric transposition associated with coledochoduodenostomy in patients without distal duodenum obstruction. Although the use of the duodenum for the anastomosis carries a higher risk of jaundice recurrence, due to secondary duodenal obstruction, it is still the method of choice in different centers with good results (Potts et al. 1990). For this group, choledoco-(hepatico)-enteric bypass is nowadays the method of choice for drainage as it provides longer palliation and avoids cholangitis. According to different reports, this procedure seems to be the gold standard for biliary bypass (Tao et al. 2002; Sarfeh et al. 1988; Egrari and O'Connell 1995). It is true that this represents a more demanding technique as it requires an extensive dissection of the biliary tree, but this could be balanced by its use in cases with longer life expectancy. According to other centers' experience (Dervenis 2000), "Roux-en-Y" anastomosis, at present, is associated with colecistectomy whenever possible, as it was found more effective and safe in jaundice palliation without adding any operative risk and slightly increasing operative time.

One out of three patients with pancreatic cancer presents symptoms caused by a degree of gastric outlet obstruction (Smith et al. 1994; Egrari and O'Connell 1995). There is large debate concerning the role of prophylactic gastric bypass in patients with unresectable pancreatic cancer operated for obstructive jaundice.

Therefore, a double bypass is generally not yet accepted as standard treatment. The reluctance to perform a prophylactic gastroenterostomy is routinely based on the occurrence of additional postoperative complications: delayed gastric emptying and gastrointestinal bleeding have been reported (Weaver et al. 1987; Schantz et al. 1984). The authors conclude that gastrojejunostomy should be performed routinely when a patient is undergoing surgical palliation for unresectable periampullary carcinoma (Smith et al. 1994). In the absence of confirmed obstruction, the gastrointestinal anastomosis tends not to function because of a vicious circle between the stomach, duodenum, and anastomosis. This can in fact worsen the patient's quality of life with symptoms of dyspepsia, slowed digestion, regurgitation, and even vomiting (Slim et al. 1996). In some cases, the anastomosis actually occludes (Roost et al. 1989).

In the Verona group, a retrocolic construction technique is routinely used combining an omega loop with an entero-entero anastomosis between the afferent and efferent limbs to decrease the problem of delayed gastric emptying (with a "Roux-en-Y" reconstruction for the biliary bypass). Since 1997, this group, observing a low incidence of delayed gastric emptying (<4%) after pylorus-preserving pancreaticoduodenectomy, has used whenever possible pylorus-preserving gastric retrocolic transposition (Dervenis 2000). After the gastrocolic and hepatogastric ligaments were opened, elective ligature of both right gastric and gastroepiploic arteries and veins was undertaken. The first 3–4 cm of duodenum distal to the pylorus was dissected, and duodenum was transected. Nevertheless, tumor growth can occlude the duodenum below the papillary region, thus creating a closed "loop" consisting of the duodenal stump and biliary tract. In case of biliary anastomosis, this results in cholangitis. This occurred after one operation and required a second operation to drain the duodenal stump exclusively.

Palliation of pain in patients with unresectable pancreatic cancer was attempted in the past with surgical drainage of the dilated pancreatic duct over a T-tube or with a pancreatico-enteroanastomosis with little or no success. Recently, promising results (60% of the patients remained pain-free after the procedure) were obtained with pancreatic stenting (Costamagna et al. 1999). Surgery for pain relief is limited to thorascopic splanchnicectomy or to perioperative coeliac plexus block, which appears to be an important part of palliative surgery.

Surgical palliation for unresectable pancreatic cancer is in selected patients the method of choice as it is the only one having the advantage of treating in a single procedure the three major symptoms: jaundice, duodenal obstruction, and pain. Patients in stage III with local vascular involvement have a longer expectation of life than patients in stage IV, so they ought to receive a surgical palliation as it is safe, gives better quality of life, and is cost effective.

2.1 Radiofrequency Thermo Ablation

Radiofrequency thermo ablation (RFTA) represents a local treating methodology possibly capable of cell destroying through thermal coagulation and proteins denaturation. RFTA is nowadays used with good results in the treatment of solid, nonresectable tumors such as those of liver, lung, kidney, brain, breast, prostate, adrenal gland, bone, and spleen (Lencioni and Crocetti 2005; Simon and Dupuy 2005; Boss et al. 2005; Shariat et al.

2005; Noguchi 2003; Martel et al. 2009; Gananadha et al. 2004; Milicevic et al. 2002).

RFTA application on pancreas presents, though critical aspects related to the peculiar organ's anatomy, disease's biology, and pancreatic parenchyma properties.

The ablation of neoplastic mass is indeed contraindicated in the presence of previously misdiagnosed liver metastases or peritoneal carcinosis (Date and Siriwardena 2005; Matsui et al. 2000; Spiliotis et al. 2007; Elias et al. 2004; Varshney et al. 2006; Lygidakis et al. 2007; Goldberg et al. 1999; Date et al. 2005).

Accurate patients' selection is fundamental. RFTA can in fact be taken into consideration in case of locally advanced pancreatic adenocarcinoma (stage III).

Intraoperative monitoring of coagulative effect is checked with ultrasounds. When RFTA is feasible, a bilio-digestive bypass should always be performed for cephalic tumors.

RFTA's possible complications are represented by acute pancreatitis, portal vein thrombosis, gastroduodenal or intraabdominal bleeding, and bilio-pancreatic fistulas. However, the risk of developing acute pancreatitis as well as biliary fistula has been demonstrated to be very low. In order to preserve surrounding structures from heat injury, a "security distance" must be maintained. Moreover, to reduce the effect of thermal conduction, the whole area should be continuously kept under the temperature of 40° with cold saline solution. In addition, a cold lint is properly placed above the inferior vena cava and the duodenum is perfused with cold physiological solution via a nasogastric probe placed in the second portion of the duodenum. Recent evidences suggested to lower the method temperature from 105 to 90° in order to minimize the already mentioned risks.

After this analysis, the "total" treatment of the pancreatic mass with RFTA appears unlikely, difficult, not secure, and thus not indicated. Residual neoplastic tissue infiltrating surrounding structures such as mesenteric vessels, duodenal walls, or retroperitoneum is obviously not removed. For this reason, it is indicated to complete RFTA citoreduction with chemotherapy alone or in association with radiotherapy.

3 Adjuvant and Neoadjuvant Therapy

The majority of patients who underwent surgical resection for pancreatic adenocarcinoma develop, during the follow-up, both hepatic and lymphatic metastasis. For this reason, adjuvant treatment is a rationale approach.

The results from the European Study Group for the Pancreatic Cancer (ESPAC1) (Neoptolemos et al. 2004) demonstrated that adjuvant therapy prolongs survival rate in this setting of patients. Following studies, e.g., ESPAC 3 and CONKO 001, tried to found the most suitable treatment to apply (Oettle et al. 2005).

Therefore, at this time, no definite standard has been established in the adjuvant treatment of pancreatic cancer, and both 5-FU-based chemoradiation with additional gemcitabine-chemotherapy and chemotherapy alone with gemcitabine, 5-FU, or capecitabine are listed in the guidelines as options for adjuvant treatment.

However, when chemotherapy alone is the choice of adjuvant therapy, gemcitabine is preferred over either 5-FU or capecitabine for most patients, and systemic gemcitabine should be administered with adjuvant 5-FU-based chemoradiation when chemoradiation is the adjuvant therapy choice.

Treatment should be initiated within 4–8 weeks from surgery and should go on 6 month.

Nevertheless, with the emergence of new agents to treat pancreatic cancer, particularly biologics, adjuvant clinical trials designed to incorporate principles of molecular biology and new imaging methods, may be more beneficial than those focused on a comparison of chemotherapy vs. chemoradiation.

A number of studies have investigated the use of neoadjuvant chemoradiation in patients with resectable disease (Wollf et al. 2002; Talamonti et al. 2006; Hoffman et al. 1998; Breslin et al. 2001; Spitz et al. 1997). Putative advantages of administering neoadjuvant therapy include treatment of micrometastases at a earlier stage, the potential to select for surgery those patients with more stable disease or disease that has not been subjected to surgery and may be more sensitive to chemoradiation, and the potential to downsize tumors so as to increase the likelihood of a margin-free resection (Varadhachary et al. 2006; Quiros et al. 2007; White et al. 2001).

In fact, emerging evidence suggests that there is a better chance of margin-negative resection with preoperative therapy (Pingpank et al. 2001).

Further, the optimal neoadjuvant regimen has not been established yet.

4 Conclusions

Although there have been substantial improvements in the management of pancreatic cancer, the correct treatment of this complex disease still represents an open challenge for the surgeon.

The gold standard for the therapy of malignant pancreatic neoplastic forms remains radical surgery. Once a complete eradication of the disease can be achieved, major pancreatic resections such as DPa and TP should be performed for head, body-tail, and whole organ neoplasms, respectively.

Recent world literature data and our experience attest how both adjuvant and neoadjuvant chemotherapy and radiotherapy play a major role in the multidisciplinary treatment of the disease, with a resulting better outcome than surgery alone.

A new perspective is represented by the still experimental RFTA of nonresectable tumors, which can provide good results in association or not with standard protocols of chemotherapy.

Despite the improvements in diagnostic preoperative imaging, the majority of patients are still unfortunately found eligible neither for radical surgery nor for cytoreductive therapies. In these cases palliative surgery plays a fundamental role, allowing good quality of life in both short and long-term results.

References

Aldridge MC, Williamson RCN (1991) Distal pancreatectomy with and without splenectomy. Br J Surg 78:976–979

Billings BJ, Christein JD, Harmsen WS, Harrington JR, Chari ST, Que FG, Farnell MB, Nagorney DM, Sarr MG (2005) Quality-of-life after total pancreatectomy: is it really that bad on long-term follow-up? J Gastrointest Surg 9(8): 1059–1067

Boss A, Clasen S, Kuczyk M, Anastasiadis A, Schmidt D, Graf H et al (2005) Magnetic resonance-guided percutaneous radiofrequency ablation of renal cell carcinoma: a pilot clinical study. Invest Radiol 40:583–590

Breslin TM, Hess KR, Harbison DB et al (2001) Neoadjuvant chemoradiotherapy for adenocarcinoma of the pancreas: treatment variables and survival duration. Ann Surg Oncol 8:123–132

Butturini G, Stocken DD, Wente MN, Jeekel H, Klinkenbijl JH, Bakkevold KE, Takada T, Amano H, Dervenis C, Bassi C, Büchler MW (2008) Neoptolemos JP; Pancreatic Cancer Meta-Analysis Group in patients with pancreatic cancer: meta-analysis of randomized controlled trials. Arch Surg 143(1):75–83

Costamagna G, Alevras P, Palladino F, Rainoldi F, Mutignani M, Morganti A (1999) Endoscopic pancreatic stenting in pancreatic cancer. Can J Gastroenterol 13(6):481–487

Date RS, Siriwardena AK (2005) Radiofrequency ablation of the pancreas. II: Intra-operative ablation of non-resectable pancreatic cancer. A description of technique and initial outcome. JOP 6:588–592

Date RS, McMahon RF, Siriwardena AK (2005) Radiofrequency ablation of the pancreas: definition of optimal thermal kinetic parameters and the effect of simulated portal venous circulation in an ex-vivo porcine model. JOP 6:581–587

Dervenis CG (2000) SD, Avgerinos C, Hatzitheoklitos E. Surgical palliation in unresectable pancreatic cancer. In: Dervenis C, Bassi C (eds) Pancreatic tumors. Georg Thieme, Stuttgart, NY, pp 251–256

Deziel DJ, Wilhelmi B, Staren ED, Doolas A (1996) Surgical palliation for ductal adenocarcinoma of the pancreas. Am Surg 62(7):582–588

Egrari S, O'Connell TX (1995) Role of prophylactic gastroenterostomy for unresectable pancreatic carcinoma. Am Surg 61(10):862–864

Elias D, Baton O, Sideris L, Lasser P, Pocard M (2004) Necrotizing pancreatitis after radiofrequency destruction of pancreatic tumors. Eur J Surg Oncol 30:85–87

Falconi M, Hilal MA, Salvia R, Sartori N, Bassi C, Pederzoli P (2004) Prophylactic pylorus-preserving gastric transposition in unresectable carcinoma of the pancreatic head. Am J Surg 187(4):564–566

Fernandez-Cruz L (2006) Distal pancreatic resection: technical differences between open and laparoscopic approaches. HPB 8:49–56

Fernandez-Cruz L, Orduna D et al (2005) Distal pancreatectomy: en block splenectomy vs spleen preserving pancreatectomy. HPB (Oxford) 7(2):93–98

Gananadha S, Wulf S, Morris DL (2004) Safety and efficacy of radiofrequency ablation of brain: a potentially minimally invasive treatment for brain tumors. Minim Invasive Neurosurg 47:325–328

Geer RJ, Brennan MF (1993) Prognostic indicators for survival after resection of pancreatic adenocarcinoma. Am J Surg 165:68–72

Goldberg SN, Mallery S, Gazelle GS, Brugge WR (1999) EUS-guided radiofrequency ablation in the pancreas: results in a porcine model. Gastrointest Endosc 50:392–401

Heidt DG, Burant C, Simeone DM (2007) Total pancreatectomy: indications, operative technique, and postoperative sequelae. J Gastrointest Surg 11:209–216

Hoffman JP, Lipsitz S, Pisanky T et al (1998) Phase II trial of preoperative radiation therapy and chemotherapy for patients with localized, respectable adenocarcinoma of the pancreas: an Eastern Cooperative Oncology Group Study. J Clin Oncol 16:317–323

Jaeck D, Boudjema K, Bachellier P, Weber JC, Asensio TE, Wolf P (1998) Exeresi pancreatiche cefaliche: duodeno-cefalo-pancreasectomie (DCP). Encycl Méd Chir (Elsevier, Parigi), Tecniche chirurgiche-Addominale 40-880-B:17

Jaeck D, Boudjema K, Bachellier P, Weber Jc, Asensio TE, Wolf P (1998) Pancreasectomie di sinistra o distali. Encycl Méd

Chir (Elsevier, Parigi), Tecniche chirurgiche-Addominale 40-880-D:6

Lencioni R, Crocetti L (2005) A critical appraisal of the literature on local ablative therapies for hepatocellular carcinoma. Clin Liver Dis 9:301–314

Lillemoe KD, Sauter PK, Pitt HA, Yeo CJ, Cameron JL (1993) Current status of surgical palliation of periampullary carcinoma. Surg Gynecol Obstet 176(1):1–10

Lillemoe KD, Cameron JL, Hardacre JM, Sohn TA, Sauter PK, Coleman J et al (1999) Is prophylactic gastrojejunostomy indicated for unresectable periampullary cancer? A prospective randomized trial. Ann Surg 230(3):322–328; discussion 328–330

Luque-de Leon E, Tsiotos GG, Balsiger B, Barnwell J, Burgart LJ, Sarr MG (1999) Staging laparoscopy for pancreatic cancer should be used to select the best means of palliation and not only to maximize the resectability rate. J Gastrointest Surg 3(2):111–117; discussion 117–118

Lygidakis NJ, Sharma SK, Papastratis P, Zivanovic V et al (2007) Microwave ablation in locally advanced pancreatic carcinoma – a new look. Hepatogastroenterology 54(77): 1305–1310

Martel J, Bueno A, Nieto-Morales ML, Ortiz EJ (2009) Osteoid osteoma of the spine: CT-guided monopolar radiofrequency ablation. Eur J Radiol 71(3):564–569

Matsui Y, Nakagawa A, Kamiyama Y et al (2000) Selective thermocoagulation of unresectable pancreatic cancers by using radiofrequency capacitive heating. Pancreas 20:14–20

Milicevic M, Bulajic P, Zuvela M, Raznatovic Z, Obradovic V, Lekic N et al (2002) Elective resection of the spleen: Overview for resection techniques and description for a new technique based on radiofrequency coagulation and dissection. Acta Chir Iugosl 49:19–24

Muller MW, Friess H, Kleeff J, Dahmen R, Wagner M, Hinz U, Breisch-Girbig D, Buchler MW (2007) Is there still a role for total pancreatectomy? Ann Surg 246:966–975

Neoptolemos JP et al (2004) A randomized trial of chemoradiotherapy a nd chemotherapy after resection of pancreatic cancer. N Engl Med 350:1200–1210

Noguchi M (2003) Minimally invasive surgery for small breast cancer. J Surg Oncol 84:94–101

Oettle H, Pelzer U, Stieler J et al (2005) Oxaliplatin/folic acid/5-fluorouracil [24h] (OFF) plus best supportive care versus best supportive care alone (BSC) in second-line therapy of gemcitabine-refractory advance advanced pancreatic cancer (CONKO 003). J Clin Oncol 23:4031

Pingpank JF, Hoffman JP, Ross EA et al (2001) Effect of preoperative chemoradiation on surgical margin status of resected adenocarcinoma of the pancreas. J Gastrointest Surg 5:121–130

Potts JR III, Broughan TA, Hermann RE (1990) Palliative operations for pancreatic carcinoma. Am J Surg 159(1):72–77; discussion 77–78

Quiros RM, Brown KM, Hoffman JP (2007) Neoadjuvant therapy in pancreatic cancer. Cancer Invest 25:267–273

Richardson DQ, Scott-Conner CEH (1989) Distal pancreatectomy with and without splenectomy. Am Surg 55:21–25

Roost HM, Ackermann C, Harder F (1989) Palliative biliodigestive anastomosis in non-resectable cancer of the head of the pancreas–with or without preventive gastroenterostomy? Helv Chir Acta 55(5):619–621

Sarfeh IJ, Rypins EB, Jakowatz JG, Juler GL (1988) A prospective, randomized clinical investigation of cholecystoenterostomy and choledochoenterostomy. Am J Surg 155(3): 411–414

Schantz SP, Schickler W, Evans TK, Coffey RJ (1984) Palliative gastroenterostomy for pancreatic cancer. Am J Surg 147(6): 793–796

Schmidt CM, Glant J, Winter JM, Dixon J, Zhao Q, Howard TJ, Madura JA, Nakeeb A, Pitt HA, Cameron JL, Yeo CJ, Lillemoe KD (2007) Total pancreatectomy (R0 resection) improves survival over subtotal pancreatectomy in isolated neck margin positive pancreatic adenocarcinoma. Surgery 142(4):572–578

Schwarz A, Beger HG (2000) Biliary and gastric bypass or stenting in nonresectable periampullary cancer: analysis on the basis of controlled trials. Int J Pancreatol 27(1):51–58

Sener SF, Fremgen A, Menck HR, Winchester DP (1999) Pancreatic cancer: a report of treatment and survival trends for 100, 313 patients diagnosed from 1985–1995, using the National Cancer Database. J Am Coll Surg 189:1–7

Shariat SF, Raptidis G, Masatoschi M, Bergamaschi F, Slawin KM (2005) Pilot study of radiofrequency interstitial tumor ablation (RITA) for the treatment of radio-recurrent prostate cancer. Prostate 65:260–267

Simon CJ, Dupuy DE (2005) Current role of image-guided ablative therapies in lung cancer. Expert Rev Anticancer Ther 5:657–666

Slim K, Pezet D, Riff Y, Richard JF, Chipponi J (1996) [Antral exclusion. A complement to palliative gastrojejunal shunt in pancreatic cancer]. Presse Med 25(14):674–676

Smith AC, Dowsett JF, Russell RC, Hatfield AR, Cotton PB (1994) Randomised trial of endoscopic stenting versus surgical bypass in malignant low bileduct obstruction. Lancet 344(8938):1655–1660

Sohn TA, Lillemoe KD, Cameron JL, Huang JJ, Pitt HA, Yeo CJ (1999) Surgical palliation of unresectable periampullary adenocarcinoma in the 1990s. J Am Coll Surg 188(6):658–666; discussion 666–669

Sohn TA, Yeo CJ, Cameron JL et al (2000) Resected adenocarcinoma of the pancreas-616 patients: results, outcomes, and prognostic indicators. J Gastrointest Surg 4:567–579

Spiliotis JD, Datsis AC, Michalopoulos NV, Kekelos SP, Vaxevanidou A et al (2007) Radiofrequency ablation combined with palliative surgery may prolong survival of patients with advanced cancer of the pancreas. Langenbecks Arch Surg 392:55–60

Spitz FR, Abruzzese JL, Lee JE et al (1997) Preoperative and postoperative chemoradiation strategies in patients treated with Pancreaticoduodenectomy for adenocarcinoma of the pancreas. J Clin Oncol 15:928–937

Talamonti MS, Small W Jr, Mulchay MF et al (2006) A multi-institutional phase II trial of preoperative full-dose gemcitabine and concurrent and concurrent radiation for patients with potentially respectable pancreatic carcinoma. Ann Surg Oncol 13:150–158

Tao KS, Lu YG, Dou KF (2002) Palliative operation procedures for pancreatic head carcinoma. Hepatobiliary Pancreat Dis Int 1(1):133–136

Trede M (1985) The surgical treatment of pancreatic carcinoma. Surgery 97(1):28–35

Varadhachary GR, Tamm EP, Abruzzese JL et al (2006)
    Borderline respectable pancreatic cancer: definitions, man-
    agement, and role of preoperative therapy. Ann Surg Oncol
    13: 1035–1046

Varshney S, Sewkani A, Sharma S, Kapoor S, Naik S et al (2006)
    Radiofrequency ablation of unresectable pancreatic carci-
    noma: feasibility, efficacy and safety. JOP 7:74–78

Wagner M, Redaelli C, Lietz M, Seiler CA, Friess H, Buchler MW
    (2004) Curative resection ist he single most important factor
    determining outcome in patients with pancreatic adenocarci-
    noma. Br J Surg 91:586–594

Weaver DW, Wiencek RG, Bouwman DL, Walt AJ (1987)
    Gastrojejunostomy: is it helpful for patients with pancreatic
    cancer? Surgery 102(4):608–613

White RR, Hurwitz HI, Morse MA et al (2001) Neoadjuvant
    chemoradiation for localized adenocarcinoma of the pan-
    creas. Ann Surg Oncol 8:758–765

Wollf RA, Evans DB, Crane CH et al (2002) Initial results of
    preoperative gemcitabine (GEM)-based chemoradiation for
    respectable pancreatic adenocarcinoma. Proc Am Soc Clin
    Oncol 21:abstract 516

The Locally Advanced Nonmetastatic Cancer

Florence Huguet

Contents

Abstract

> At the time of diagnosis, around 20% of patients present with a resectable tumor, 50% with a metastatic disease, and 30% with a locally advanced tumor, unresectable because of superior mesenteric artery (SMA) or celiac encasement but nonmetastatic. Despite advances in chemoradiation (CRT) and improved systemic chemotherapeutic agents, those who present with locally advanced disease suffer both from high rates of distant metastatic failure and local progression, with median survival time ranging from 5 to 11 months. In the past 30 years, modest improvements in median survival have been attained for patients with locally advanced tumors treated by CRT or chemotherapy (CT) protocols. However, no significant impact on long-term survival has been accomplished. Optimal therapy for patients with locally advanced pancreatic carcinoma remains controversial. A recent systematic review concluded that there is no standard for the treatment of locally advanced pancreatic cancers, but two options: gemcitabine-based CT or CRT. These approaches are complementary and both should be considered. An induction CT followed by a CRT for nonprogressive patients is a promising strategy whose validation is ongoing in a phase III trial.

F. Huguet
Service d'Oncologie Radiothérapie, Hôpital Tenon, Assistance
Publique – Hôpitaux de Paris, 4 rue de la Chine, 75020 Paris,
France
e-mail: florence.huguet@tnn.aphp.fr

A. Laghi (ed.), *New Concepts in Diagnosis and Therapy of Pancreatic Adenocarcinoma*,
Medical Radiology, DOI: 10.1007/174_2010_2, © Springer-Verlag Berlin Heidelberg 2011

1 Introduction

At the time of diagnosis, around 20% of patients with pancreatic cancer presents with a resectable tumor, 30% with a locally advanced tumor, and 50% with a metastatic disease. Patients with locally advanced carcinoma of the pancreas comprise a group of patients with an intermediate prognosis between resectable and metastatic patients with median survival time ranging from 5 to 11 months (Yeo et al. 2002). These patients have pancreatic tumors that are defined as surgically unresectable, but have no evidence of distant metastases. A tumor is considered to be unresectable if it has one of the following features:

- Encasement or occlusion of the superior mesenteric vein (SMV) or SMV/portal vein confluence
- Direct involvement of the SMA, inferior vena cava, aorta, or celiac axis

However, recent advances in surgical technique may allow for the resection of selected patients with tumors involving the SMV (Leach et al. 1998).

Optimal therapy for patients with locally advanced pancreatic carcinoma remains controversial. Currently, there are two therapeutic options. In the early 1980s, 5-fluorouracil (5-FU)-based concomitant chemoradiation (CRT) was shown to be better than radiotherapy alone (Moertel et al. 1981). Moreover, gemcitabine has improved the outcome of patients with advanced disease (26% locally advanced, 74% metastatic) by improving survival with a clinical benefit (Burris et al. 1997). The results of four randomized trials comparing CRT vs. chemotherapy (CT) were contradictory (GITSG 1988; Klaassen et al. 1985; Chauffert et al. 2008; Loehrer et al. 2008). A recent systematic review concluded that there is no standard for the treatment of locally advanced pancreatic cancer, but two options: gemcitabine-based CT or CRT (Huguet et al. 2009). Other therapeutic options of patients with locally advanced pancreatic cancer include intraoperative radiation therapy (IORT), stereotactic body radiation therapy (SBRT), intensity-modulated radiation therapy (IMRT), and more recently, external beam radiation therapy (EBRT) with novel chemotherapeutic and targeted agents. Another approach is to consider that CRT and CT are complementary and should be associated. An induction CT followed by a CRT for nonprogressive patients is a promising strategy whose validation is ongoing in a phase III trial. In evaluating the results of these various therapies, it is useful to remember that a median survival of 6 months has been reported for this subset of patients undergoing best supportive care (Shinchi et al. 2002).

2 Prospective Trials (Table 1)

2.1 Chemoradiation vs. Best Supportive Care

Only one recent randomized trial compared CRT to best supportive care in 31 patients with locally advanced pancreatic cancer (Shinchi et al. 2002). CRT was delivered in 16 patients using a standard fractionation scheme to a planned total dose of 50.4 Gy concurrently, with a continuous infusion of 5-FU at 200 mg/m^2/day. Fifteen patients were assigned to receive best supportive care. Despite a high heterogeneity in the effectively delivered dose of radiation (ranging from 25.2 to 60 Gy), results demonstrated a significant benefit of CRT, both on overall survival ($p < 0.001$) and quality of life, which was evaluated with the quality-adjusted life-months score ($p < 0.001$).

2.2 Chemoradiation vs. Radiation Therapy Alone

With the exception of one trial, CRT for locally advanced pancreatic cancer has been shown to improve survival compared to conventional EBRT alone in several prospective randomized trials. The first trial was published in 1969 by a team of the Mayo Clinic and included various types of gastrointestinal cancers, in which there were 64 patients with locally advanced pancreatic adenocarcinoma (Moertel et al. 1969). They received 35–40 Gy EBRT combined with concurrent 5-FU or placebo. A significant survival advantage was seen for patients receiving EBRT with 5-FU vs. EBRT only (10.4 vs. 6.3 months). The Gastrointestinal Tumors Study Group (GITSG) followed with a similar study comparing EBRT alone to EBRT with concurrent and maintenance 5-FU (Moertel et al. 1981). One hundred and ninety-four eligible patients with locally advanced

Table 1 Prospective randomized trials for locally advanced pancreatic cancer

References	Treatment	n	Disease free survival (months)	Overall survival (months)	1-Year survival (%)
Moertel et al. (1969)	RT 35–40 Gy	32		6.3 $p<0.05$	6[a]
	CRT 35–40 Gy + 5-FU	32		10.4	25[a]
Moertel et al. (1981)	RT 60 Gy	25	2.9 $p<0.01$ 7	5.3 $p<0.01$ 8.4	10
	CRT 40 Gy + 5-FU then 5-FU	117	$p=0.14$	$p=0.19$	35
	CRT 60 Gy + 5-FU then 5-FU	111	7.6	11.4	46
Hazel et al. (1981)	5-FU + methylCCNU	30		7.8 n.s.	
	CRT 46 Gy + 5-FU then 5-FU + methylCCNU			7.3	
GITSG (1985)	CRT 60 Gy + 5-FU then 5-FU	73		8.5 n.s.	33
	CRT 40 Gy + adria then 5-FU	70		7.6	27
Klaassen et al. (1985)	5-FU	44		8.2	32[a]
	CRT 40 Gy + 5-FU then 5-FU	47		n.s. 8.3	26[a]
GITSG (1988)	SMF	21		7.4	19
	CRT 54 Gy + 5-FU then SMF	22		n.s. 9.7	$p<0.02$ 41
Earle et al. (1994)	CRT 55 Gy + 5-FU	87		7.8	
	CRT 50 Gy + hycanthone			n.s. 7.8	
Shinchi et al. (2002)	Best supportive care	31		6.4	0
	CRT 50.8 Gy + 5-FU then 5-FU			$p<0.001$ 13.2	$p<0.001$ 53
Li et al. (2003)	CRT + 5-FU then gem	34	2.7	6.7	
	CRT + gem then gem		$p=0.019$ 7.1	$p=0.027$ 14.5	
Chung et al. (2004)	CRT 45 Gy + gem + doxifluridine then gem + doxi	46	12	12	
	CRT 45 Gy + docetaxel + doxi then gem + doxi		n.s. 12.5	n.s. 14	
Cohen et al. (2005)	RT 59.4 Gy	108	5	7.1	
	CRT 59.4 Gy + 5-FU + mito C		n.s. 5.1	n.s. 8.4	
Chauffert et al. (2008)	Gem	60		13	53
	CRT 60 Gy + 5-FU + cisplatine then gem	59		$p=0.03$ 8.6	32
Loehrer et al. (2008)	Gem × 7	35	6.1	9.2	30[a]
	CRT 50.4 Gy + gem then gem × 5	34	n.s. 6.3	$p=0.04$ 11	45[a]

n number of patients; *GISTG* Gastrointestinal Study Group; *ECOG* Eastern Cooperative Oncology Group; *RT* radiation therapy; *CRT* chemoradiation; *5-FU* 5-fluorouracil; *SMF* streptozocin, mitomycin C, and 5-flurouracil; *gem* gemcitabine; *doxi* doxifluridine; *mito C* mitomycine C; *n.s.* nonsignificant

[a]Extrapolated from survival curve

pancreatic adenocarcinoma were randomized to receive 60 Gy of split course EBRT alone, 40 Gy of split course EBRT with concurrent bolus 5-FU CT (500 mg/m^2 on the first 3 days of each 20 Gy radiation), or 60 Gy split course EBRT using a similar CT regimen. Patients in the latter groups received maintenance 5-FU after EBRT completion. The EBRT-alone arm was closed early after an interim analysis as a result of an inferior survival rate. The median overall survival in the two combined modality therapy arms was 8.4 and 11.4 months, respectively, vs. 5.3 months in the EBRT-alone arm ($p < 0.01$). No significant differences were seen between the high- and low-dose EBRT in the CRT arms ($p = 0.19$). Most recently, another phase III trial compared CRT to EBRT alone. In this study, standard EBRT to a total dose of 59.4 Gy was compared to CRT with 5-FU and mitomycin C (Cohen et al. 2005). This trial enrolled 114 patients. No significant difference in terms of overall survival was reported between the two arms (8.4 vs. 7.1 months, respectively; $p = 0.16$). CRT was associated in the last two studies with higher hematological and digestive toxicity rates.

Two metaanalyses compared CRT to exclusive radiotherapy in locally advanced pancreatic carcinoma (Sultana et al. 2007b; Yip et al. 2007). The metaanalysis reported by Sultana et al. included the randomized trials described above, whereas the Cochrane Collaboration study analyzed only the trial by Moertel et al., together with ancient historical studies. However, the two met12aanalyses concluded a significant benefit of CRT on overall survival, with, in the Sultana's study, a 31%-decrease in tumor-related deaths following CRT, when compared with radiotherapy.

2.3 Chemoradiation vs. Chemotherapy Alone

CRT was compared with CT in five randomized trials. Three studies were published in the 1980s (Hazel et al. 1981; GITSG 1988; Klaassen et al. 1985). In these trials, CRT consisted of the combination of standard radiotherapy, delivering total doses ranging from 40 to 54 Gy, and 5-FU. CRT was compared to various CT regimens: 5-FU, methylCCNU and 5-FU, or SMF (streptomycin, mitomycin C, 5-FU). A GITSG trial compared CT alone to CRT, again in surgically confirmed unresectable tumors. Forty-three patients were randomized to receive the combination streptozocin,

mitomycin C, and 5-FU (SMF) CT or 54 Gy of EBRT with two cycles of concurrent bolus 5-FU CT, followed by adjuvant SMF CT. The CRT arm demonstrated a significant survival advantage over the CT alone arm (1-year survival 41 vs. 19%, respectively; $p < 0.02$) (GITSG 1988). In the two other trials, CT and CRT had same results. A most recent randomized trial addressing this question was reported in 2008 by the French FFCD-SFRO trial (Chauffert et al. 2008). In this study, CRT was delivered to a total dose of 60 Gy concurrently with cisplatin (20 mg/m^2 during the first and fifth weeks of radiotherapy) and 5-FU (continuous infusion at 300 mg/m^2/day). The CT arm was gemcitabine (1,000 mg/m^2/week), which has become the standard treatment of advanced pancreatic carcinoma (Burris et al. 1997). In contrast to the initial hypothesis of the trial, overall survival was shorter in the CRT arm. Higher grade 3–4 toxicity rates were observed in the CRT arm compared to the CT arm (66 vs. 40%, respectively).

More recently, the results of another phase III trial (ECOG E4201) comparing CRT and CT alone were presented at the annual ASCO meeting 2008. In this trial, patients with locally unresectable pancreatic cancer were randomized between a CRT with concurrent gemcitabine followed by gemcitabine vs. gemcitabine alone (Loehrer et al. 2008). In the CRT arm, the total dose was 50.4 Gy with concurrent gemcitabine (600 mg/m^2/week). The inclusion of 316 patients was planned to have an 88% power to detect a 50% improvement in median overall survival. The study closed after the inclusion of 74 patients only because of low accrual rate. Median overall survival was better in the CRT arm (11 vs. 9.2 months, $p = 0.044$). Grade 4 toxicity was more common in CRT arm (41.2 vs. 5.7%, $p < 0.0001$). These results should be considered cautiously because of the limited number of patients included.

Metaanalysis of the four first studies, including preliminary data of the FFCD-SFRO but not those of ECOG E4201, concluded that the overall survival was not significantly different following CRT or CT (HR = 0.79; IC 95%: 0.32–1.95) (Sultana et al. 2007a, b).

2.4 Chemotherapy Alone

The results of CT alone for this stage of pancreatic cancer are often difficult to evaluate in the literature as most trials pool patients with locally advanced and metastatic cancers. Table 2 summarizes the main

Table 2 Summary of phase II and III trials of gemcitabine-based chemotherapy in locally advanced pancreatic adenocarcinoma

References	Type of trial	Treatment	n	Median PFS (months)	Median OS (months)	1-Year survival (%)
Louvet et al. (2001)	II	Gem/5-FU	22	7	11.5	46
Reni et al. (2001)	II	Gem/5-FU/cisplatin/ epirubicine	18	10.5	18.5	–
Stathopoulos et al. (2001)	II	Gem/irinotecan	9	–	8.5	26.7
Louvet et al. (2002)	II	Gem/oxaliplatin	30	6.2	11.5	47
El-Rayes et al. (2003)	II	Gem/cisplatin/5-FU	16	7.2	10.3	35
Van Cutsem et al. (2004)	III	Gem Gem / tipifarnib	164	4.5 6.6	8.7 10.4	– –
Rocha Lima et al. (2004)	III	Gem Gem/irinotecan	24 27	3.9 7.7	11.7 9.8	– –
Louvet et al. (2005)	III	Gem Gem/oxaliplatin	47 51	5.3 7.4	10.3 10.3	– –
Heinemann et al. (2006)	III	Gem Gem/cisplatin	20 20	3.2 8.6	10.4 10.3	– –
Poplin et al. (2009)	III	Gem Gem FDR Gem/oxaliplatine	86	5.4	9.2	

n number of patients; *Gem* gemcitabine; *FDR* fixed-dose rate infusion; *5-FU* 5-fluorouracil; *PFS* progression-free survival; *OS* overall survival

results of gemcitabine-based CT phase II and III trials which have individualized patients with LA tumors.

3 Modalities of Chemoradiation

3.1 Type of Concurrent Chemotherapy

Numerous CT regimens have been combined with radiotherapy in locally advanced pancreatic carcinoma: 5-FU, 5-FU and cisplatin, 5-FU and mitomycin, gemcitabine, oxaliplatine, paclitaxel, docetaxel, and tyrosine kinase inhibitors.

3.1.1 Continuous Infusional 5-Fluorouracil

The idea that continuous infusion 5-FU allows for increased cumulative drug dose to be given without a significant increase in toxicity and for a more protracted radiosensitization effect relative to bolus 5-FU has prompted its study in locally advanced pancreatic cancer. Trials of other gastrointestinal sites have shown an increased survival using continuous infusion 5-FU

(O'Connell et al. 1994). Rich et al. (1985) first reported the use of concurrent radiotherapy and 5-FU by protracted venous infusion (PVI) in nine patients with locally advanced or resected pancreatic cancer. With a median radiotherapy dose of 46 Gy and concurrent 5-FU at doses ranging from 200 to 300 mg/m²/day, 7 of 9 patients experienced mild treatment-related gastointestinal toxicity and 2 of 9 moderate toxicity requiring a treatment interruption. A phase I trial from ECOG found the maximal tolerated dose (MTD) of PVI 5-FU to be 250 mg/m²/day with the dose-limiting toxicity being gastrointestinal. The progression-free survival at 1 year was 40% with a median survival of 11.9 months (Whittington et al. 1995). A retrospective study compared treatment intensity and toxicity of CRT with 5-FU bolus or PVI (Poen et al. 1998). Concurrent radiation therapy with PVI 5-FU was well-tolerated and permitted greater CT and radiation therapy dose intensity with reduced hematologic toxicity and fewer treatment interruptions compared with concurrent radiation therapy and bolus 5-FU. Numerous phase II trials have been performed showing that the use of concurrent infusional 5-FU is effective without excessive treatment-related toxicity (Ishii et al. 1997; Andre et al. 2000; Boz et al. 2001).

Although no randomized trials have been published, combined radiation therapy with PVI 5-FU is now commonly used.

In addition, capecitabine, an oral 5-FU analog, in combination with radiation therapy for the treatment of pancreatic cancer has been reported (Ben-Josef et al. 2004; Saif et al. 2005; Crane et al. 2006). Dosing of capecitabine has been extrapolated from combined modality trials in rectal cancer to be about 1,600 mg/m^2/day divided twice a day during radiation treatment (Vaishampayan et al. 2002; Rich et al. 2004b; De Paoli et al. 2006). No randomized trial has been reported with this combination.

3.1.2 Doxorubicin

One of the GITSG trials randomized 157 patients with locally advanced pancreatic adenocarcinoma to 60-Gy split course EBRT with concurrent and maintenance 5-FU as in the trial published by Moertel et al. vs. 40-Gy continuous course radiation with weekly concurrent doxorubicin CT, followed by maintenance doxorubicin and 5-FU. A significant increase in treatment-related toxicity was seen in the doxorubicin arm. However, no survival difference was observed between the two groups (median survival 8.5 vs. 7.6 months) (p=0.8) (GITSG 1985). The addition of hycanthone, an alkylating agent, to 5-FU led to similar overall survival in a randomized phase II trial (Earle et al. 1994).

3.1.3 Gemcitabine

Because of the high incidence of metastases and poor results with standard CRT, current and future research efforts include evaluation of EBRT with newer systemic agents including gemcitabine. Interest in this agent is based on both its systemic cytotoxic effects and its radiosensitizing properties. Following several phase I studies, gemcitabine-based CRT was evaluated in four studies. Chung et al. (2004) reported similar overall survival with gemcitabine (1,000 mg/m^2/week) or paclitaxel (50 mg/m^2/week), both in combination with oral doxifluridin and radiotherapy to a total dose of 45 Gy. Three subsequent studies compared 5-FU-based chemoradiotherapy to gemcitabine-based chemoradiotherapy: a retrospective analysis with radiotherapy to a total dose of 30 Gy (ten fractions) in the two arms

reported similar overall survival, and local and metastatic time-to-progression rates (p=0.19, 0.68, and 0.7, respectively) (Crane et al. 2002); a prospective study compared 5-FU to cisplatin-gemcitabine, concurrently with standard radiotherapy to a total dose of 50 Gy, and did not demonstrate any difference in the overall survival (Wilkowski et al. 2006); a third study, reported by Li et al. (2003), showed a survival benefit with gemcitabine at weekly doses of 600 mg/m^2 (14.5 vs. 6.7 months in the 5-FU arm; p=0.027), concurrently with radiotherapy to a total dose of 50.4 Gy.

3.1.4 Paclitaxel

In a phase I trial at Brown University evaluating paclitaxel and 50 Gy of EBRT for patients with unresectable pancreatic and gastric cancers, the maximum tolerated dose of weekly paclitaxel with conventional irradiation was 50 mg/m^2 (Safran et al. 1999). The response rate was 31% among 13 evaluable pancreatic cancer patients. In the Brown University phase II study employing 50 Gy of EBRT with 50 mg/m^2/week of paclitaxel, 6/18 (33%) evaluable pancreatic cancer patients had a partial response, stable disease was observed in seven patients (39%), only one patient (6%) had local tumor progression after completion of treatment, and four (22%) have developed distant metastases. These data have led to an RTOG phase II study evaluating paclitaxel with EBRT for patients with unresectable pancreatic cancer (Rich et al. 2004a). The median survival of the 109 patients in this study was 11.2 months (95% CI, 10.1–12.3) with estimated 1- and 2-year survival rates of 43 and 13%, respectively. External irradiation plus concurrent weekly paclitaxel was well-tolerated. Chung et al. (2004) reported similar overall survival with gemcitabine (1,000 mg/m^2/week) or paclitaxel (50 mg/m^2/week), both in combination with oral doxifluridin and radiotherapy to a total dose of 45 Gy.

3.1.5 Molecular-Targeted Therapies

As the biological basis of cancer is better understood, the use of cancer-specific targeted therapies is being increasingly investigated. There is preclinical evidence for either additive or synergistic effects of several of these approaches, such as antibodies against epidermal growth factor receptor (EGFR) and vascular endothelial factor receptor (VEGF), with both CT and radiation therapy, making these approaches especially promising. These targeted agents have been studied most extensively in the metastatic disease. Currently, the only targeted agent that has shown a statistically significant survival benefit in the metastatic setting compared to CT alone is erlotinib, an anti-EGFR tyrosine kinase inhibitor. However, the survival benefit is small, improving slightly the overall survival from 5.91 months for the gemcitabine plus placebo arm to 6.37 months for the gemcitabine plus erlotinib arm ($p = 0.025$) (Moore et al. 2007). A phase I study from Brown University has established an MTD of 50 mg for the combination of erlotinib, gemcitabine, paclitaxel, and radiation therapy at the dose of 50.4 Gy for patients with locally advanced pancreatic cancer followed by maintenance treatment with erlotinib (Iannitti et al. 2005). The median survival was 14 months. Another phase I study of erlotinib, gemcitabine, and radiation therapy for patients with locally advanced pancreatic cancer has found an MTD of erlotinib 100 mg daily, gemcitabine 40 mg/m^2 biweekly, and radiation therapy to 50.4 Gy (Duffy et al. 2008). The median survival was 18.7 months. Two small trials have reported preliminary results using another EGFR inhibitor, cetuximab, in combination with gemcitabine and radiation therapy for localized pancreatic cancer (Krempien et al. 2006; Pipas et al. 2006). These studies have found that cetuximab can be given at full dose with CT and radiation therapy without significantly increased toxicity. Efficacy results are pending.

Preclinical data have shown that inhibition of VEGF has radiosensitizing effects. The mechanisms of this radiosensitization are not well-understood, but could include enhanced lethality of endothelial cells, tumor cells, or normalization of tumor vasculature leading to a reduction in tumor hypoxia (Gorski et al. 1999; Garcia-Barros et al. 2003; Jain 2005). A phase I study from MDACC has studied the combination of bevacizumab, capecitabine, and radiation therapy at the dose of 50.4 Gy for patients with locally advanced pancreatic cancer followed by maintenance treatment with bevacizumab (Crane et al. (2006). Significant acute gastrointestinal (43% grade 2; 4% grade 3), hand and foot syndrome (21% grade 2), and transient hematologic (8% grade 3 or greater) events were uncommon with protocol mandated dose reductions of capecitabine grade 2 toxicity (43% of patients). Among the first 30 patients treated, three

patients had tumor-associated bleeding duodenal ulcers and one had a contained duodenal perforation. No additional bleeding events occurred among the final 18 patients after patients with duodenal involvement by tumor were excluded. The median survival was 11.6 months. In a RTOG phase II trial, 82 patients with locally advanced pancreatic cancer without duodenal invasion were treated with 50.4 Gy radiation therapy with concurrent capecitabine and bevacizumab followed by maintenance gemcitabine and bevacizumab (Crane et al. 2009). The median survival was 11.9 months. Overall, 35.4% of patients had grade 3 or greater treatment-related gastrointestinal toxicity. These results are not good enough to recommend further study of this regimen.

Several molecular abnormalities have been implicated in contributing to the development of pancreatic cancer. At this time, four tumor suppressor genes have been implicated (p16, p53, DPC4, and BRCA2), with incidences of 50–95% in all pancreatic tumors. Among oncogenes, K-ras activation is observed in 90% of these tumors. A better knowledge of the role of these genes in the pancreatic carcinogenesis could allow the development of more efficient molecular-targeted therapies.

3.2 Increased EBRT Dosing

Because of the limited tolerance of normal tissue in the upper abdomen (liver, kidney, spinal cord, and bowel) to EBRT, total doses of only 45–54 Gy in 25–30 Gy fractions have usually been given. For an unresectable tumor, this dose of radiation seems inadequate, as demonstrated by the high rates of local tumor progression and poor survival seen in both prospective and retrospective studies. An attempt has been made to evaluate whether an increased dose of radiation may improve outcomes. The effect on survival of a higher total dose has been studied in the phase III trial by Moertel et al. (1981). In the arm B, patients received a total dose of 40 Gy, whereas they received 60 Gy in the arm C. Survival was not different between the two arms ($p = 0.16$). However, these results were observed with a split course technique that is no longer used. In a report from Thomas Jefferson University Hospital, 46 evaluable patients with unresectable disease by laparotomy were treated with 63–70 Gy EBRT with or without CT. Despite high-dose EBRT, the local failure rate was 78% (Whittington et al. 1984).

The limitation of irradiated volumes to the gross tumor volume (GTV), without prophylactic irradiation of the peri-pancreatic regional lymph nodes, was reported in one retrospective study and one prospective noncontrolled trial (Figs. 1 and 2). In a retrospective study, Murphy et al. (2007) evaluated the feasibility of chemoradiotherapy with gemcitabine (1,000 mg/m^2/week) and radiotherapy to a total dose of 36 Gy. The planed target volume (PTV) covered the GTV with a limited 1-cm margin. A prospective phase II trial with 5-FU-based chemoradiotherapy used similar margins for the PTV (Goldstein et al. 2007). These two studies reported similar local recurrence rates to previously reported studies. However, digestive toxicity was lower and significantly correlated to the PTV.

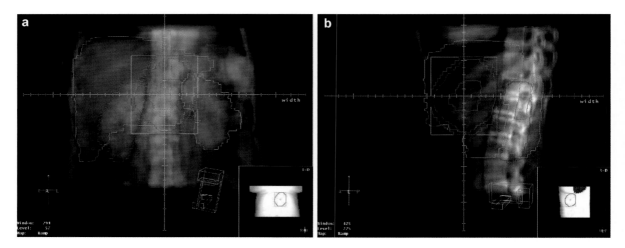

Fig. 1 Typical treatment volumes for locally advanced pancreatic cancer. (**a**) Anterioposterior digitally reconstructed radiograph (DRR) with in *red* the GTV (gross tumor volume) and in *blue* the PTV (planning target volume). (**b**) Left lateral DRR

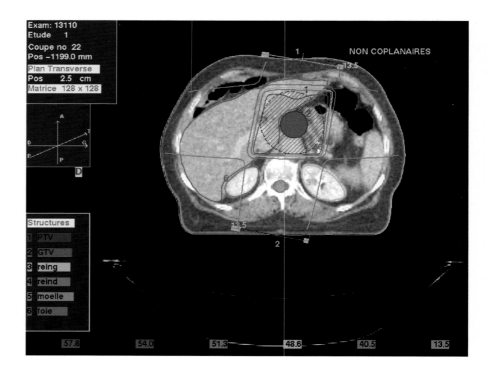

Fig. 2 Three-dimensional axial dosimetry of locally advanced pancreatic carcinoma

3.3 Other Radiation Therapy Techniques

The other modalities of radiotherapy for locally advanced pancreatic carcinoma, including IMRT, IORT, SBRT, are promising but have not been evaluated in phase III randomized trials.

3.3.1 Intraoperative Radiation Therapy

Because of the poor local control and results achieved with conventional EBRT and CT, specialized radiation therapy techniques that increase the radiation dose to the tumor volume have been used to improve local tumor control without significantly increasing normal tissue morbidity. These include iodine-125 implants and IORT as a dose escalation technique in combination with EBRT and CT. A lower incidence of local failure in most series and improved median survival in some have been reported with these techniques when compared with conventional external beam irradiation, but it is uncertain whether this is due to superior treatment or case selection (Roldan et al. 1988).

A recent study from investigators of the Massachusetts General Hospital reported the results of 150 patients treated with IORT and EBRT and CT (Willett et al. 2005). Although the study spanned nearly 25 years, it is relevant because it shows for the first time that long-term survival is possible for patients with unresectable pancreatic cancer. Although the 3- and 5-year survival rates (7 and 4%, respectively) are modest, they are not markedly different from the results reported in contemporary trials of resected pancreatic cancer patients (20 and 10%, respectively) or patients undergoing palliative pancreaticoduodenectomy (6.3 and 1.6%, respectively), especially when taking into account those patients with smaller tumors. For 25 patients treated with a small diameter applicator (5 or 6 cm), the 2- and 3-year actuarial survival rates were 27 and 17%, respectively. Furthermore, this study shows that postoperative and late treatment-related toxicity rates were acceptable. These study results support further study of selected patients with small, unresectable tumors into innovative protocols employing IORT.

3.3.2 Stereotactic Body Radiation Therapy

Stereotactic body radiation therapy (SBRT) is capable of precisely delivering high doses of radiation to small tumor volumes. SBRT using the Cyberknife system with compensation for organ motion following metallic marker implantation has been evaluated in a phase I dose escalation trial using a single fraction of radiation therapy at Stanford University (Koong et al. 2004). The final dose of 25 Gy was well-tolerated and has been recommended for further study. The phase II study that followed used 45 Gy IMRT with concurrent 5-FU followed by a 25 Gy SBRT boost to the primary tumor (Koong et al. 2005). Sixteen patients completed the planned therapy. Two patients experienced grade 3 toxicity. Fifteen of these 16 patients were free from local progression until death. Median overall survival was 5.6 months. The authors concluded that concurrent IMRT and 5-FU followed by SBRT resulted in excellent local control, but did not improve the overall survival and was associated with more toxicity than SBRT alone. Another phase II study from Stanford University evaluated the efficacy of a single fraction of 25 Gy SBRT delivered between cycles 1 and 2 of gemcitabine CT in 16 patients (Schellenberg et al. 2008). The median survival was 11.4 months. Acute gastrointestinal toxicity was mild, with one case of grade 3 toxicity (6%). Late gastrointestinal toxicity was more common, with five ulcers (grade 2), one duodenal stenosis (grade 3), and one duodenal perforation (grade 4). In the same time, a Danish phase II trial enrolled 22 patients with locally advanced pancreatic carcinoma (Hoyer et al. 2005). SBRT was given on standard linear accelerator with three fractions of 15 within 5–10 days. Only two patients (9%) were found to have a partial response. The median survival was 5.7 months. Acute toxicity was pronounced with deterioration in performance status, nausea, and pain. Four patients suffered from severe mucositis or ulceration of the stomach or duodenum and one of the patients had a nonfatal ulcer perforation of the stomach. The authors concluded that "SBRT was associated with poor outcome, unacceptable toxicity and questionable palliative effect and cannot be recommended for patients with advanced pancreatic carcinoma."

3.3.3 IMRT

Since its introduction into clinical use, IMRT has generated widespread interest. IMRT optimally assigns nonuniform intensities to tiny subdivisions of beams, which have been called rays or "beamlets." The ability to optimally manipulate the intensities of individual rays within each beam permits greatly increased control over the radiation fluence, enabling custom design of optimum dose distributions. These improved dose distributions may potentially lead to improved tumor control and reduced normal tissue toxicity. IMRT requires the settings of the relative intensities of tens of thousands of rays comprising an intensity-modulated treatment plan. This task cannot be accomplished manually and requires the use of specialized computer-aided optimization methods. The optimum beamlet intensities are determined using a systematic iterative process during which the computer sequentially generates intensity-modulated plans one by one, evaluates each of them according to user-selected criteria, and makes incremental changes in the ray intensities based on the deviation from the desired objectives. Several groups have demonstrated the feasibility of using IMRT in the treatment of pancreatic tumors. First, Crane et al. (2001) reported the results of a phase I dose-escalation study of radiotherapy with concurrent gemcitabine CT. The aim of this study was to alternate escalating the radiation dose by 3 Gy and the gemcitabine dose by 50 mg/m^2. The starting dose of gemcitabine was 350 mg/m^2 and 33 Gy per 11 fractions of IMRT to the regional lymphatics and primary disease. All three patients in the first cohort who were treated suffered dose-limiting toxicity, and the trial was ultimately closed because of excessive myelosuppression and upper gastrointestinal toxicity. Then, Milano et al. (2004) reported on 25 patients with pancreatic and bile duct carcinomas, comparing IMRT with conventional four-field 3D-CRT plans. The dose received by critical structures such as right kidney, liver, and small bowel was significantly reduced with the use of IMRT plans. Treatment was well-tolerated in this series. Ben-Josef et al. (2004) treated 15 patients with pancreatic adenocarcinoma with IMRT and concurrent capecitabine. Treatment was well-tolerated. Only 1 patient (7%) had grade 3 toxicity, a gastric ulceration that responded to medical management. Brown et al. (2006) performed a dosimetric analysis of 15 patients with pancreatic cancer and compared 3DCRT, IMRT with sequential boost, and IMRT with integrated boost, and found that IMRT with integrated boost allowed dose escalation up to 64.8 Gy to the primary tumor. More recently, a team from Amsterdam compared conformal radiotherapy to IMRT and respiration-gated radiotherapy (RGRT) for pancreatic cancers (Van der Geld et al. 2008). IMRT significantly reduced the mean doses to

kidneys, liver, stomach, and small bowel. The additional dosimetric benefits from RGRT appeared limited in this study. A recent study showed that there were substantial respiratory-associated movements of pancreatic tumors that were not predicted by 4D-CT planning scans (Minn et al. 2009).

3.4 A New Strategy: Induction Chemotherapy Followed by Chemoradiation

Optimal treatment of patients with locally advanced pancreatic cancer is still under debate. Another approach is to consider that CRT and CT are complementary and should be associated. Indeed, an important concern about administering CRT on the first intention in patients with locally advanced pancreatic cancer is that about 30% of them have occult metastatic disease at diagnosis and will clearly not benefit from this local-regional treatment. Induction CT can potentially help to select a subgroup of patients without early metastatic course who can potentially benefit from CRT. An induction CT followed by a CRT for nonprogressive patients is a promising strategy. In a phase II trial, 25 patients received an induction CT with six cycles of fixed-dose rate gemcitabine associated to low-dose cisplatin, followed by a CRT with concurrent 5-FU (Ko et al. 2007). The median survival was 13.5 months for all the patients and 17 months for the patients who received the two phases of the treatment. Two retrospective studies evaluated the interest of induction CT before concurrent chemoradiotherapy in locally advanced pancreatic carcinoma (Huguet et al. 2007; Krishnan et al. 2007). The first study retrospectively compared induction CT followed by CRT to exclusive CT (Huguet et al. 2007). One hundred eighty-one patients received induction CT with gemcitabine, gemcitabine, and oxaliplatine, or gemcitabine, 5-FU, and leucovorin; 128 patients without tumor progression at first evaluation received either CRT to a total dose of 55 Gy with 5-FU ($n = 72$), or the same CT regimen as during the induction phase ($n = 56$). For the patients who received induction CT and CRT, median survival was 15 months. The second study compared induction CT (gemcitabine alone or combined with cisplatin) to exclusive CRT in 323 patients (Krishnan et al. 2007). CRT consisted of the association of conformal EBRT to total doses ranging from 30 to 50 Gy, with concurrent 5-FU or gemcitabine. For the patients who received induction CT and CRT, median survival was 11.9 months. In these two studies, induction CT before chemoradiotherapy produced significantly prolonged survival, when compared with chemoradiotherapy alone or exclusive CT. An international phase III trial is ongoing to validate prospectively this promising strategy.

4 Conclusion

Treatment of locally advanced pancreatic cancer is one of the most formidable challenges that clinical and translational researchers face today. In the last 10 years, few progresses had been done despite numerous trials. In the absence of a therapeutic effect in any phase III trial, there is currently no standard treatment. The use of CRT for locally advanced pancreatic adenocarcinoma is based on few randomized trials. CRT, even if superior to best supportive care and exclusive radiotherapy alone, leads to a similar outcome when compared to modern CT with gemcitabine and may produce higher rates of toxicity. Even if gemcitabine-based CT could be considered as a standard of care in many clinical situations, the addition of chemoradiotherapy in nonprogressing patients after 3–4 months of induction CT is a promising strategy that has to be validated in prospective randomized trial. Reduction of the conformal fields to gross disease results in a better tolerance of radiation therapy. Optimal radiation dose to the tumor and better concurrent CT are discussed. Moreover, a better understanding of the molecular mechanisms underlying pancreatic carcinogenesis is essential to improve the outcome of the patients with new adapted targeted therapies.

References

Andre T, Balosso J et al (2000) Combined radiotherapy and chemotherapy (cisplatin and 5-fluorouracil) as palliative treatment for localized unresectable or adjuvant treatment for resected pancreatic adenocarcinoma: results of a feasibility study. Int J Radiat Oncol Biol Phys 46:903–911

Ben-Josef E, Shields AF, Vaishampayan U, Vaitkevicius V, El-Rayes BF, McDermott P, Burmeister J, Bossenberger T, Philip PA (2004) Intensity-modulated radiotherapy (IMRT) and concurrent capecitabine for pancreatic cancer. Int J Radiat Oncol Biol Phys 59:454–459

Boz G, De Paoli A, Innocente R, Rossi C, Tosolini G, Pederzoli P, Talamini R, Trovo MG (2001) Radiotherapy and continuous infusion 5-fluorouracil in patients with nonresectable pancreatic carcinoma. Int J Radiat Oncol Biol Phys 51:736–740

Brown MW, Ning H, Arora B, Albert PS, Poggi M, Camphausen K, Citrin D (2006) A dosimetric analysis of dose escalation using two intensity-modulated radiation therapy techniques in locally advanced pancreatic carcinoma. Int J Radiat Oncol Biol Phys 65:274–283

Burris HA III, Moore MJ et al (1997) Improvements in survival and clinical benefit with gemcitabine as first-line therapy for patients with advanced pancreas cancer: a randomized trial. J Clin Oncol 15:2403–2413

Chauffert B, Mornex F et al (2008) Phase III trial comparing intensive induction chemoradiotherapy (60 Gy, infusional 5-FU and intermittent cisplatin) followed by maintenance gemcitabine with gemcitabine alone for locally advanced unresectable pancreatic cancer. Definitive results of the 2000-01 FFCD/SFRO study. Ann Oncol 19:1592–1599

Chung HW, Bang SM, Park SW, Chung JB, Kang JK, Kim JW, Seong JS, Lee WJ, Song SY (2004) A prospective randomized study of gemcitabine with doxifluridine versus paclitaxel with doxifluridine in concurrent chemoradiotherapy for locally advanced pancreatic cancer. Int J Radiat Oncol Biol Phys 60:1494–1501

Cohen SJ, Dobelbower R Jr, Lipsitz S, Catalano PJ, Sischy B, Smith TJ, Haller DG (2005) A randomized phase III study of radiotherapy alone or with 5-fluorouracil and mitomycin-C in patients with locally advanced adenocarcinoma of the pancreas: Eastern Cooperative Oncology Group study E8282. Int J Radiat Oncol Biol Phys 62:1345–1350

Crane CH, Antolak JA et al (2001) Phase I study of concomitant gemcitabine and IMRT for patients with unresectable adenocarcinoma of the pancreatic head. Int J Gastrointest Cancer 30:123–132

Crane CH, Abbruzzese JL et al (2002) Is the therapeutic index better with gemcitabine-based chemoradiation than with 5-fluorouracil-based chemoradiation in locally advanced pancreatic cancer? Int J Radiat Oncol Biol Phys 52:1293–1302

Crane CH, Ellis LM et al (2006) Phase I trial evaluating the safety of bevacizumab with concurrent radiotherapy and capecitabine in locally advanced pancreatic cancer. J Clin Oncol 24:1145–1151

Crane CH, Winter K, Regine WF, Safran H, Rich TA, Curran W, Wolff RA, Willett CG (2009) Phase II study of bevacizumab with concurrent capecitabine and radiation followed by maintenance gemcitabine and bevacizumab for locally advanced pancreatic cancer: Radiation Therapy Oncology Group RTOG 0411. J Clin Oncol 27:4096–4102

De Paoli A, Chiara S et al (2006) Capecitabine in combination with preoperative radiation therapy in locally advanced, resectable, rectal cancer: a multicentric phase II study. Ann Oncol 17:246–251

Duffy A, Kortmansky J, Schwartz GK, Capanu M, Puleio S, Minsky B, Saltz L, Kelsen DP, O'Reilly EM (2008) A phase I study of erlotinib in combination with gemcitabine and radiation in locally advanced, non-operable pancreatic adenocarcinoma. Ann Oncol 19:86–91

Earle JD, Foley JF, Wieand HS, Kvols LK, McKenna PJ, Krook JE, Tschetter LK, Schutt AJ, Twito DI (1994) Evaluation of external-beam radiation therapy plus 5-fluorouracil (5-FU) versus external-beam radiation therapy plus hycanthone (HYC) in confined, unresectable pancreatic cancer. Int J Radiat Oncol Biol Phys 28:207–211

El-Rayes BF, Zalupski MM, Shields AF, Vaishampayan U, Heilbrun LK, Jain V, Adsay V, Day J, Philip PA (2003) Phase II study of gemcitabine, cisplatin, and infusional fluorouracil in advanced pancreatic cancer. J Clin Oncol 21: 2920–2925

Garcia-Barros M, Paris F, Cordon-Cardo C, Lyden D, Rafii S, Haimovitz-Friedman A, Fuks Z, Kolesnick R (2003) Tumor response to radiotherapy regulated by endothelial cell apoptosis. Science 300:1155–1159

Gastrointestinal Tumor Study Group (1985) Radiation therapy combined with Adriamycin or 5-fluorouracil for the treatment of locally unresectable pancreatic carcinoma. Cancer 56:2563–2568

Gastrointestinal Tumor Study Group (1988) Treatment of locally unresectable carcinoma of the pancreas: comparison of combined-modality therapy (chemotherapy plus radiotherapy) to chemotherapy alone. J Natl Cancer Inst 80:751–755

Goldstein D, Van Hazel G et al (2007) Gemcitabine with a specific conformal 3D 5FU radiochemotherapy technique is safe and effective in the definitive management of locally advanced pancreatic cancer. Br J Cancer 97:464–471

Gorski DH, Beckett MA et al (1999) Blockage of the vascular endothelial growth factor stress response increases the antitumor effects of ionizing radiation. Cancer Res 59: 3374–3378

Hazel JJ, Thirlwell MP, Huggins M, Maksymiuk A, MacFarlane JK (1981) Multi-drug chemotherapy with and without radiation for carcinoma of the stomach and pancreas: a prospective randomized trial. J Can Assoc Radiol 32:164–165

Heinemann V, Quietzsch D et al (2006) Randomized phase III trial of gemcitabine plus cisplatin compared with gemcitabine alone in advanced pancreatic cancer. J Clin Oncol 24:3946–3952

Hoyer M, Roed H et al (2005) Phase-II study on stereotactic radiotherapy of locally advanced pancreatic carcinoma. Radiother Oncol 76:48–53

Huguet F, Andre T et al (2007) Impact of chemoradiotherapy after disease control with chemotherapy in locally advanced pancreatic adenocarcinoma in GERCOR phase II and III studies. J Clin Oncol 25:326–331

Huguet F, Girard N, Guerche CS, Hennequin C, Mornex F, Azria D (2009) Chemoradiotherapy in the management of locally advanced pancreatic carcinoma: a qualitative systematic review. J Clin Oncol 27:2269–2277

Iannitti D, Dipetrillo T et al (2005) Erlotinib and chemoradiation followed by maintenance erlotinib for locally advanced pancreatic cancer: a phase I study. Am J Clin Oncol 28:570–575

Ishii H, Okada S et al (1997) Protracted 5-fluorouracil infusion with concurrent radiotherapy as a treatment for locally advanced pancreatic carcinoma. Cancer 79:1516–1520

Jain RK (2005) Normalization of tumor vasculature: an emerging concept in antiangiogenic therapy. Science 307:58–62

Klaassen DJ, MacIntyre JM, Catton GE, Engstrom PF, Moertel CG (1985) Treatment of locally unresectable cancer of the stomach and pancreas: a randomized comparison of 5-fluorouracil alone with radiation plus concurrent and maintenance 5-fluorouracil–an Eastern Cooperative Oncology Group study. J Clin Oncol 3:373–378

Ko AH, Quivey JM, Venook AP, Bergsland EK, Dito E, Schillinger B, Tempero MA (2007) A phase II study of fixed-dose rate gemcitabine plus low-dose cisplatin followed by consolidative chemoradiation for locally advanced pancreatic cancer. Int J Radiat Oncol Biol Phys 68:809–816

Koong AC, Le QT et al (2004) Phase I study of stereotactic radiosurgery in patients with locally advanced pancreatic cancer. Int J Radiat Oncol Biol Phys 58:1017–1021

Koong AC, Christofferson E et al (2005) Phase II study to assess the efficacy of conventionally fractionated radiotherapy followed by a stereotactic radiosurgery boost in patients with locally advanced pancreatic cancer. Int J Radiat Oncol Biol Phys 63:320–323

Krempien RC, Munter MW et al (2006) Phase II study evaluating trimodal therapy with cetuximab intensity modulated radiotherapy (IMRT) and gemcitabine for patients with locally advanced pancreatic cancer [ISRCTN56652283]. J Clin Oncol (Meeting Abstracts) 24:4100

Krishnan S, Rana V et al (2007) Induction chemotherapy selects patients with locally advanced, unresectable pancreatic cancer for optimal benefit from consolidative chemoradiation therapy. Cancer 110:47–55

Leach SD, Lee JE, Charnsangavej C, Cleary KR, Lowy AM, Fenoglio CJ, Pisters PW, Evans DB (1998) Survival following pancreaticoduodenectomy with resection of the superior mesenteric-portal vein confluence for adenocarcinoma of the pancreatic head. Br J Surg 85:611–617

Li CP, Chao Y, Chi KH, Chan WK, Teng HC, Lee RC, Chang FY, Lee SD, Yen SH (2003) Concurrent chemoradiotherapy treatment of locally advanced pancreatic cancer: gemcitabine versus 5-fluorouracil, a randomized controlled study. Int J Radiat Oncol Biol Phys 57:98–104

Loehrer PJ, Powell ME, Cardenes HR, Wagner L, Brell JM, Ramanathan RK, Crane CH, Alberts SR, Benson AB (2008) A randomized phase III study of gemcitabine in combination with radiation therapy versus gemcitabine alone in patients with localized, unresectable pancreatic cancer: E4201. J Clin Oncol (Meeting Abstracts) 26:4506

Louvet C, Andre T et al (2001) Phase II trial of bimonthly leucovorin, 5-fluorouracil and gemcitabine for advanced pancreatic adenocarcinoma (FOLFUGEM). Ann Oncol 12:675–679

Louvet C, Andre T et al (2002) Gemcitabine combined with oxaliplatin in advanced pancreatic adenocarcinoma: final results of a GERCOR multicenter phase II study. J Clin Oncol 20:1512–1518

Louvet C, Labianca R et al (2005) Gemcitabine in combination with oxaliplatin compared with gemcitabine alone in locally advanced or metastatic pancreatic cancer: results of a GERCOR and GISCAD phase III trial. J Clin Oncol 23:3509–3516

Milano MT, Chmura SJ, Garofalo MC, Rash C, Roeske JC, Connell PP, Kwon OH, Jani AB, Heimann R (2004) Intensity-modulated radiotherapy in treatment of pancreatic and bile duct malignancies: toxicity and clinical outcome. Int J Radiat Oncol Biol Phys 59:445–453

Minn AY, Schellenberg D et al (2009) Pancreatic tumor motion on a single planning 4D-CT does not correlate with intrafraction tumor motion during treatment. Am J Clin Oncol 32:364–368

Moertel CG, Childs DS Jr, Reitemeier RJ, Colby MY Jr, Holbrook MA (1969) Combined 5-fluorouracil and super-voltage radiation therapy of locally unresectable gastrointestinal cancer. Lancet 2:865–867

Moertel CG, Frytak S et al (1981) Therapy of locally unresectable pancreatic carcinoma: a randomized comparison of high dose (6000 rads) radiation alone, moderate dose radiation (4000 rads + 5-fluorouracil), and high dose radiation + 5-fluorouracil: The Gastrointestinal Tumor Study Group. Cancer 48:1705–1710

Moore MJ, Goldstein D et al (2007) Erlotinib plus gemcitabine compared with gemcitabine alone in patients with advanced pancreatic cancer: a phase iii trial of the National Cancer Institute of Canada Clinical Trials Group. J Clin Oncol 25:1960–1966. doi:10.1200/JCO.2006.07.9525

Murphy JD, Adusumilli S, Griffith KA, Ray ME, Zalupski MM, Lawrence TS, Ben-Josef E (2007) Full-dose gemcitabine and concurrent radiotherapy for unresectable pancreatic cancer. Int J Radiat Oncol Biol Phys 68:801–808

O'Connell MJ, Martenson JA, Wieand HS, Krook JE, Macdonald JS, Haller DG, Mayer RJ, Gunderson LL, Rich TA (1994) Improving adjuvant therapy for rectal cancer by combining protracted-infusion fluorouracil with radiation therapy after curative surgery. N Engl J Med 331:502–507

Pipas JM, Zaki B et al (2006) Cetuximab, intensity-modulated radiotherapy (IMRT), and twice-weekly gemcitabine for pancreatic adenocarcinoma. J Clin Oncol (Meeting Abstracts) 24:14056

Poen JC, Collins HL et al (1998) Chemo-radiotherapy for localized pancreatic cancer: increased dose intensity and reduced acute toxicity with concomitant radiotherapy and protracted venous infusion 5-fluorouracil. Int J Radiat Oncol Biol Phys 40:93–99

Poplin E, Feng Y et al (2009) Phase III, randomized study of gemcitabine and oxaliplatin versus gemcitabine (fixed-dose rate infusion) compared with gemcitabine (30-minute infusion) in patients with pancreatic carcinoma E6201: a trial of the Eastern Cooperative Oncology Group. J Clin Oncol 27:3778–3785

Reni M, Passoni P, Panucci MG, Nicoletti R, Galli L, Balzano G, Zerbi A, Di Carlo V, Villa E (2001) Definitive results of a phase II trial of cisplatin, epirubicin, continuous-infusion fluorouracil, and gemcitabine in stage IV pancreatic adenocarcinoma. J Clin Oncol 19:2679–2686

Rich TA, Lokich JJ, Chaffey JT (1985) A pilot study of protracted venous infusion of 5-fluorouracil and concomitant radiation therapy. J Clin Oncol 3:402–406

Rich T, Harris J, Abrams R, Erickson B, Doherty M, Paradelo J, Small W Jr, Safran H, Wanebo HJ (2004a) Phase II study of external irradiation and weekly paclitaxel for nonmetastatic, unresectable pancreatic cancer: RTOG-98-12. Am J Clin Oncol 27:51–56

Rich TA, Shepard RC, Mosley ST (2004b) Four decades of continuing innovation with fluorouracil: current and future approaches to fluorouracil chemoradiation therapy. J Clin Oncol 22:2214–2232

Rocha Lima CM, Green MR et al (2004) Irinotecan plus gemcitabine results in no survival advantage compared with gemcitabine monotherapy in patients with locally advanced or metastatic pancreatic cancer despite increased tumor response rate. J Clin Oncol 22:3776–3783

Roldan GE, Gunderson LL, Nagorney DM, Martin JK, Ilstrup DM, Holbrook MA, Kvols LK, McIlrath DC (1988) External beam versus intraoperative and external beam irradiation for locally advanced pancreatic cancer. Cancer 61:1110–1116

Safran H, Akerman P, Cioffi W, Gaissert H, Joseph P, King T, Hesketh PJ, Wanebo H (1999) Paclitaxel and concurrent radiation therapy for locally advanced adenocarcinomas of the pancreas, stomach, and gastroesophageal junction. Semin Radiat Oncol 9:53–57

Saif MW, Eloubeidi MA et al (2005) Phase I study of capecitabine with concomitant radiotherapy for patients with locally advanced pancreatic cancer: expression analysis of genes related to outcome. J Clin Oncol 23:8679–8687

Schellenberg D, Goodman KA et al (2008) Gemcitabine chemotherapy and single-fraction stereotactic body radiotherapy for locally advanced pancreatic cancer. Int J Radiat Oncol Biol Phys 72:678–686

Shinchi H, Takao S, Noma H, Matsuo Y, Mataki Y, Mori S, Aikou T (2002) Length and quality of survival after external-beam radiotherapy with concurrent continuous 5-fluorouracil infusion for locally unresectable pancreatic cancer. Int J Radiat Oncol Biol Phys 53:146–150

Stathopoulos GP, Mavroudis D et al (2001) Treatment of pancreatic cancer with a combination of docetaxel, gemcitabine and granulocyte colony-stimulating factor: a phase II study of the Greek Cooperative Group for Pancreatic Cancer. Ann Oncol 12:101–103

Sultana A, Smith CT, Cunningham D, Starling N, Neoptolemos JP, Ghaneh P (2007a) Meta-analyses of chemotherapy for locally advanced and metastatic pancreatic cancer. J Clin Oncol 25:2607–2615

Sultana A, Tudur Smith C, Cunningham D, Starling N, Tait D, Neoptolemos JP, Ghaneh P (2007b) Systematic review, including meta-analyses, on the management of locally advanced pancreatic cancer using radiation/combined modality therapy. Br J Cancer 96:1183–1190

Vaishampayan UN, Ben-Josef E, Philip PA, Vaitkevicius VK, Du W, Levin KJ, Shields AF (2002) A single-institution experience with concurrent capecitabine and radiation therapy in gastrointestinal malignancies. Int J Radiat Oncol Biol Phys 53:675–679

Van Cutsem E, van de Velde H et al (2004) Phase III trial of gemcitabine plus tipifarnib compared with gemcitabine plus placebo in advanced pancreatic cancer. J Clin Oncol 22:1430–1438

van der Geld YG, van Triest B, Verbakel WF, van Sornsen de Koste JR, Senan S, Slotman BJ, Lagerwaard FJ (2008) Evaluation of four-dimensional computed tomography-based intensity-modulated and respiratory-gated radiotherapy techniques for pancreatic carcinoma. Int J Radiat Oncol Biol Phys 72:1215–1220

Whittington R, Solin L, Mohiuddin M, Cantor RI, Rosato FE, Biermann WA, Weiss SM, Pajak TF (1984) Multimodality therapy of localized unresectable pancreatic adenocarcinoma. Cancer 54:1991–1998

Whittington R, Neuberg D, Tester WJ, Benson AB 3rd, Haller DG (1995) Protracted intravenous fluorouracil infusion with radiation therapy in the management of localized pancreaticobiliary carcinoma: a phase I Eastern Cooperative Oncology Group Trial. J Clin Oncol 13:227–232

Wilkowski R, Rau H, Bruns C, Wagner A, Sauer R, Hohenberger W, Koelbl O, Heinemann V (2006) Randomized phase II trial comparing gemcitabine/cisplatin-based chemoradiotherapy (CRT) to 5-FU-based CRT in patients with locally advanced pancreatic cancer. J Clin Oncol (Meeting Abstracts) 24:4038

Willett CG, Del Castillo CF et al (2005) Long-term results of intraoperative electron beam irradiation (IOERT) for patients with unresectable pancreatic cancer. Ann Surg 241:295–299

Yeo TP, Hruban RH et al (2002) Pancreatic cancer. Curr Probl Cancer 26:176–275

Yip D, Karapetis C, Strickland A, Steer CB, Goldstein D (2007) Chemotherapy and radiotherapy for inoperable advanced pancreatic cancer. Cochrane Library 4:1–72

Metastatic Pancreatic Cancer: Systemic Therapy

Jennifer Brown and T. R. Jeffry Evans

Contents

Abstract

> Infiltrating ductal adenocarcinoma of the pancreas has an aggressive nature. Approximately 90% of patients have surgically unresectable disease at the time of diagnosis. In addition, the majority of the selected patients who undergo potentially curative resection for small, localised lesions inevitably develop recurrent or metastatic disease. Most systemic therapies have limited efficacy in patients with metastatic disease. Gemcitabine, with or without erlotinib, has modest clinical benefit and a marginal survival advantage in patients with metastatic pancreatic cancer and has become a standard of care for these patients. However, the median survival of patients with metastatic pancreatic cancer remains poor and is less than 6 months. This chapter gives an overview of the various monotherapy and combination chemotherapy regimens that have been evaluated in this disease, discusses the studies which have incorporated molecularly targeted agents into the treatment regimens, and highlights the challenges in developing therapeutic strategies to improve survival in metastatic pancreatic cancer.

J. Brown
Beatson West of Scotland Cancer Centre,
1053 Great Western Road, Glasgow, G12 OYN, UK

T.R.J. Evans (✉)
Beatson West of Scotland Cancer Centre,
1053 Great Western Road, Glasgow, G12 OYN, UK and
Beatson Laboratories, University of Glasgow, Garscube Estate,
Switchback Road, Glasgow, G61 1BD, UK
e-mail: j.evans@beatson.gla.ac.uk

1   Metastatic Pancreatic Cancer: The Clinical Problem

Pancreatic ductal adenocarcinoma shows a characteristic aggressive invasion and early metastases are common manifestation of the disease, such that 90% of

A. Laghi (ed.), *New Concepts in Diagnosis and Therapy of Pancreatic Adenocarcinoma*,
Medical Radiology, DOI: 10.1007/174_2010_3, © Springer-Verlag Berlin Heidelberg 2011

patients are surgically unresectable at the time of diagnosis. In addition, the majority of the selected patients who undergo potentially curative resection for small, localised lesions inevitably develop recurrent or metastatic disease (Yeo et al. 2002), presumably due to the presence of distant micro-metastases at initial diagnosis. Adjuvant (post-operative) chemotherapy can improve outcome, although overall survival remains disappointing (Neoptolemos et al. 2004; Stocken et al. 2005). Furthermore, most systemic therapies have limited efficacy in patients with metastatic disease, and the median survival of patients with metastatic pancreatic cancer remains poor and is less than 6 months (Li et al. 2004). Consequently, the development of more effective strategies for patients with metastatic pancreatic cancer is of paramount importance.

2 Chemotherapy Studies

Pancreatic ductal adenocarcinoma responds poorly to most single-agent chemotherapy regimens. Prior to the introduction of gemcitabine, the best response rates were seen with 5-fluorouracil (5-FU) (21–26%) (Carter 1975; Moertel 1976), ifosfamide (26%) (Bernard et al. 1986), epirubicin (22%) (Wils et al. 1985) and cisplatin (21%) (Wils et al. 1993). The results of combination chemotherapy regimens had been equally disappointing with objective responses of only 10% using a combination of 5-FU with BCNU (Kovach et al. 1974), 10% with 5-FU and mitomycin C (Buroker et al. 1979), 14% with FAM (5-FU, doxorubicin and mitomycin C) or SMF (5-FU, streptozotocin and mitomycin C) (Oster et al. 1986), and only 17% with a combination of continuous infusional 5-FU, epirubicin and cisplatin (Evans et al. 1996), which had demonstrated significant activity in gastro-oesophageal cancer at that time.

Furthermore, many of these studies were performed prior to the introduction of robust tools to assess objective responses such as the RECIST criteria (Therasse et al. 2000), and it is, therefore, likely that these studies may have resulted in enhanced response rates, especially as they were predominantly non-randomised trials in selected patients. Prior to the introduction of gemcitabine, 5-FU was the most extensively studied agent and was considered the agent of choice, although no consistent effect on disease-related symptoms or survival had been demonstrated (Hausen et al. 1988).

Nevertheless, two small studies at that time had demonstrated improved overall survival with combination chemotherapy compared to no treatment, without impairing quality of life, thereby encouraging researchers to continue to explore novel therapeutic approaches (Mallinson et al. 1980; Palmer et al. 1994).

2.1 Gemcitabine Monotherapy

Gemcitabine (difluorodeoxycytidine, dFdC) is a nucleoside analogue with a broad spectrum of anti-tumour activity in preclinical solid tumour models (Grindey et al. 1990; Hertel et al. 1990). It requires intracellular phosphorylation, resulting in the accumulation of difluorodeoxyctidine triphosphate (dFdCTP) (Heinemann et al. 1988). dFdCTP competes with deoxycytidine triphosphate (dTP) for incorporation into DNA, in turn inhibiting DNA synthesis (Heinemann et al. 1988; Huang et al. 1991). Gemcitabine also reduces intracellular deoxynucleoside triphosphate pools, presumably by inhibiting ribonucleotide reductase (Ghandi and Plunkett 1990).

The development of novel anti-cancer therapies traditionally includes three phases of clinical studies. The optimal dose and schedule of the novel agent are determined in phase I clinical trials based on the toxicity and safety assessments and pharmacokinetic analyses. Phase II trials are designed to determine a level of efficacy for the drug in question, with subsequent comparison with standard therapies performed in phase III studies, usually with overall survival as the primary endpoint (Vasey and Evans 2002). The classical endpoint of efficacy with cytotoxic agents in phase II trials is objective tumour reduction of measurable disease as determined using radiological techniques based on anatomical, non-functional, imaging. However, reproducible, reliable disease measurements of pancreatic cancer are often difficult in the absence of distant metastases. Patients with measurable distant, e.g. liver, metastases often have a poor performance status and a dismal prognosis such that these may not be the optimal patient population in which to determine the efficacy of a novel agent. In addition, the statistical basis of many phase II clinical trial designs is dependent on detecting a threshold response rate, often of 20%, above which further study is warranted within phase III clinical trials. However, an objective response rate of 20% with a single-agent chemotherapy drug in advanced pancreatic cancer has been rarely achievable since the introduction of robust criteria for response assessments and appropriate radiological techniques. Consequently, agents that may have a palliative benefit in this disease could be abandoned at the phase II stage of clinical development because they are considered to be "inactive" by these conventional end points.

The initial phase II study of single-agent gemcitabine found that a number of patients, including some who did not experience substantial tumour reduction, had stabilisation or improvement in performance status and a reduction in pain and daily analgesia consumption (Casper et al. 1994). Consequently, the concept of clinical benefit response was developed as a method to assess the palliative effect of gemcitabine chemotherapy in early phase studies in patients with advanced pancreatic cancer. Clinical benefit response was defined as a composite assessment of pain, performance status, and weight (Rothenberg et al. 1996), and a clinical benefit responder was defined as a patient with a sustained improvement in these parameters.

The effect of gemcitabine on cancer symptoms was subsequently formally assessed in a further phase II study of 74 patients (Rothenberg et al. 1996). Of these patients, 63 completed a pain stabilisation period and were treated with gemcitabine. Clinical benefit response – defined as a $\geq 50\%$ reduction in pain intensity, $\geq 50\%$ reduction in daily analgesic consumption, or ≥ 20 – point improvement in Karnofsky performance status, sustained for at least 4 consecutive weeks – was observed in 27% of patients, with a median duration of clinical benefit response of 14 weeks (Rothenberg et al. 1996). The significance of a clinical benefit response of 27% in a non-randomised phase II study was uncertain. However, these observations did allow for the rational design of a phase III trial (Burris et al. 1997) to determine the role of gemcitabine in palliating advanced disease.

In this randomised phase III study (Burris et al. 1997), 126 patients with symptoms of advanced pancreas cancer completed an initial observation period to characterise and stabilise pain and were randomised to receive either gemcitabine or 5-FU by weekly intravenous bolus (600 mg/m^2). The primary efficacy measure, clinical benefit response, was superior in the patients treated with gemcitabine (23.8%) compared to those treated with 5-FU (4.8%; $p = 0.0022$). Although the objective response rate with gemcitabine was only 5.4%, this modest activity was sufficient to result in a

significantly superior median survival (5.65 vs. 4.41 months; $p = 0.0025$) and 1-year survival (18 vs. 2%) with gemcitabine compared to 5-FU (Burris et al. 1997). On the basis of this study, single-agent gemcitabine is now considered a standard of care for advanced pancreatic cancer.

2.2 Combination Chemotherapy Regimens

2.2.1 Gemcitabine and Fluoropyrimidines

In an attempt to develop therapeutic strategies that will improve the overall survival in advanced pancreatic cancer, several cytotoxic chemotherapy agents have been evaluated, either alone or in combination with gemcitabine. Fluoropyrimidines, including 5-FU, have been among the agents most frequently studied in combination with gemcitabine. Objective response rates have been observed in phase II studies including 12–29% with gemcitabine and 5-FU (Kanat et al. 2004; Murad et al. 2003; Barone et al. 2003), 21–26% with gemictabine and 5-FU and leucovorin (Correale et al. 2003; Marantz et al. 2001; Louvet et al. 2001), 22–33% with gemcitabine and UFT (Lee et al. 2004; Feliu et al. 2003), and 17% with gemcitabine and UFT/leucovorin (Kim et al. 2002). The response rates for these combinations are variable yet encouraging, with a median overall survival for patients treated in these studies of 5–11 months. In a phase III randomised trial of gemcitabine with 5-FU vs. gemcitabine alone in patients with biopsy-proven inoperable pancreatic cancer ($n = 327$), objective responses were uncommon in both treatment arms (Berlin et al. 2002). Although there was an improvement in progression-free survival with the combination regimen (3.4 vs. 2.2 months; $p = 0.022$), there was no improvement in the primary end point of median overall survival (6.7 months for gemcitabine + 5-FU; 5.4 months for gemcitabine alone, $p = 0.09$), and further studies of the combination are not likely to improve the poor survival of these patients (Berlin et al. 2002).

2.2.2 Gemcitabine and Capecitabine

Capecitabine is an orally-available tumour-selective fluoropyrimidine carbamate, which is bioactivated by a 3-enzyme process to provide prolonged high levels of the active moiety, 5-FU, in tumour cells. After oral administration, capecitabine passes unchanged from the gastrointestinal tract and is metabolised in the liver by 60 Kd carboxylesterase (previously known as acylamidase isozyme A) to 5′-deoxy-5-fluorocytidine (5′-DFCR). This is then converted to 5′-deoxy-5-fluorouridine (5′-DFUR) by cytidine deaminase located in the liver and also in tumour tissues. Further metabolism of 5′-DFUR then occurs at the site of the tumour under the action of thymidine phosphorylase (dThdPase) to 5-FU. The exposure of healthy body tissues to systemic 5-FU is, therefore, minimised.

Capecitabine is widely used as the fluoropyrimidine of choice in patients with colorectal, breast and gastric cancer. Single-agent activity has been observed with capecitabine, in patients with pancreatic cancer, with objective responses of 7% (Cartwright et al. 2002), and an objective response of 19% has been observed for the combination of gemcitabine and capecitabine (Hess et al. 2003; Stathopoulos et al. 2004). In a subsequent phase III trial (Cunningham et al. 2005), patients with previously untreated locally advanced or metastatic adenocarcinoma of the pancreas were randomised to gemcitabine ($n = 266$) (1,000 mg/m^2 weekly for 7 weeks followed by a 1-week drug holiday, and then weekly for 3 consecutive weeks every 4-weekly cycle) or to GEM-CAP ($n = 267$) (gemcitabine 1,000 mg/m^2 weekly for 3 consecutive weeks every 4-weekly cycle and capecitabine 1,660 mg/m^2/day for 21 days followed by 7 days' drug holiday every 4-weekly cycle). Treatment continued until disease progression or intolerable toxicities. At the time of the interim analysis, 373 (70%) deaths had occurred. GEM-CAP significantly improved the overall survival over gemcitabine alone (hazard ratio (HR): 0.80; $p = 0.026$). The median overall survival for gemcitabine and GEM-CAP was 6 and 7.4 months, respectively, and 1-year survival rates were 19 and 26%, respectively. After adjusting for baseline stratification factors (disease extent and performance status), the survival advantage for GEM-CAP remains (HR: 0.77; $p = 0.014$). The objective response rates were 7 and 14% with gemcitabine and GEM-CAP, respectively ($p = 0.008$). NCI-CTC grades 3/4 toxicities were similar in the two treatment groups.

This finding of a survival benefit with gemcitabine in combination with capecitabine in this study is in contrast to previous studies of fluoropyrimidines in combination with gemcitabine which have not demonstrated a survival benefit. However, the final results of this study have yet to be published. Furthermore, gemcitabine in combination with capecitabine has been compared with gemcitabine monotherapy in another study (Herrmann et al. 2007). Patients with metastatic or locally advanced pancreatic cancer ($n = 319$) were randomised to receive either GEM-CAP (capecitabine 650 mg/m^2 twice daily days 1–14 plus gemcitabine 1,000 mg/m^2 on days 1 and 8 every 3 weeks) or gemcitabine 1,000 mg/m^2 weekly for 7 weeks, followed by a 1-week drug holiday, then weekly for 3 weeks every 4-weekly cycle. The combination of capecitabine with gemcitabine did not give an improvement in the overall survival for the study population. However, there was a significant improvement in the overall survival in a sub-set of patients with good performance status (10.1 vs. 7.4 months). However, the dose of capecitabine used in this study was significantly lower than that used in the UK study (Cunningham et al. 2005).

2.2.3 Other Combination Chemotherapy Regimens

Objective responses have also been observed with other gemcitabine-containing combination chemotherapy regimens including gemcitabine with oxaliplatin (11–30%) (Alberts et al. 2002, 2003; Louvet et al. 2002), gemcitabine with irinotecan (24%) (Stathopoulos et al. 2003; Rocha Lima et al. 2002), gemcitabine with docetaxel (12–27%) (Shepard et al. 2004; Schneider et al. 2003; Ryan et al. 2002), gemcitabine with cisplatin (9–26%) (Cascinu et al. 2003; Philip et al. 2001), gemictabine with epirubicin (20–25%) (Neri et al. 2002; Ianniello et al. 2001), and similar response rates have also been observed with gemcitabine in combination with either raltitrexed (12%) (Kralidis et al. 2003), tamoxifen (11%) (Tomao et al. 2002), or flutamide (15%) (Corrie et al. 2002). Several groups have also reported response rates from phase II studies for 3-drug or 4-drug combination regimens including G-FLIP (24–27%) (Rachamalla et al. 2004; Kozuch et al. 2001), gemcitabine with cisplatin and 5-FU (19–26%) (Novarino et al. 2004; El-Rayes et al. 2003), and MCF (46%) (Petty et al. 2003). However, the survival of patients treated in these studies remains poor.

A number of phase III trials have been reported comparing gemcitabine monotherapy with regimens consisting of gemcitabine-containing combinations of cytotoxic chemotherapy agents. In a phase III randomised comparison ($n = 107$), the combination of gemcitabine with cisplatin gave a superior objective response rate than gemcitabine alone (26 vs. 9%; $p = 0.02$) and also a superior median time to progression (20 vs. 8 weeks; $p = 0.048$), but did not yield any improvement in clinical benefit or overall survival (Colucci et al. 2002). A randomised multi-centre phase III trial compared PEFG (cisplatin, epirubicin, gemcitabine, and 5-FU; $n = 52$) with gemcitabine monotherapy ($n = 40$) (Reni et al. 2005). PEFG yielded a superior response rate, 1-year overall survival, and 4-month profession-free survival, but was associated with greater toxicity.

Gemcitabine and oxaliplatin (GemOx) has also been compared with gemcitabine monotherapy in a phase III randomised trial ($n = 326$) (Louvet et al. 2005). GemOx was superior to gemcitabine in terms of response rate (26.8 vs. 17.3%, respectively; $p = 0.04$), progression-free survival (5.8 vs. 3.7 months, respectively; $p = 0.04$), and clinical benefit (38.2 vs. 26.9%, respectively; $p = 0.03$). However, median overall survival for GemOx and gemcitabine was 9.0 and 7.1 months, respectively ($p = 0.13$). Thus, this study failed to demonstrate a statistically significant overall survival advantage for the combination compared with gemcitabine. Similarly, gemcitabine combined with irinotecan has been compared with gemcitabine ($n = 360$) (Rocha Lima et al. 2004). Although a superior response rate (16.1%) was observed for the combination compared with gemcitabine monotherapy (4.4%), there was no difference in the median overall survival (6.3 months for gemcitabine plus irinotecan; 6.6 months for gemcitabine). Furthermore, gemcitabine plus pemetrexed has been compared with gemcitabine ($n = 565$) (Oettle et al. 2005) and demonstrated no difference in the median overall survival for the combination regimen (6.2 months) compared with gemcitabine (6.3 months).

Thus, it can be concluded that despite encouraging response rates in selected patients in phase II studies, no study has yet demonstrated a survival advantage for cytotoxic chemotherapy combination regimens in phase III studies in comparison with gemcitabine, except for one of the studies combining gemcitabine with capecitabine (Cunningham et al. 2005) for which the final results have not yet been published. Any superiority in response rate that does not improve either clinical benefit or overall survival is of questionable benefit given the additional toxicity within the context of a patient population that has such a poor prognosis. Nevertheless, there is likely to be a sub-set of patients who might benefit from a combination chemotherapy regimen.

2.2.4 Combination Chemotherapy Regimens: A Meta-Analysis

Meta-analysis provides a useful tool for analysis when research results have been conflicting or the apparent benefits are marginal (Sacks et al. 1987). A meta-analysis of 51 trials of chemotherapy involving 9,970 patients with locally advanced and metastatic pancreatic cancer has reported the HR and its variance for the primary outcome measure of the overall survival (Sultana et al. 2007). This meta-analysis confirmed that chemotherapy improves overall survival compared with best supportive care (HR = 0.64). Nineteen studies involving 4,697 patients were included in the comparison of gemcitabine vs. gemcitabine-based combination chemotherapy. The overall survival was significantly better, with a reduction of 9% in the risk of death for gemcitabine-based combination chemotherapy (HR = 0.91). In the sub-group analysis for the overall survival, platinum-based compounds (3 trials; 1,077 patients) (HR = 0.85) and capecitabine (3 trials; 935 patients) (HR = 0.83) in combination with gemcitabine consistently performed better than single-agent gemcitabine, unlike irinotecan-based (2 trials; 486 patients) (HR = 1.01) and 5-FU-based combinations (3 trials; 879 patients) (HR = 0.98). This suggests that gemcitabine-based combination chemotherapy regimens may be of benefit in patients with advanced pancreatic cancer. Efforts are currently ongoing to identify sub-sets of patients who are most likely to benefit from this approach.

3 Targeted Therapies

3.1 Targeting the Epidermal Growth Factor Receptor

The current generation of novel anti-cancer agents in development is based on exploiting our increasing understanding of the molecular and cellular basis of the development and progression of malignant disease and is often referred to as molecularly targeted therapies. One example of these agents is erlotinib which is an oral HER1/EGFR tyrosine kinase inhibitor.

Human epidermal growth factor receptor type 1 (HER1/EGFR) is over-expressed in many pancreatic cancers (Fjallskog et al. 2003; Tobita et al. 2003) and is associated with poor prognosis and tumour progression (Ueda et al. 2004). Blocking HER1/EGFR tyrosine kinase signalling decreases the growth and metastasis of human pancreatic cancer xenografts (Bruns et al. 2000) and improves the anti-cancer effects of gemcitabine (Ng et al. 2002). Erlotinib plus gemcitabine resulted in a statistically superior overall survival (6.24 months) compared with gemcitabine alone (5.91 months) (HR = 0.82; $p = 0.038$) in a phase III randomised trial ($n = 569$) (Moore et al. 2007). One-year survival was also superior for the combination compared with gemcitabine monotherapy (23 vs. 17%; $p = 0.023$) as was progression-free survival (HR = 0.77; $p = 0.04$). Objective response rates were not statistically significantly different between the two treatment arms, but more patients treated with the combination therapy had disease stabilisation. This was the first phase III trial to demonstrate a statistically improved survival in advanced pancreatic cancer by adding an agent to gemcitabine. Nevertheless, the survival advantage remains modest and has not been adopted as standard of care in some parts of the world. In contrast, the addition of the anti-EGFR monoclonal antibody, cetuximab, to gemcitabine failed to demonstrate a clinically significant advantage for the overall survival (HR = 1.09; $p = 0.14$), progression-free survival (HR = 1.13) or response rate compared with gemcitabine monotherapy in patients with advanced pancreatic cancer ($n = 766$) (Philip et al. 2007).

3.2 Targeting the Vascular Endothelial Growth Factor Receptor

Pancreatic cancers commonly over-express many growth factors and their receptors, including those for the vascular endothelial growth factor (VEGF) family (Shi et al. 2001; Luo et al. 2001). The elevated activities of such receptor tyrosine kinases contribute to evasion of apoptosis, angiogenesis, invasion, and metastasis. There is some rationale for using a VEGFR inhibitor in pancreatic cancer, since VEGF can have autocrine effects on pancreatic cancer cells that express VEGF receptors and paracrine effects on microvascular endothelial cells (Luo et al. 2001; Itakura et al. 2000; Von Marschall et al. 2000). Inhibitors of VEGF tyrosine kinases, as well as anti-VEGF and anti-KDR antibodies, inhibit growth and angiogenesis of established pancreatic tumours (Baker et al. 2002; Solorzano et al. 2001; Bockhorn et al. 2003; Tsuzuki et al. 2001; Bruns et al. 2002) and can potentiate the anti-tumour effect of gemcitabine (Baker et al. 2002; Solorzano et al. 2001; Bruns et al. 2002).

The results of a non-randomised phase II study of gemcitabine in combination with bevacizumab, a recombinant humanised anti-VEGF monoclonal antibody, were very encouraging (Kindler et al. 2005). Disappointingly, the subsequent phase III trial of the combination compared with gemcitabine monotherapy failed to demonstrate any survival advantage for the combination ($n = 602$) (Kindler et al. 2007). Furthermore, the addition of bevacizumab to a gemcitabine and erlotinib doublet did not significantly improve the median overall survival compared with gemcitabine-erlotinib (HR = 0.89; $p = 0.21$; $n = 607$) (Van Cutsem et al. 2009). Further studies of other novel targeted therapies are, therefore, required to improve the dismal survival for patients with advanced pancreatic cancer.

4 Future Strategies

In human pancreatic cancer, development, progression, and metastases arise via the accumulation of multiple genetic and epigenetic changes, including inactivation of tumour-suppressor genes and activation or over-expression of proto-oncogenes. A progression model for the precursor lesions of pancreatic cancer has been proposed (Cubilla and Fitzgerald 1975, 1976; Hruban et al. 2000a; Klimstra and Longnecker 1994). These lesions, given the collective term pancreatic intra-epithelial neoplasia (PanIN), are grouped into three histological stages based on increasing degrees of architectural and nuclear atypia (Kern et al. 2001). Activating mutations of the *k-ras* proto-oncogene are found in around 90% of invasive pancreatic cancers (Almoguerra et al. 1998). Genetic and epigenetic inactivations of a number of tumour-suppressor genes also occur, including p16^{INK4a}, p53, DPC4 and BRCA2, and increase in frequency in progressively higher PanIN stages (Hruban et al. 2000b).

In a recently developed model of pancreatic cancer, endogenous K-Ras^{G12D} is targeted to progenitor cells of the mouse pancreas, resulting in ductal lesions that recapitulate the full spectrum of human PanIN, likely precursors to invasive pancreatic cancer (Hingorani et al. 2003). The PanINs that develop are highly proliferative, show evidence of histological progression, and activate signalling pathways normally quiescent in ductal epithelium (Hingorani et al. 2003). At low frequency, these lesions progress spontaneously to invasive and metastatic adenocarcinomas (Hingorani et al. 2003). However, by also targeting endogenous expression of Trp53^{R172H} and Kras^{G12D} to the mouse pancreas, adult mice develop invasive and widely metastatic pancreatic carcinoma (after loss of function of the remaining p53 allele), and this recapitulates the human disease (Hingorani et al. 2005). The full spectrum of pre-invasive lesions is evident in these mice, with significant malignant disease burden becoming apparent in animals by 10 weeks of age. The primary carcinomas and metastases demonstrate genomic instability and the mice have a significantly reduced survival due to locally advanced and metastatic cancer, similar to the human disease (Hingorani et al. 2005). Consequently, this mouse model will enable us to better study potential therapeutic targets and their inhibitors in the future and develop more rational therapeutic strategies, with the ultimate aim of improving quality of life and overall survival in patients with metastatic pancreatic cancer.

References

Alberts SR, Townley PM, Goldberg RM et al (2002) Gemcitabine and oxaliplatin for patients with advanced or metastatic pancreatic cancer: a North Central Cancer Treatment Group Phase I study. Ann Oncol 13:553–557

Alberts SR, Townley PM, Goldberg RM et al (2003) Gemcitabine and oxaliplatin for metastatic pancreatic adenocarcinoma: a North Central Cancer Treatment Group phase II study. Ann Oncol 14:580–585

Almoguerra C, Shibata D, Forrester K et al (1998) Most human carcinomas of the exocrine pancreas contain mutant c-K-ras genes. Cell 53:549–554

Baker CH, Solorzano CC, Fidler IJ (2002) Blockade of vascular endothelial growth factor receptor and epidermal growth factor receptor signaling for therapy of metastatic human pancreatic cancer. Cancer Res 62:1996–2003

Barone C, Cassano A, Corsi DC et al (2003) Weekly gemcitabine and 24-hour infusional 5-fluorouracil in advanced pancreatic cancer: a phase I–II study. Oncology 64:139–145

Berlin JD, Catalano P, Thomas JP et al (2002) Phase III study of gemcitabine in combination with fluorouracil versus gemcitabine alone in patients with advanced pancreatic carcinoma: Eastern Cooperative Oncology Group Trial E2297. J Clin Oncol 20:3270–3275

Bernard S, Noble S, Wilcosky T et al (1986) A phase II study of ifosfamide (IFOS) plus N-acetyl cysteine (NAC) in metastatic measurable pancreatic adenocarcinoma (abstract). Proc Am Soc Clin Oncol 5:328

Bockhorn M, Hsuzuki Y, Xu L et al (2003) Differential vascular and transcriptional responses to anti-vascular endothelial growth factor antibody in orthotopic human pancreatic cancer xenografts. Clin Cancer Res 9:4221–4226

Bruns CJ, Solorzano CC, Harbison MT et al (2000) Blockade of the epidermal growth factor receptor signalling by a novel tyrosine kinase inhibitor leads to apoptosis of endothelial cells and therapy of human pancreatic carcinoma. Cancer Res 60:2926–2935

Bruns CJ, Shrader M, Harbison MT et al (2002) Effect of the vascular endothelial growth factor receptor-2 antibody DC-101 plus gemcitabine on growth, metastasis, and angiogenesis of human pancreatic cancer growing orthotopically in nude mice. Int J Cancer 102:101–108

Buroker T, Kim PN, Groppe C et al (1979) 5-FU infusion with mitomycin C versus 5-FU infusion with methyl CCNU in the treatment of advanced upper gastrointestinal cancer. Cancer 44:1215–1221

Burris HA, Moore MJ, Andersen J et al (1997) Improvements in survival and clinical benefit with gemcitabine as first-line therapy for patients with advanced pancreas cancer: a randomised trial. J Clin Oncol 15:2403–2413

Carter SK (1975) The integration of chemotherapy into a combined modality approach for cancer treatment: VI. Pancreatic adenocarcinoma. Cancer Treat Rev 3:193–214

Cartwright TH, Cohn A, Varkey JA et al (2002) Phase II study of oral capecitabine in patients with advanced or metastatic pancreatic cancer. J Clin Oncol 20:160–164

Cascinu S, Labianca R, Catalano V et al (2003) Weekly gemcitabine and cisplatin chemotherapy: a well-tolerated but ineffective chemotherapeutic regimen in advanced pancreatic cancer patients. A report from the Italian Group for the Study of Digestive Tract Cancer (GESCAD). Ann Oncol 14:205–208

Casper ES, Green MR, Kelsen DP et al (1994) Phase II trial of gemcitabine (2′2-difluorodeoxycytidine) in patients with adenocarcinoma of the pancreas. Invest New Drugs 12: 29–34

Colucci G, Guiliani F, Gebbia V et al (2002) Gemcitabine alone or with cisplatin for the treatment of patients with locally advanced and/or metastatic pancreatic carcinoma: a prospective, randomised phase III study of the Gruppo Oncoliga del'Italia Meridionale. Cancer 94:902–910

Correale P, Messinese S, Marsili S et al (2003) A novel bi weekly pancreatic cancer treatment schedule with gemcitabine, 5-fluorouracil and folinic acid. Br J Cancer 89:239–242

Corrie P, Mayer A, Shaw J et al (2002) Phase II study to evaluate combining gemcitabine with flutamide in advanced pancreatic cancer patients. Br J Cancer 87:716–719

Cubilla AL, Fitzgerald PJ (1975) Morphological patterns of primary nonendocrine human pancreas carcinoma. Cancer Res 35:2234–2248

Cubilla AL, Fitzgerald PJ (1976) Morphological lesions associated with human primary invasive nonendocrine pancreas cancer. Cancer Res 36:2690–2698

Cunningham D, Chau I, Stocken D et al (2005). Phase III randomised comaprison of gemcitabine versus gemcitabine plus capecitabine in patients with advanced pancreatic cancer. Eur J Cancer Suppl 3:4(abstract 4)

El-Rayes BF, Zalupski MM, Shields AF et al (2003) Phase II study of gemcitabine, cisplatin and infusional fluorouracil in advanced pancreatic cancer. J Clin Oncol 21:2920–2925

Evans TRJ, Lofts FJ, Mansi JL et al (1996) A phase II study of continuous-infusion 5-fluorouracil with cisplatin and epirubicin in inoperable pancreatic cancer. Br J Cancer 73:1260–1264

Feliu J, Mel R, Borrega P et al (2003) Phase II study of a fixed dose-rate infusion of gemcitabine associated with uracil/tegafur in advanced carcinoma of the pancreas. Ann Oncol 13:1756–1762

Fjallskog MLH, Lejonklou MH, Oberg KE et al (2003) Expression of molecular targets for tyrosine kinase receptor antagonists in malignant endocrine pancreatic tumors. Clin Cancer Res 9:1469–1473

Ghandi V, Plunkett W (1990) Modulatory activity of 2′2′-difluorodeoxycytidine on the phosphorylation and cytotoxicity of arabinosyl nucleosides. Cancer Res 50: 3675–3680

Grindey GB, Hertel LW, Plunkett W (1990) Cytotoxicity and anti-tumour activity of 2′2′-difluorodeoxycytidine (Gemcitabine). Cancer Invest 8:313–318

Hausen R, Quebbman E, Ritch P et al (1988) Continous 5-fluorouracil infusion in carcinoma of the pancreas. Am J Med Sci 295:91–93

Heinemann V, Hertel L, Grindey GB (1988) Comparison of the cellular pharmacokinetics and toxicity of 2′2′-difluorodeoxycytidine and 1-b-D-arabinofuranasyl cytosine. Cancer Res 48:4024–4031

Herrmann R, Bodoky G, Ruhstaller T et al (2007) Gemcitabine plus capecitabine compared with gemcitabine alone in advanced pancreatic cancer: A randomized, multicenter, phase III trial of the Swiss Group for Clinical Cancer Research and the Central European Cooperative Oncology Group. J Clin Oncol 25:2212–2217

Hertel W, Boder GB, Kroin JS et al (1990) Evaluation of the anti-tumour activity of gemcitabine (2′2′-difluorodeoxycytidine). Cancer Res 50:4417–4422

Hess V, Salzberg M, Borner M et al (2003) Combining capecitabine and gemcitabine in patients with advanced pancreatic carcinoma: a phase I/II trial. J Clin Oncol 21:66–68

Hingorani SR, Petricoin EF, Maitra A et al (2003) Preinvasive and invasive ductal pancreatic cancer and its early detection in the mouse. Cancer Cell 4:437–449

Hingorani SR, Wang L, Multani AS et al (2005) Trp53[R172H] and Kras[G12D] cooperate to promote chromosomal instability and widely metastatic pancreatic ductal adenocarcinoma in mice. Cancer Cell 7:469–483

Hruban RH, Goggins M, Parsons J et al (2000a) Progression model for pancreatic cancer. Clin Cancer Res 6:2969–2972

Hruban RH, Wilentz RE, Kern SE (2000b) Genetic progression in the pancreatic ducts. Am J Pathol 156:1821–1825

Huang P, Chubb S, Hertel W et al (1991) Action of 2′2′-difluorodeoxycytidine on DNA synthesis. Cancer Res 51:6110–6117

Ianniello GP, Orditura M, Rossi A et al (2001) Gemcitabine plus epirubicin in advanced pancreatic cancer: a phase II multicenter trial. Oncol Rep 8:1111–1115

Itakura J, Ishiwata T, Shen B et al (2000) Concomitant overexpression of vascular endothelial growth factor and its receptors in pancreatic cancer. Int J Cancer 85:27–34

Kanat O, Eurensel T, Kurt E et al (2004) Treatment of metastatic pancreatic cancer with a combination of gemcitabine and 5-fluorouracil: a single center phase II study. Tumori 90: 192–195

Kern S, Hruban R, Hollingsworth MA et al (2001) A white paper: the product of a pancreas cancer think tank. Cancer Res 61:4923–4932

Kim TW, Kang HJ, Ahn JH et al (2002) Phase II study of gemcitabine, UFT and leucovorin in patients with advanced pancreatic cancer. Acta Oncol 41:689–694

Kindler HL, Friberg G, Singh DA et al (2005) Phase II trial of bevacizumab plus gemcitabine in patients with advanced pancreatic cancer. J Clin Oncol 23:8033–8040

Kindler HL, Niedzwiecki D, Hollis D et al (2007) A double-blind, placebo-controlled, randomized phase III trial of gemcitabine (G) plus bevacizumab (B) versus gemcitabine plus placebo (P) in patients (pts) with advanced pancreatic cancer (PC): a preliminary analysis of Cancer and Leukemia Group B (CALGB). J Clin Oncol 25:18s(abstact 4508)

Klimstra DS, Longnecker DS (1994) K-ras mutations in pancreatic ductal proliferative lesions. Am J Pathol 145:1547–1550

Kovach JS, Moertel CG, Schuft AJ et al (1974) A controlled study of combined 1, 3-bio(2-chloroethyl)-1-nitrosurea and 5-fluorouracil therapy for advanced gastric and pancreatic cancer. Cancer 33:563–567

Kozuch P, Grossbard ML, Barzdins A et al (2001) Irinotecan combined with gemcitabine, 5-fluorouracil, leucovorin, and cisplatin (G-FLIP) is an effective and non cross-resistant treatment for chemotherapy refractory metastatic pancreatic cancer. Oncologist 6:488–495

Kralidis E, Aebi S, Friess H et al (2003) Activity of raltitrexed and gemcitabine in advanced pancreatic cancer. Ann Oncol 14:574–579

Lee J, Park JO, Kim WS et al (2004) Phase II study of gemcitabine combination with uracil – tegafur in metastatic pancreatic cancer. Oncology 66:32–37

Li D, Xie K, Wolff R et al (2004) Pancreatic cancer. Lancet 363:1049–1057

Louvet C, Andre T, Hammel P et al (2001) Phase II trial of bimonthly leucovorin, 5-fluorouracil and gemcitabine for advanced pancreatic adenocarcinoma (FOLFUGEM). Ann Oncol 12:675–679

Louvet C, Andre T, Lledo G et al (2002) Gemcitabine combined with oxaliplatin in advanced pancreatic adenocarcinoma: final results of a GERCOR multicenter phase II study. J Clin Oncol 20:1512–1518

Louvet C, Labianca R, Hammel P et al (2005) Gemcitabine in combination with oxaliplatin compared with gemcitabine alone in locally advanced or metastatic pancreatic cancer: results of a GERCOR and GISCARD phase III trial. J Clin Oncol 23:3509–3516

Luo J, Guo P, Matsuda K et al (2001) Pancreatic cancer cell-derived vascular endothelial growth factor is biologically active in vitro and enhances tumorigenicity in vivo. Int J Cancer 92:361–369

Mallinson GN, Rake MO, Cocking JB et al (1980) Chemotherapy in pancreatic cancer: results of a controlled, prospective, randomised, multicentre trial. Br Med J 281:1589–1591

Marantz A, Jovtis S, Almira E et al (2001) Phase II study of gemcitabine, 5-fluorouracil, and leucovorin in patients with pancreatic cancer. Semin Oncol 28:44–49

Moertel CG (1976) Chemotherapy for gastrointestinal cancer. Clin Gastroenterol 5:777–793

Moore MJ, Goldstein D, Hamm J et al (2007) Erlotinib plus gemcitabine compared with gemcitabine alone in patients with advanced pancreatic cancer: a phase III trial of the National Cancer Institute of Canada Clinical Trials Group. J Clin Oncol 25:1960–1966

Murad AM, Guimaeres RC, Aragao BC et al (2003) Phase II trial of the use of gemcitabine and 5-fluorouracil in the treatment of advanced pancreatic and biliary tract cancer. Am J Clin Oncol 26:151–154

Neoptolemos JP, Stocken DD, Freiss H et al (2004) A randomized trial of chemoradiotherapy and chemotherapy after resection of pancreatic cancer. N Engl J Med 350:1200–1210

Neri B, Cini G, Doni L et al (2002) Weekly gemcitabine plus epirubicin as effective chemotherapy for advanced pancreatic cancer: a multicenter phase II study. Br J Cancer 87:497–501

Ng SSW, Tsao MS, Nicklee T et al (2002) Effects of the epidermal growth factor receptor inhibitor OSI-774, Tarceva, on downstream signalling pathways and apoptosis in human pancreatic adenocarcinoma. Mol Cancer Ther 1:777–783

Novarino A, Chiappino I, Bertelli GF et al (2004) Phase II study of cisplatin, gemcitabine and 5-fluorouracil in advanced pancreatic cancer. Ann Oncol 15:474–477

Oettle H, Richards D, Ramanathan R et al (2005) A phase III trial of pemetrexed plus gemcitabine versus gemcitabine in patients with unresectable or metastatic pancreatic cancer. Ann Oncol 16:1639–1645

Oster MW, Gray R, Panasci L et al (1986) Chemotherapy for advanced pancreatic cancer: A comparison of 5-fluorouracil, adriamycin and mitomycin C (FAM) with 5-fluorouracil, streptozotcin and mitomycin C (FSM). Cancer 57:29–33

Palmer KR, Kerr M, Knowles G et al (1994) Chemotherapy prolongs survival in inoperable pancreatic carcinoma. Br J Surg 81:882–885

Petty RD, Nicolson MC, Skaria S et al (2003) A phase II study of mitomycin-C, cisplatin and protracted infusional 5-fluorouracil in advanced pancreatic carcinoma: efficacy and low toxicity. Ann Oncol 14:1100–1105

Philip PA, Zalupski MM, Vaitkevicius VK et al (2001) Phase II study of gemcitabine and cisplatin in the treatment of patients with advanced pancreatic carcinoma. Cancer 92:569–577

Philip PA, Benedetti C, Fenoglio-Preiser M et al (2007) Phase III study of gemcitabine [G] plus cetuximab [C] versus gemcitabine in patients [pts] with locally advanced or metastatic pancreatic adenocarcinoma [PC]: SWOG S0205 study. J Clin Oncol 25:18s(absract 4509)

Rachamalla R, Malamud S, Grossbard ML et al (2004) Phase I dose-finding study of biweekly irinotecan in combination with fixed doses of 5-fluorouracil/leucovorin, gemcitabine and cisplatin (G-FLIP) in patients with advanced pancreatic cancer or other solid tumors. Anticancer Drugs 15:211–217

Reni M, Cordio S, Milandri C et al (2005) Gemcitabine versus cisplatin, epirubicin, fluorouracil, and gemcitabine in advanced pancreatic cancer: a randomised controlled multicentre phase III trial. Lancet Oncol 6:369–376

Rocha Lima CM, Savarese D, Bruckner H et al (2002) Irinotecan plus gemcitabine induces both radiographic and CA19-9 tumor marker responses in patients with previously untreated advanced pancreatic cancer. J Clin Oncol 20:1182–1191

Rocha Lima C, Green M, Rotche R et al (2004) Irinotecan plus gemcitabine results in no survival advantage compared with gemcitabine monotherapy in patients with locally advanced or metastatic pancreatic cancer despite increased tumor response rate. J Clin Oncol 18:3776–3783

Rothenberg ML, Moore MJ, Cripps MC et al (1996) A phase II trial of gemcitabine in patients with 5-FU-refractory pancreas cancer. Ann Oncol 7:347–535

Ryan DP, Kulke MH, Fuchs CS et al (2002) A phase II study of gemcitabine and docetaxel in patients with metastatic pancreatic carcinoma. Cancer 94:97–103

Sacks H, Berrier J, Reitman D et al (1987) Meta-analysis of randomised controlled trials. N Engl J Med 316:450–455

Schneider BP, Ganjoo KN, Seitz OE et al (2003) Phase II study of gemcitabine plus docetaxel in advanced pancreatic cancer: a Hoosier Oncology Group study. Oncology 65:218–223

Shepard LC, Levy DE, Berlin JD et al (2004) Phase II study of gemcitabine in combination with docetaxel in patients with advanced pancreatic carcinoma (E1298). A trial of the Eastern Cooperative Oncology Group. Oncology 66:303–309

Shi Q, Le X, Peng Z et al (2001) Constitutive Sp1 activity is essential for differential constitutive expression of vascular endothelial growth factor in human pancreatic adenocarcinoma. Cancer Res 61:4143–4154

Solorzano CC, Baker CH, Bruns CJ et al (2001) Inhibition of growth and metastasis of human pancreatic cancer growing in nude mice by PTK787/K222584, an inhibitor of the vascular endothelial growth factor receptor tyrosine kinase. Cancer Biother Radiopharm 16:359–370

Stathopoulos GP, Rigatos SK, Dimopoulos MA et al (2003) Treatment of pancreatic cancer with a combination of irinotecan (CPT-11) and gemcitabine: a multicenter phase II study by the Greek Cooperative Group for Pancreatic Cancer. Ann Oncol 14:388–394

Stathopoulos GP, Syrigos K, Polyzos A et al (2004) Front-line treatment of inoperable or metastatic pancreatic cancer with gemcitabine and capecitabine: an intergroup, multicenter, phase II study. Ann Oncol 15:224–229

Stocken DD, Buchler MW, Dervenis C et al (2005) Meta-analysis of randomized adjuvant therapy trials for pancreatic cancer. Br J Cancer 92:1372–1381

Sultana A, Tudor Smith C, Cunningham D et al (2007) Meta-Analyses of chemotherapy for locally advanced and metastatic pancreatic cancer. J Clin Oncol 25:2607–2615

Therasse P, Arbuck SG, Eisenhauer EA et al (2000) New guidelines to evaluate the response to treatment in solid tumors: European Organization for Research and Treatment of Cancer, National Cancer Institute of the United States, National Cancer Institute of Canada. J Natl Cancer Inst 92:205–216

Tobita K, Kijima H, Dowaki S et al (2003) Epidermal growth factor receptor expression in human pancreatic cancer: significance for liver metastasis. Int J Mol Med 11:305–309

Tomao S, Romiti A, Massidda B et al (2002) A phase II study of gemcitabine and tamoxifen in advanced pancreatic cancer. Anticancer Res 22:2361–2364

Tsuzuki Y, Mouta Carreira C, Bockborn M et al (2001) Pancreas microenvironment promotes VEGF expression and tumor growth: novel window models for pancreatic tumor angiogenesis and microcirculation. Lab Invest 81:1439–1451

Ueda S, Ogata S, Tsuda H et al (2004) The correlation between cytoplasmic overexpression of epidermal growth factor receptor and tumor aggressiveness: poor prognosis in patients with pancreatic ductal adenocarcinoma. Pancreas 29:E1–E8

van Cutsem E, Vervenne WL, Bennouna J et al (2009) Phase III trial of bevacizumab in combination with gemcitabine and erlotinib in patients with metastatic pancreatic cancer. J Clin Oncol 27:2231–2237

Vasey PA, Evans J (2002) Principles of chemotherapy and drug development. In: Price P, Sikora K (eds) Treatment of cancer. Arnold, London, pp 103–129

von Marschall Z, Cramer T, Hocker M et al (2000) De novo expression of vascular endothelial growth factor in human pancreatic cancer: evidence for an autocrine mitogenic loop. Gastroenterology 119:1358–1372

Wils J, Bleiberg H, Blijham G et al (1985) Phase II study of epirubicin in advanced adenocarcinoma of the pancreas. Eur J Cancer Clin Oncol 21:191–194

Wils J, Kok T, Wagener OJ et al (1993) Activity of cisplatin in adenocarcinoma of the pancreas. Eur J Cancer 29:203–204

Yeo CJ, Cameron JL, Lillemoe KD et al (2002) Pancreaticoduodenectomy with or without distal gastrectomy and extended retroperitoneal lymphadenectomy for peri-ampullary adenocarcinoma, part 2: Randomised controlled trial evaluating survival, morbidity, and mortality. Ann Surg 236:355–366

The Role of Interventional Endoscopy

Guido Costamagna, Pietro Familiari, Andrea Tringali, and Ivo Boškoski

Contents

G. Costamagna (✉), P. Familiari, A. Tringali, and I. Boškoski
Digestive Endoscopy Unit, Gemelli University Hospital,
Università Cattolica del Sacro Cuore, Largo Gemelli 8,
00167 Rome, Italy

Abstract

> Interventional endoscopy has a key role in the palliation of pancreatic cancer.

> Biliary obstruction leading to jaundice and hitching can be safely resolved by endoscopic plastic or metal stenting. Metal stents have a longer patency than plastic, and are cost-effective in patients with 4-6 months life expectancy. Endoscopic palliation of jaundice improves the quality of life, is mini-invasive, safe and effective and is preferred to surgery or interventional radiology. The main problem of biliary stents is cholangitis recurrence due to stent clogging: the development of new drug-eluting stent maybe will improve stent patency in the near future.

> Also pain in pancreatic cancer can be reduced by endoscopic pancreatic stenting or EUS-guided celiac plexus block/neurolysis in selected cases.

> A late complication of pancreatic cancer is the developmant of a duodenal stricture and Gastric Outlet Obstruction Symptoms. This complication, which usually occurs in end-stage and fragile patients, can be resolved by endoscopic insertion of a duodenal metal stents. Duodenal stenting is preferred to surgery due to its lower morbidity and mortality, shorter hospitalization and earlier symptoms relief.

> ERCP and EUS are also a tool for intraluminal brachytherapy and delivery of cytotoxic agents directly into the pancreatic tumor. This latest possibility can represent a future approach to pancreatic and other tumors.

A. Laghi (ed.), *New Concepts in Diagnosis and Therapy of Pancreatic Adenocarcinoma*,
Medical Radiology, DOI: 10.1007/174_2010_60, © Springer-Verlag Berlin Heidelberg 2011

1 Introduction

Gastrointestinal endoscopy, especially Endoscopic Retrograde Cholangio-Pancreatography (ERCP) and Endoscopic Ultrasound (EUS), plays an important role in the management of patients affected by pancreatic adenocarcinoma.

Most endoscopic therapies are centered on the palliation of jaundice and other complications of advanced pancreatic disease (including pain and gastric outlet obstruction).

Recently, novel EUS-guided endoscopic therapeutic procedures have been developed, which include interstitial brachytherapy and injection of other therapeutic agents into the tumor (Pausawasdi & Scheiman 2007).

The improvement of existing accessories for ERCP and techniques, and the development of novel procedures, may significantly expand the role of endoscopy in the management of pancreatic carcinoma.

2 Preoperative Biliary Drainage

The majority of patients with pancreatic cancer presents at the time of the diagnosis with clinical signs of biliary obstruction, that is, jaundice, itching, and cholangitis (Warshaw & Fernandez-del 1992). This is especially true for tumors located in the pancreatic head, because of the intrapancreatic location of the lower third of the common bile duct.

The value of biliary drainage before pancreatoduodenectomy is controversial. In experimental models, preoperative biliary drainage is usually associated with important benefits, including improved liver function and nutritional status, reduction of systemic endotoxemia and improved immune response, and reduction of perioperative mortality.

On the contrary, human studies showed conflicting results, and preoperative biliary drainage (either endoscopic or percutaneous-transhepatic) is no longer routinely recommended (Wang et al. 2008).

Proponents of preoperative biliary drainage might argue that it facilitates referral to high-volume tertiary centers. Biliary drainage does not significantly affect the surgical operation, in terms of fluid and transfusion requirements, or surgery duration (Wang et al. 2008; Coates et al. 2009), but it may increase the post-operative morbidity rate (Mezhir et al. 2009).

Cultures of bile collected during pancreatoduodenectomy are positive in the majority of patients who undergo preoperative biliary drainage (up to 98%), and in a minority of patients who do not undergo biliary drainage (up to 7%). Consequently, the incidence of infectious complications including wound infections and intra-abdominal abscess has been found to be increased up to two fold after preoperative biliary drainage (Mezhir et al. 2009; Herzog et al. 2009; Lermite et al. 2008).

Because of the lack of demonstrated benefits, biliary drainage before pancreatoduodenenctomy should not be routinely performed. However, it might still be indicated in special clinical situations, such as acute cholangitis, severe jaundice and itching, and impaired hepatic function due to prolonged biliary obstruction.

Current therapies for patients with locally advanced pancreatic neoplasm might be modified in future (i.e., neoadjuvant chemo-radiotherapy). Consequently, the role of preoperative endoscopic biliary drainage may be re-evaluated in the future.

When a preoperative drainage is strictly indicated, plastic stents are preferred to Self Expanding Metal Stents (SEMS), because of lower costs, and because surgery is usually performed within the stent-patency time. In patients who will receive neoadjuvant therapies, the placement of covered SEMS (regardless of tumor resectability), might be appropriated, because a prolonged stent patency can ensure the continuity of the treatment. In any case, surgical resection is possible and safe also when a (short) transpapillary SEMS has been placed. Conversely, surgical resection and hepatico-jejunostomy might be very difficult or precluded if the proximal end of the SEMS raises the main biliary confluence or reaches the intrahepatic ducts.

3 Palliation of Biliary Obstruction

In inoperable patients, biliary drainage reduces dyspeptic symptoms, and improves anorexia and indigestion (Ballinger et al. 1994). Relief of jaundice is associated with a prolonged survival and improved quality of life in patients with inoperable pancreatic cancer (Sarr & Cameron 1982); furthermore, jaundice and itching resolution provides a much needed psychological boost to the patient and family members.

Palliation of jaundice and biliary drainage can be obtained by surgery or by biliary stent insertion (either percutaneous or endoscopic). In expert hands, surgery, endoscopy and interventional radiology are equally effective for the palliation of symptoms secondary to biliary obstruction. However, specific considerations should be done when choosing a technique or another, and include complication rate, patient's expected survival, co-morbidities, local availability and patients' preferences.

3.1 Patient Selection: Surgery, Endoscopy, or Radiology?

Before considering either an operative or conservative management of jaundice, some aspects should first be considered.

The possibility of a radical surgery should be rationally excluded. Surgery, including pancreatic resection, is no longer prohibited in elderly patients. Furthermore, in some patients, the final decision on operability might be assessed only after neoadjuvant therapies. Secondly, jaundice must be caused by a bile duct obstruction. Usually, pancreatic head cancer directly invades and constricts the common bile duct, causing obstruction to the bile flow and jaundice. However, extensive liver metastases may cause both a functional liver failure and obstruction of the intrahepatic bile ducts. These latter conditions might not benefit from any kind of endoscopic or surgical drainage or bypass, and should be promptly identified when planning the treatment. Increased serum bilirubin, alkaline phosphatase and gamma-glutamyl transferase levels do not automatically indicate the need for a biliary decompression. On the contrary, non-invasive imaging studies, especially trans-abdominal ultrasonography, are usually necessary and permit to easily and quickly separate patients who may benefit from a biliary drainage from those who may not.

Surgical bypass (hepatico-jejunostomy, choledocho-jejunostomy or cholecysto-jejunostomy) was the preferred approach for jaundice palliation until non-operative techniques became popular (Sarr & Cameron 1982). Despite the efficacy, the mortality rate after operative palliation of biliary obstruction is quite elevated (up to 20%), even in referral centers (Sarr & Cameron 1982; Watanapa & Williamson 1992).

Some randomized controlled trials have compared surgical bypass and endoscopic stenting for the management of malignant obstructive jaundice (Smith et al. 1994; Shepherd et al. 1988; Andersen et al. 1989). Endoscopic stenting is effective as surgical bypass for the relief of clinical signs of biliary obstruction, but it is associated with a lower thirty-day mortality rate and early treatment-related complication rate. On the contrary, many patients receiving endoscopic palliation may suffer from recurrent attacks of cholangitis or recurrence of jaundice due to stent occlusion, requiring endoscopic re-treatment. However, most of the leading papers comparing surgical and endoscopic management of malignant biliary obstruction, were published 15–20 years ago, before the development of self-expanding metal stents (SEMS). Therefore, current endoscopic palliation of malignant biliary obstruction might be substantially better than surgery, providing improved quality of life and effectiveness.

Percutaneous transhepatic biliary drainage (PTBD) became popular in the past for the management of malignant biliary strictures. Bile duct decompression, by means of either internal, internal-external and external biliary drainage, is a direct competitor of endoscopy in the field of non-operative management of malignant biliary strictures. In expert hands, the percutaneous transhepatic route is as effective as the endoscopic transoral one. However, severe complications are more frequent after PTBD (Speer et al. 1987). Where available, ERCP is considered as the procedure of choice for the management of inoperable distal common bile duct strictures. On the contrary, when the papilla of Vater is not accessible because of a surgically-altered gastrointestinal anatomy (i.e., gastric resection, Roux-en-Y gastric bypass, total gastrectomy), or extended duodenal strictures, the percutaneous route may be easier and safer than the transoral route.

Some patients may still benefit from a conventional surgical palliation of biliary obstruction, for example the patients found inoperable during a surgical exploration. In developing countries, surgery is still widely used for the palliation of biliary strictures, and might be an effective option due to the relatively low initial cost of surgery and the lack of endoscopic facilities (Artifon et al. 2006; Sunpaweravong et al. 2005).

3.2 Types of Biliary Stents

Two different types of stents are available for the endoscopic treatment of malignant biliary strictures: plastic stents and SEMS.

Plastic stents were the first to be made, and they are still the most used. A variety of plastic stents are currently available: they differ in size, shape and polymer composition.

Plastic stents used for biliary indications are available in different lengths (5–18 cm), diameters (3F to 11.5F) and shapes. Most straight stents are slightly bent, to conform to the anatomy of the bile ducts. They may have side holes to improve the flow of bile, and are provided with side flaps at each end for anchoring and to reduce the chances of stent migration.

Three different polymers are used for biliary and pancreatic stents. They include Polyethylene, Teflon and Polyurethane. The most used plastic stents are made in polyethylene. In the early 1980s, homemade stents were pretty popular. Polyethylene was chosen because it is relatively cheap, and sufficiently soft and malleable to be easily shaped, molded and cut according to clinical need.

The Soehendra-Tannenbaum stents are made of Teflon which has a lower coefficient of friction compared to polyethylene. Sohendra-Tannenbaum stents have no side holes, and four anchoring flaps at each end are cut into the thickness of the stent wall. Theoretically this polymer and shape should help prevent sludge accumulation in the stent lumen, and thus prolong patency, but clinical trials have not demonstrated such an advantage in comparison to the standard stents (Raijman 2003; Catalano et al. 2002; Schilling et al. 2003; van Berkel et al. 1998).

Other materials have also been used. However, clinical studies have not been able to show any definite advantage in terms of longer patency of Teflon, polyurethane, polyamidoamine cross-linked to polyurethane chains, hydromer-coated polyurethane or perfluoro-aloxy combined with polyamide elastomer stents when compared to standard polyethylene stents (Catalano et al. 2002; Schilling et al. 2003; van Berkel et al. 1998; Cetta et al. 1999; Costamagna et al. 2000; Tringali et al. 2003; Landoni et al. 2000).

The diameter of biliary stents varies between 7F and 11.5F. Having larger stents means longer patency (Pedersen 1993); for this reason most endoscopists prefer the placement of 10F or 11.5F stents for the palliation of malignant distal biliary obstructions.

Unfortunately, sooner or later, plastic stents will occlude leading to recurrent signs of biliary obstruction. The average plastic stent effective duration is 3 months. SEMS were developed to overcome the problem of early clogging of plastic stents and improve biliary drainage in patients with malignant biliary obstruction. SEMS that are inserted into the bile duct in a constrained state may expand after deployment to a diameter of up to 30F.

The vast majority of SEMS are made of Nitinol. Nitinol SEMS have a low magnetic susceptibility and are completely Magnetic Resonance Imaging (MRI) compatible. Nitinol has at least two very important properties: thermal shape-memory effect and superelasticity. Thermal shape-memory enables Nitinol SEMS to be constrained into a small calibre introducer. Upon deployment in situ, SEMS are restored to their original shape and diameter.

The overall proper characteristics of a SEMS also depend on stent mesh design. Many SEMS are made with a woven braided mesh. A braided mesh combines good flexibility and radial force with resistance to longitudinal traction. Usually the thinner the mesh-wire, the more flexible the stent. The current available SEMS made with a braided mesh varies because of the mesh-wire size, material and design of the stent edges. Theoretically, a soft and flexible end could reduce the epithelial reactivity and thus tissue overgrowth. Flared and barbed ends could prevent stent migration but may induce tissue overgrowth (Raijman 2003).

Biliary SEMS can also be made by a single Nitinol wire, laser cut (from a single Nitinol tube) with a spiral, "zig-zag" design. The special design of the stent mesh offers superior flexibility and a good radial force. Most stents for cardiac use have this special design. SEMS with this mesh design usually do not shorten after deployment, leading to a more precise stent positioning across the stricture.

SEMS are currently available in two versions – uncovered or covered with a plastic coating. "Covered" SEMS are designed to reduce tumor ingrowth into the stent mesh and thus prolong patency.

SEMS have shown to have a longer patency than plastic stents (Kaassis et al. 2003; Schmassmann et al. 1996; Yeoh et al. 1999), minimizing the need for periodic stent exchange. However, the high cost of these devices still limits their use in routine practice.

3.3 Plastic or Metal Stents for the Palliation of Malignant Biliary Strictures?

Plastic and metal stents are equally efficient for the prompt resolution of clinical signs of biliary obstruction (jaundice and itching), and for the palliation of malignant biliary obstruction during the first three months after placement (Davids et al. 1992). However, the overall patency of biliary SEMS is significantly longer than the patency of plastic biliary stents. A prolonged stent patency limits the need for periodical stent exchange, and thus improves the quality of palliation and the quality-of-life of patients. However, the cost of plastic and metal stents are significantly different. The cost analysis of health care is a matter of debate worldwide, and the cost-effectiveness of plastic vs. metal stents, has been studied.

SEMS compared to plastic stents showed longer patency, reduced hospitalization and use of antibiotics, number of ERCPs and transabdominal US, leading to a lower overall cost in selected patients (Moss et al. 2007) (Fig. 1).

Because of the 3 months expected patency of plastic stents, SEMS should be theoretically considered only for those patients with a longer life-expectancy. Patients with large tumors (>2.5–3 cm), severe comorbidities or with liver metastases are likely to have a bad prognosis and short survival duration (Kaassis et al. 2003; Moss et al. 2007; Moss et al. 2006)

Comparative studies demonstrated that SEMS placement is an appropriate and cost-effective palliative procedure for patients without metastases and at least a 4 to 6 months life-expectancy at initial stent placement (Kaassis et al. 2003; Moss et al. 2007; Moss et al. 2006).

Despite the cost-effectiveness studies, biliary SEMS may be the treatment of choice also in few patients with a short expected survival. This is the case of patients with synchronous duodenal and biliary strictures, or with a difficult access to the papilla of Vater and bile ducts (i.e., previous gastric resection), to eventually avoid repeated, difficult, endoscopic procedures. Furthermore, SEMS may be indicated whenever the patients have early clogging of plastic stents, because

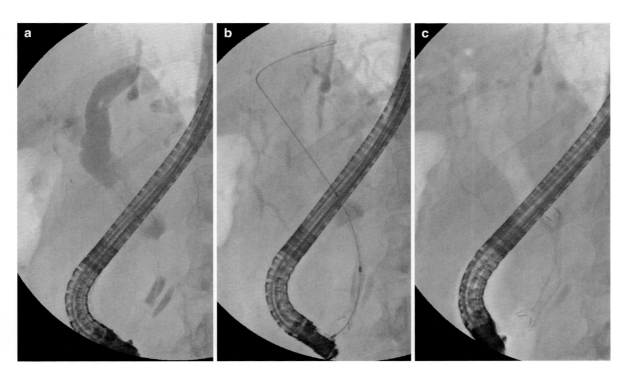

Fig. 1 (**a**) ERCP shows a distal common bile duct stricture, associated with a stricture of the pancreatic duct ("double duct" sign). (**b**) Insertion of a guidewire into the common bile duct, with the proximal end into the left hepatic duct. (**c**) Deployment of a Nitinol, biliary Self Expanding Metal Stent (NITI-S D-Type, Taewoong Medical Co., Korea)

of biliary sludge, pus and clots: the large SEMS diameter allows the passage of large amount of sludge and clots, and thus reduces the risk of early re-clogging.

In developing countries (but also in low-volume hospitals in industrialized countries), SEMS may still have prohibitive costs, and the choice may ineluctably fall on the plastic stents, despite the expected survival of patients and the cost-effectiveness studies (Yoon et al. 2009).

3.4 Clinical Outcomes

Although the endoscopic drainage of obstructed bile ducts is now a well-established procedure, its technical feasibility and clinical effectiveness may vary between the different centers. Local facilities and endoscopic skills can be partially responsible for this variability. Furthermore, patient selection might impair significantly the bile duct cannulation rate and the clinical efficacy. In expert hands, plastic stent placement is feasible in about 80–95% of cases with a clinical success rate (decline in total bilirubin levels and cholestasis) of 90% (Fig. 2).

Selective biliary cannulation still remains the most challenging part of ERCP. In the majority of cases, technical failures of biliary drainage are due to a difficult cannulation. Duodenal diverticula, duodenal strictures, previous gastric surgery, and neoplastic spreading with distortion of the papillary area contribute to make the cannulation more difficult.

Patency duration of endoprosthesis is usually one of the indicators of clinical effectiveness of endoscopic biliary drainage. However, calculation of the median functioning time of a plastic or metal stent is not meaningful as the majority of the patients die with an indwelling and functioning endoprosthesis. Thirty-day mortality after endoscopic palliation of malignant jaundice is very high (up to 10%); the median survival of patients after endoscopic palliation is about 80–150 days (Smith et al. 1994; Andersen et al. 1989). Nevertheless, when the patients survive enough to have experience of stent clogging, a recurrent attack of jaundice or cholangitis usually occurs after a median of 3–4 months after stent placement. Stent occlusion can be found in about 30% of cases after 3 months, and definitely in more than 45% of patients 6 months after ERCP. When a plastic stent becomes occluded it can be easily exchanged. However, the patency duration of the second and third stent significantly and progressively decreases (Ballinger et al. 1994; Smith et al. 1994; Shepherd et al. 1988; Andersen et al. 1989; Speer et al. 1987; Davids et al. 1992; Yoon et al. 2009; Matsuda et al. 1991; Abraham et al. 2002; Luman et al. 1997).

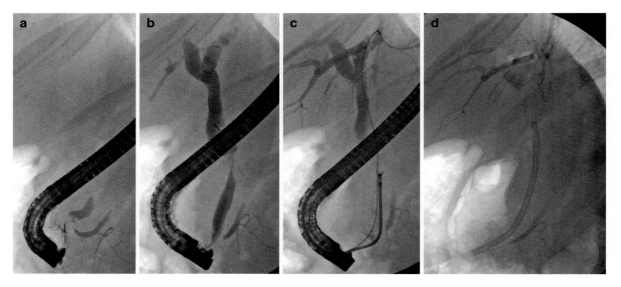

Fig. 2 Endoscopic Retrograde Cholangiopanceratography and drainage of the bile ducts in a patients with pancreatic cancer. (**a**, **b**) "double duct sign". ERCP shows two strictures on the bile duct and on the pancreatic duct. (**c**) X-ray guided forceps biopsy of the biliary stricture. (**d**) A plastic stent has been inserted into the common bile duct

SEMS have been shown to be superior to plastic stents with respect to patency and are being used more and more. The larger diameters are thought to contribute to the longer patency observed with SEMSs as compared to that of plastic stents (Kaassis et al. 2003; Schmassmann et al. 1996; Moss et al. 2007; Huibregtse 1993; Perdue et al. 2008; Soderlund & Linder 2006).

In expert hands, SEMS placement is feasible and successful in more than 90–95% of cases. With the currently available SEMS, complete stent expansion is likely to be obtained in all the patients, and again, the major technical limit to SEMS deployment, is failed deep cannulation of the common bile duct.

Because of the short survival of patients with pancreatic cancer, SEMS occlusion is a relatively rare event. The majority of the patients die with a patent stent (up to 85% of cases). Overall, median SEMS patency interval is 7 months, and does not significantly differ between covered and uncovered SEMS. Similarly, cumulative SEMS patency at 3-, 6-, and 12-months after deployment, and SEMS occlusion rate (between 10% and 38%) in most series do not significantly differ when comparing covered and uncovered SEMS (Kaassis et al. 2003; Davids et al. 1992; Yoon et al. 2009; Huibregtse 1993; Chen et al. 2006; Ferlitsch et al. 2001; Fumex et al. 2006; Isayama et al. 2004; Kahaleh et al. 2005; Katsinelos et al. 2008; Leung & Rahim 2006; Nakai et al. 2005; Park et al. 2006; Weber et al. 2009; Yang et al. 2009; Yoon et al. 2006; Ornellas et al. 2009; Kim et al. 2002) (Table 1).

3.5 Complication of Biliary Stenting and Management of Malfunctioning Stents

Complications of stent placement include ERCP-related complications and some specific complications related to stent insertion. Most common adverse events after ERCP are bleeding after sphincterotomy (1–2% of cases), acute pancreatitis (1–7% of cases), acute cholecystitis (0.2–0.5%) and duodenal perforation (0.3–0.6%) (Freeman 2002).

The commonest specific stent-related complications are recurrent cholangitis (clinical signs of stent occlusion or dysfunction) (Dowidar et al. 1991), stent migration, duodenal perforation (Lo et al. 2008; Storkson et al. 2000), and more rarely, pancreatitis and

cholecystitis. Any stent malfunctioning is usually clinically significant, and will ineluctably lead to recurrent signs of biliary obstruction, including jaundice and cholangitis. A prompt intervention is always necessary in case of cholangitis to resolve symptoms and avoid more severe complications.

Sooner or later, all biliary endoprosthesis, plastic or SEMS, will occlude. Bile is normally sterile in the bile ducts, but after sphincterotomy or stent placement a variety of bacteria colonizes the biliary system. Bacteria adhere to the inner surface of the stents and create a biofilm that represents the primary event in stent clogging. Bacterial enzymes promote bilirubin deconjugation and precipitation of biliary salts and calcium bilirubinate, forming biliary sludge and stones (van Berkel et al. 2005). Microscopic irregularities on the inner surface of plastic stents have been advocated as being one of the causes of bacterial adhesion and biofilm creation. Ultra-smooth polymers, including Teflon or Polyurethane, or bactericidal agents, bile salts or antibiotics, have been used to prevent or delay stent clogging, but they were eventually proved inefficacious (Raijman 2003).

The risk of occlusion of standard polyethylene stents increases significantly after 3 months. A routine three-monthly stent exchange may theoretically reduce the incidence of cholangitis due to stent clogging. However, because of the usually short survival of patients with advanced pancreatic cancer, routine plastic stent exchange is no longer recommended.

Plastic stents may also malfunction for other reasons. They may impact into the bile duct wall, leading to poor bile drainage, especially in case of the C-curved bile ducts or when inappropriately long stents have been placed (Raijman 2003).

The second most common complication, is stent migration, that may occur in about 5–6% of patients with a malignant stricture (Johanson et al. 1992; Arhan et al. 2009). Migration, both proximal or distal, is symptomatic in the vast majority of cases. Complications associated with stent migration have also been reported and include penetration, intestinal perforation, and small bowel obstruction (Lo et al. 2008; Storkson et al. 2000).

The management of malfunctioning or occluded stent is relatively simple. When a biliary plastic stent occludes or malfunctions it can usually be easily removed and replaced with a new one or with a SEMS. Usually, plastic stent replacement does not require special skills.

Table 1 Reported results of uncovered and covered Self Expandable Metal Stents for Jaundice palliation in pancreatic cancer

Author, year	No. of patients	SEMS type	Median survival (days)	SEMS patency (days)	SEMS occlusion/malfunctioning					% patency, 3-months	% patency, 6-months	% patency, 12-months
					SEMS occlusion n (%)	Ingrowth (%)	Overgrowth (%)	Sludge (%)				
Ornellas, 2009 (Ornellas et al. 2009)	104	Covered	129	n/a	19 (18.3)	–	26.3	73.7	94	84	58
Yang, 2009 (Yang et al. 2009)	60	Uncovered	148	124	17 (28, 3)	64.7	11.8	23.5	89	68	39
	41	Uncovered	160	153	11 (26.8)	72.2	9.1	18.2	91	79	26
Katsinelos, 2008 (Katsinelos et al. 2008)	44	Uncovered	347	328	11 (25)	81.8	18.2	–	n/a	n/a	n/a
	45	Uncovered	307	289	14 (31.1)	78.6	14.3	7.14	n/a	n/a	n/a
Fumex, 2006 (Fumex et al. 2006)	61	Covered	167	142	9/54 (16.6)	–	55.5	33.3	n/a	n/a	n/a
Park, 2006 (Park et al. 2006)	98	Covered	209	149	21 (21.4)	–	4.8	95.2	72	56	47
	108	Uncovered	207	143	20 (18.5)	85	–	15	77	54	37
Yoon, 2006 (Yoon et al. 2006)	36	Covered	392	242	9 (25%)	–	55.5	22.2	83	78	54
	41	Uncovered	308	202	15 (36.6)	33.3	53.3	6.6	83	66	36
Nakai, 2005 (Nakai et al. 2005)	69	Covered	201	139	7 (10.1%)	–	14.3	85.7	94	88	83
Isayama, 2004 (Isayama et al. 2004)	57	Covered	255	255	8 (14)	–	50	25	100	91	74
	55	Uncovered	237	193	21 (38)	76.2	9.5	9.5	81	68	55
Shah, 2003 (Shah et al. 2003)	68	Uncovered	n/a	154	13 (19.1)	92.3%	15.4%	23.1	n/a	n/a	n/a
	64	Uncovered	n/a	152	8 (12.6)	100%	–	62.5	n/a	n/a	n/a
Kim, 2002 (Kim et al. 2002)	68	Uncovered	n/a	231	28 (41)	82.1%	14.3%	7.1	83	56	n/a
Ferlitsch, 2001 (Ferlitsch et al. 2001)	126	Uncovered	173	477	28 (22.2)	88%	12%	–	97%	92%	34%

When the plastic stents is still visible beyond the papilla of Vater, the stent may be grasped with a foreign body forceps or a snare, and removed through the accessory channel of the endoscope or by removing the endoscope from the patient's mouth. Stent removal through the endoscope's accessory channel is feasible and very easy for small calibre stents (7F–8.5F), but can be very tricky or impossible in the case of large bore stents (10F–11.5F).

When the stent has migrated into the CBD, stent removal may be more difficult. Many endoscopists prefer to use a foreign body forceps, a Dormia basket, or a snare, that can be opened inside the bile duct to grasp the migrated stent (Chaurasia et al. 1999). Others might prefer the Soehendra Stent Retriever, a special accessory developed for the "over-the-wire" stent exchange (Soehendra et al. 1990), that consists of a flexible metal catheter with a threaded tip that is screwed into the stent to be removed.

More rarely, plastic stent placement may directly cause acute pancreatitis and this complication is more likely to occur in patients who did not receive a prior biliary sphincterotomy. Acute pancreatitis may be caused by the occlusion of the intra-ampullary part of the pancreatic duct by the stent decubitus. However, this complication is usually mild and requires conservative treatment only (Simmons et al. 2008). Obviously, acute pancreatitis may complicate the placement of SEMS (van Steenbergen et al. 1992), and the need for a biliary sphincterotomy before biliary stent placement should be carefully considered.

As the plastic counterpart, SEMS may become occluded over time, or may migrate. In contrast with plastic stents, management of malfunctioning SEMS is usually more difficult and technically demanding. The majority of the available SEMS have not been designed to be removed.

Mechanisms of occlusion of covered and uncovered SEMS may be different (Bueno et al. 2003; Menon & Barkun 1999; Rogart et al. 2008; Tham et al. 1998). Ingrowth is the main cause of occlusion of uncovered SEMS. With time, the neoplasm may grow within the meshes of the SEMS, until the latter becomes almost completely occluded. The placement of a new SEMS or of a plastic stent inside the occluded one is usually considered the best approach for the management of occluded SEMS. Because of the larger diameter, the placement of a new SEMS is recommended when the biliary obstruction of contaminated bile ducts has been complicated by sludge and stone formation or by suppurative cholangitis, because in such situations a plastic stent can quickly become occluded.

Covered SEMS become occluded because of sludge and debris or neoplastic overgrowth (Fumex et al. 2006; Yoon et al. 2006). Bacterial colonization of the inner surface of the SEMS and bio-film creation (similarly to plastic stents) are probably the primary cause of covered SEMS occlusion due to sludge and stones. Duodeno-biliary reflux contributes and accelerates covered SEMS occlusion. Sludge and stones may be extracted by using balloons or Dormia baskets. Although the plastic covering of covered SEMS has been designed to prevent neoplastic ingrowth, most covered SEMS have uncovered proximal and distal ends, in order to prevent migration. Over time, the tumor may grow between the meshes of these uncovered ends (ingrowth) or above the covered SEMS (overgrowth) contributing to its malfunction (Fumex et al. 2006; Yoon et al. 2006). Again, the placement of a new plastic stent or a SEMS inside an occluded covered SEMS is probably the most cost-effective treatment (Bueno et al. 2003; Menon & Barkun 1999; Rogart et al. 2008; Tham et al. 1998).

SEMS migration accounts for 4% of SEMS complications (Ferlitsch et al. 2001; Fumex et al. 2006; Isayama et al. 2004; Kahaleh et al. 2005; Katsinelos et al. 2008; Nakai et al. 2005; Park et al. 2006; Yang et al. 2009; Yoon et al. 2006; Shah et al. 2003; Ho et al. 2010). Covered SEMS are likely to migrate more often than the uncovered ones, and in some cases they may impact into the duodenal wall (Fumex et al. 2006; Isayama et al. 2004; Kahaleh et al. 2005; Park et al. 2006; Yoon et al. 2006; Ho et al. 2010). SEMS impaction into the duodenal wall may lead to recurrent biliary obstruction, or more severe complications, including perforation or bleeding. Migrated SEMS or those that impact into the duodenal wall should be removed and exchanged with a new SEMS (Familiari et al. 2005) or trimmed by using Argon Plasma Coagulation (Christiaens et al. 2008).

Less frequently, SEMS may impact into the medial bile duct wall. SEMS impaction may cause biliary obstruction and cholangitis. This complication might be related to the high axial force of some SEMS (Isayama et al. 2009). Theoretically, those SEMS with a lower axial force should be preferred in case of distorted and curved bile ducts, where the risk of impaction is higher. However, the current published data do not support this hypothesis (Yang et al. 2009).

SEMS placement may induce acute cholecystitis. Incidence of acute cholecystitis after SEMS placement varies between 1% and 10%, in the published series (Fumex et al. 2006; Park et al. 2006; Yoon et al. 2006; Ho et al. 2010; Isayama et al. 2006). Acute cholecystitis may be caused by the occlusion of the cystic duct by SEMS. Some clinical trials showed that acute cholecystitis occurs more frequently in patients with a covered SEMS (Fumex et al. 2006; Park et al. 2006; Ho et al. 2010). Occurring in frail neoplastic patients, acute cholecystitis may become a life threatening complication. Its management includes percutaneous gallbladder drainage, surgery or, in very selected cases, endoscopic transpapillary gallbladder drainage (Mutignani et al. 2009).

When treating malignant biliary strictures, it is probably safer not to cover the cystic duct insertion with the SEMS. If this is inevitable because of stricture location and extension, placement of an uncovered SEMS is preferable.

Overall, the current stent- or SEMS- related mortality is very low. Mortality after stent placement, is more likely to be related to the well known ERCP complications than to a direct effect of the stenting.

4 Endoscopic Treatment of Pancreatic Pain

4.1 Obstructive Type Pancreatic Pain: The Chance for ERCP

The so called "obstructive type" pancreatic pain in pancreatic cancer is related to ductal hypertension, is typically related to meal, and does not improve with pancreatic enzymes. Nearly all the patients with pancreatic adenocarcinoma have a stricture of the main pancreatic duct (MPD) which is symptomatic in only 15% of the cases (Costamagna et al. 1999). This small group of patients can benefit from MPD drainage by plastic stents. Crossing of a neoplastic MPD stricture may be difficult and not always possible due to angulation and/or the presence of necrosis. The technique of endoscopic pancreatic stenting does not substantially

differ from that applied on the biliary tree. Endoscopic pancreatic sphincterotomy is seldom strictly necessary to ease access to the MPD. Systematical mechanical dilation with catheters of increasing diameter is suggested before pancreatic stent insertion because the hardness of the stricture is unpredictable. When possible, placement of ten French plastic stents is preferred. Pancreatic stenting may be obtained in more than 80% of these selected patients, with low morbidity (less than 10%) and no procedure-related mortality. About 60% of patients treated because of "obstructive pain" become symptom-free, and another 20–25% significantly reduce the amount of analgesic drugs required (Costamagna et al. 1999; Tham et al. 2000) (Fig. 3).

4.2 Celiac Block/Neurolysis: The Chance for EUS

Pancreatic pain is predominantly transmitted through the celiac plexus and the splanchnic nerve. The most common pancreatic cancer pain is the so called "non obstructive" type: chronic, continuous, dull pain, unrelated to meals, located in the upper abdominal quadrants and often radiating to the back. This kind of pain can be usually managed by NSAIDs and opiates.

Uncontrolled "non obstructive" pain can be treated by celiac plexus block or neurolysis. Anesthetics and/or corticosteroids are used for temporary plexus block, while absolute ethanol permanently destroys the plexus (neurolysis). Celiac plexus block is preferred in pain due to chronic pancreatitis, while neurolysis is generally used in patients with pancreatic cancer.

Celiac plexus *neurolysis* relieves pain, avoiding all the side effects of opioids and can be done surgically, percutaneously under CT guidance, or by endoscopic ultrasonography (EUS). EUS-guided neurolysis is effective and has a lower risk of serious complications (aortal rupture or paraplegia) than the surgical or percutaneous approaches (Gunaratnam et al. 2001).

Anatomically, the celiac plexus is composed of two ganglia, usually located anterior and lateral to the aorta at the level of the celiac trunk. With a curvilinear array echoendoscope, this region can be easily visualized from the lesser gastric curvature, by following the aorta to the origin of the main celiac artery. It also possible to directly visualize the celiac ganglia which appear as

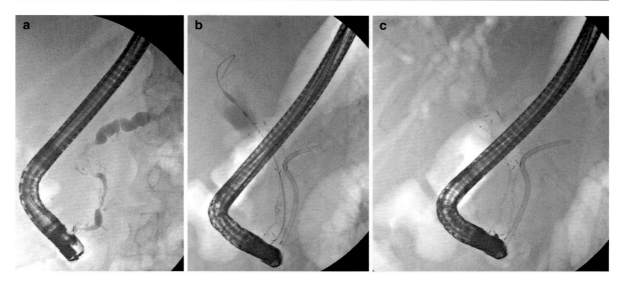

Fig. 3 Endoscopic management of obstructive-type pancreatic pain. (**a**) ERCP shows a long malignant stricture of the pancreatic duct at the level of the pancreatic head. Dilation of the main pancreatic duct above the stricture. The patient reports pancreatic-type pain, usually post-prandial. (**b**) Placement of a plastic stent in the pancreatic duct. Please, note the complete outflow of contrast medium from the pancreatic duct and the appearance of air in the duct. (**c**) Deployment of a Nitinol Self Expanding Metal Stent (NITI-S D-Type, Taewoong Medical Co., Korea) in the common bile duct for the management of a symptomatic biliary stricture. Note the massive aerobilia at the end of the procedure

one to five elongated hypoechoic structures (Levy et al. 2006). EUS-guided block/neurolysis was first described in 1996 (Wiersema & Wiersema 1996); the procedure can be done in a short time (10 min) and under conscious sedation. The procedure is usually performed with a 19-gauge needle or a dedicated 20-gauge needle with multiple side holes. The injection is performed at the base (central) or on the sides (bilateral) of the celiac axis. The major EUS related risk is the potential translocation of bacteria in the retroperitoneum; parenteral administration of antibiotics in the perioperative period has been proposed to reduce the risk of bacterial seeding (Levy et al. 2006; Gress et al. 2001). Other EUS-related risks and contraindications are the same as those for endoscopy and sedation in general.

Data from a recent meta-analysis suggest that EUS-guided celiac plexus neurolysis is effective to manage cancer pain and to reduce abdominal pain due to pancreatic cancer in 73% of the patients (Kaufman et al. 2010). Another meta-analysis of five randomized controlled trials confirms improvement of pain control, reduction of narcotic usage and constipation (Yan & Myers 2007) after EUS-guided celiac plexus neurolysis for pancreatic cancer. At present, after more than ten years from the first published report (Wiersema & Wiersema 1996), there are no available studies comparing outcomes of EUS with other procedures for celiac plexus neurolysis. EUS-guided celiac plexus block/neurolysis seems to be safe and effective but is not yet largely diffuse.

5 Gastric-Outlet Obstruction

Gastric outlet obstruction (GOO) is a late complication mostly of gastric, pancreatic, duodenal, and biliary malignancies (Lillemoe & Pitt 1996). GOO becomes symptomatic only in advanced stages of the disease when palliation is the only chance. Palliation should offer the best quality of life to pre-terminal patients.

Gastrojejunostomy is the main surgical palliative option for GOO. Surgical jejunostomy, gastric and enteral decompression are reserved for those cases with peritoneal carcinosis. In these already debilitated patients, surgery bears higher morbidity and mortality risk, with prolonged hospital stay and delayed symptoms relief (Jeurnink et al. 2007a; Siddiqui et al. 2007) than endoscopic stenting. Surgery is considered of some advantage over endoscopic stenting for GOO in patients with at least six months of life expectancy.

After the first report of stent placement for malignant GOO in 1992 by Truong and co-workers (Truong et al. 1992), endoscopic palliation has become an attractive and effective approach. Today, endoscopy is considered the first line approach to treat GOO due to its greater clinical success, reduced morbidity and mortality and shorter hospital stay, when compared to surgery (Hosono et al. 2007). The reported clinical and technical success rate of endoscopic duodenal SEMS placement is 84% and 97% respectively (Dormann et al. 2004; Holt et al. 2004; van Hooft et al. 2007).

5.1 Enteral Stents

Enteral endoscopic stenting is indicated in patients with single site obstructive malignancy of the gastric outlet, without evidence of multiple strictures of the small bowel and/or peritoneal carcinosis. Contraindications for endoscopic stent placement are the same as those for endoscopy and sedation. The through-the-scope (TTS) placement of enteral stents is the preferable stenting technique (Laasch et al. 2005; Maetani et al. 2001; Maetani et al. 2002). The procedure can be done under conscious sedation. The stenting technique consists in the passage of the stricture with a stiff, kinking resistant guide wire under fluoroscopy. Once the guide wire is placed distal to the duodenal stricture, the stent is advanced through the lesion and deployed. The stent should be at least few centimeters longer than the stricture, to guarantee disease-free margin and good extension over curves. The new designed stent delivery systems allow stent re-sheathing in case of wrong stent position during release. Nitinol wire stents have almost completely replaced other materials. This alloy is soft, flexible, with smoother wire ends reducing the trauma to the bowel wall. Nitinol stents have good axial and radial force (Isayama et al. 2009; Stoeckel et al. 2004). Stents can be also covered and uncovered. Silicone, polyurethane, and expanded polytetrafluoroethylene are materials used for the sheet of covered stents. These stents are designed to prevent tumor ingrowth that can lead to stent obstruction (Song et al. 1993). The disadvantage of covered stents is their tendency to migrate, the relative rigidity and costs (Jung et al. 2000).

Uncovered stents are more flexible, anchor better on strictures, are easier to deploy in situ, and are usually preferred for GOO palliation. Besides ingrowth, other events that can lead to stent malfunction are overgrowth, food impaction, migration and biliary obstruction. These events can be safely managed by endoscopy (Piesman et al. 2009). Re-intervention for stent malfunction is required in 20–25% of patients (Laasch et al. 2005).

5.2 Outcomes of Enteral Stents

The Adler and Baron's Gastric Outlet Obstruction Scoring System (GOOSS) assess the level of oral intake before and after the stent placement (Jeurnink et al. 2007b). This scoring system consists in assigning point scores on the basis of the level of oral intake of patients before and after stenting: 0, no oral intake; 1, liquids only; 2, soft solids; 3, low-residue or full diet. After stenting, improvements of GOOSS scale have been reported in many studies (Holt et al. 2004; van Hooft et al. 2007; Jeurnink et al. 2007b; Lee et al. 2007; Lowe et al. 2007; Maetani et al. 2007; Schiefke et al. 2003; Yim et al. 2001) ranging from 75% to 100%. Additional treatments as radio and chemotherapy can positively influence the stent patency by reducing the tumor burden, ingrowth and overgrowth (Kim et al. 2007; Telford et al. 2004). The reported median survival after enteral stenting ranges from 49 to 195 days (Holt et al. 2004; van Hooft et al. 2007; Jeurnink et al. 2007b; Lee et al. 2007; Lowe et al. 2007; Maetani et al. 2007; Schiefke et al. 2003; Yim et al. 2001; Kim et al. 2007; Adler & Baron 2002; Mittal et al. 2004; Maetani et al. 2005; Stawowy et al. 2007).

5.3 Bilioduodenal Stenting

Patients with malignant GOO often have concomitant biliary obstruction, that mainly occurs before the onset of the gastroduodenal obstruction (Baron & Harewood 2003; Maetani et al. 2004; Wong et al. 2002). In these patients, a combined biliary and duodenal metallic stent insertion is difficult and represents a technical challenge. According to the relationship of the duodenal and biliary obstruction, "bilio-duodenal" strictures are classified as: type I stenosis, involving duodenal bulb or upper duodenal genu, without involvement of the papilla, type II affecting the second part of the duodenum, with involvement of the papilla and type III involving the third part of the duodenum without involvement of the papilla (Mutignani et al. 2007). The success in "bilio-duodenal" stenting for type I and III strictures is 100% (Mutignani et al. 2007) Type II duodenal obstruction is the more difficult to treat (Baron & Harewood 2003; Bessoud et al. 2005; Kaw et al. 2003) and the reported success of double stenting is 86% (134). Access to the bile ducts can be obtained by fenestrating the meshes of the duodenal stent using argon plasma (Mutignani et al. 2007; Topazian & Baron 2009) or by percutaneous drainage techniques (Fig. 4).

6 Ongoing Researches and Future Developments

6.1 Ir^{192}-HDR Brachytherapy

High dose rate (HDR) brachytherapy allows a high dose radiation of a well-defined volume of tissue, minimizing the risks of exposure of adjacent organs. In external beam irradiation, the radiation exposure is limited due to the low tolerance of liver, kidneys and bowel. The first report of intraluminal brachytherapy with iridium-192 for extrahepatic bile duct carcinoma was published in 1979 (Ikeda et al. 1979). Iridium-192 is a gamma emitter used for radiation therapy. Intraluminal brachytherapy offers the possibility to administer high dose radiation (30–50 Gy) in a short time, within the range of 1–1.5 cm, reducing all the

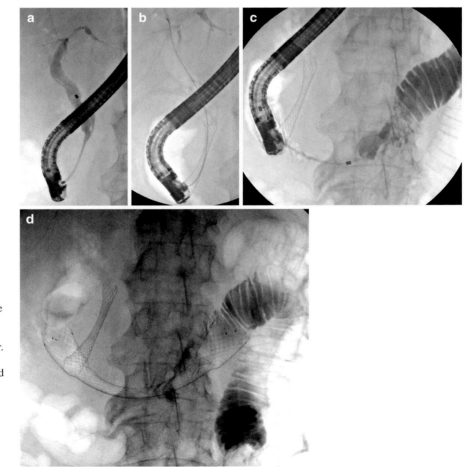

Fig. 4 Endoscopic management of gastric outlet obstruction in a patient with pancreatic cancer and a synchronous stricture of the common bile duct and duodenum. (**a**) ERCP shows a stricture of the distal common bile duct. (**b**) Placement of a biliary Self Expanding Metal Stent (WallFlex Biliary RX Stents, Boston Scientific, Natick, MA, USA). Note the massive aerobilia. (**c**) Injection of contrast medium into the duodenum through a catheter. The duodenal stricture involves the inferior genu and a large part of the third duodenum. (**d**) Deployment of a Duodenal Self-Expanding Metal Stent (Evolution Duodenal Stent, Cook Medical, Winston-Salem, NC, USA)

side effects of external beam radiotherapy. HDR intraluminal brachytherapy finds an indication in biliary tumors and can be administered percutaneously or trough naso-biliary tubes (placed by ERCP) with Iridium-192 wires of homogeneous linear activity. HDR brachytherapy for primitive bile duct tumors has been evaluated alone or in association with external beam irradiation, in a some studies (Bruha et al. 2001; Fritz et al. 1994; Shin et al. 2003; Kocak et al. 2005), showing a prolonged survival in patients with cholangiocarcinoma, and carcinoma of the papilla of Vater, but no effect in those with gallbladder carcinoma. The role of HDR in pancreatic cancer palliation has not yet been evaluated. Only one small series (Mutignani et al. 2002) reported the use of low-dose rate intraluminal brachytherapy into the pancreatic duct, through an endoscopically inserted naso-pancreatic drain. The reported median survival was 11 months without brachytherapy-related complications. Intraluminal brachytherapy in the main pancreatic duct is safe and feasible, but large prospective series are necessary to establish its possible role in pancreatic cancer.

6.2 Frontiers of Therapeutic Endoscopic Ultrasonography

EUS has a key role in the diagnosis of pancreatic cancer and will probably be a tool for direct placement of pharmaceuticals and biological agents directly into a pancreatic tumor. Delivery of cytotoxic agents, gene therapy and radioactive seeds into the tumor mass has been reported (Mishra et al. 2003; Chang et al. 2008). Feasibility and results of this new application of EUS are under evaluation.

6.3 Drug-Eluting Stents

In the past thirty years, there has been a dramatic change in the development, composition and design of stents for gastrointestinal diseases. Plastic stents, stainless still and Nitinol self-expandable metallic stents are of common use in the palliation of jaundice secondary to pancreatic cancer. Stents covered with anti-tumor agents or nano silver particles to decreased bacterial adherence are under evaluation (Leung et al. 1992).

Drug-eluting stents incorporates anti-tumor agents that should improve stent patency minimizing tumor ingrowth. Biliary insertion of metallic stents covered with a paclitaxel-incorporated membrane (Lee et al. 2005; Suk et al. 2007) resulted feasible, safe and effective in prolonging biliary stent patency. Drug-eluting stents requires a molecule to be loaded, retained, and released in a controlled manner to achieve correct delivery. Three methods for drugs delivery were described: drugs directly attached to the metal surface, drugs loaded into the pore of a porous stent, drugs incorporated into a stent coating polymer (Machan 2006). The first two ways permit drug delivery by simple diffusion. In coating polymers, the drug delivery can be controlled by the thickness of the coating polymer. Another drug delivery method is represented by biodegradable polymer, which dissolving, gradually releases the drug on adjacent tissue. Research is also focused to stents with incorporated drugs that will prevent acid, pepsin and pancreatic enzymes related-damage of the covered part, and antibiotics that will prevent the formation of biofilms responsible for stent clogging (Weickert et al. 2009). Drug-eluting stents are a challenging and promising treatment for pancreatic and bile duct cancer, exploiting its nature to grow along the lumen and to spread submucosally. It is expected that these "stents of the future" will improve stent patency and prolong patients' survival.

References

Abraham, N.S., Barkun, J.S., Barkun, A.N.: Palliation of malignant biliary obstruction: a prospective trial examining impact on quality of life. Gastrointest Endosc **56**, 835–841 (2002)

Adler, D.G., Baron, T.H.: Endoscopic palliation of malignant gastric outlet obstruction using self-expanding metal stents: experience in 36 patients. Am J Gastroenterol **97**, 72–78 (2002)

Andersen, J.R., Sorensen, S.M., Kruse, A., Rokkjaer, M., Matzen, P.: Randomised trial of endoscopic endoprosthesis versus operative bypass in malignant obstructive jaundice. Gut **30**, 1132–1135 (1989)

Arhan, M., Odemis, B., Parlak, E., Ertugrul, I., Basar, O.: Migration of biliary plastic stents: experience of a tertiary center. Surg Endosc **23**, 769–775 (2009)

Artifon, E.L., Sakai, P., Cunha, J.E., Dupont, A., Filho, F.M., Hondo, F.Y., Ishioka, S., Raju, G.S.: Surgery or endoscopy for palliation of biliary obstruction due to metastatic pancreatic cancer. Am J Gastroenterol **101**, 2031–2037 (2006)

Ballinger, A.B., McHugh, M., Catnach, S.M., Alstead, E.M., Clark, M.L.: Symptom relief and quality of life after stenting for malignant bile duct obstruction. Gut **35**, 467–470 (1994)

Baron, T.H., Harewood, G.C.: Enteral self-expandable stents. Gastrointest Endosc **58**, 421–433 (2003)

Bessoud, B., de Baere, T., Denys, A., Kuoch, V., Ducreux, M., Precetti, S., Roche, A., Menu, Y.: Malignant gastroduodenal obstruction: palliation with self-expanding metallic stents. J Vasc Interv Radiol **16**, 247–253 (2005)

Bruha, R., Petrtyl, J., Kubecova, M., Marecek, Z., Dufek, V., Urbanek, P., Kodadova, J., Chodounsky, Z.: Intraluminal brachytherapy and selfexpandable stents in nonresectable biliary malignancies – the question of long-term palliation. Hepatogastroenterology **48**, 631–637 (2001)

Bueno, J.T., Gerdes, H., Kurtz, R.C.: Endoscopic management of occluded biliary Wallstents: A cancer center experience. Gastrointest Endosc **58**, 879–884 (2003)

Catalano, M.F., Geenen, J.E., Lehman, G.A., Siegel, J.H., Jacob, L., McKinley, M.J., Raijman, I., Meier, P., Jacobson, I., Kozarek, R., Al-Kawas, F.H., Lo, S.K., Dua, K.S., Baille, J., Ginsberg, G.G., Parsons, W., Meyerson, S.M., Cohen, S., Nelson, D.B., McHattie, J.D., Carr-Locke, D.L.: "Tannenbaum" Teflon stents versus traditional polyethylene stents for treatment of malignant biliary stricture. Gastrointest Endosc **55**, 354–358 (2002)

Cetta, F., Rappuoli, R., Montalto, G., Baldi, C., Gori, M., Cetta, D., Zuckermann, M., Magnani, A., Barbucci, R.: New biliary endoprosthesis less liable to block in biliary infections: description and in vitro studies. Eur J Surg **165**, 782–785 (1999)

Chang, K.J., Lee, J.G., Holcombe, R.F., Kuo, J., Muthusamy, R., Wu, M.L.: Endoscopic ultrasound delivery of an antitumor agent to treat a case of pancreatic cancer. Nat Clin Pract Gastroenterol Hepatol **5**, 107–111 (2008)

Chaurasia, O.P., Rauws, E.A., Fockens, P., Huibregtse, K.: Endoscopic techniques for retrieval of proximally migrated biliary stents: the Amsterdam experience. Gastrointest Endosc **50**, 780–785 (1999)

Chen, J.H., Sun, C.K., Liao, C.S., Chua, C.S.: Self-expandable metallic stents for malignant biliary obstruction: efficacy on proximal and distal tumors. World J Gastroenterol **12**, 119–122 (2006)

Christiaens, P., Decock, S., Buchel, O., Bulte, K., Moons, V., D'Haens, G., Van, O.G.: Endoscopic trimming of metallic stents with the use of argon plasma. Gastrointest Endosc **67**, 369–371 (2008)

Coates, J.M., Beal, S.H., Russo, J.E., Vanderveen, K.A., Chen, S.L., Bold, R.J., Canter, R.J.: Negligible effect of selective preoperative biliary drainage on perioperative resuscitation, morbidity, and mortality in patients undergoing pancreaticoduodenectomy. Arch Surg **144**, 841–847 (2009)

Costamagna, G., Alevras, P., Palladino, F., Rainoldi, F., Mutignani, M., Morganti, A.: Endoscopic pancreatic stenting in pancreatic cancer. Can J Gastroenterol **13**, 481–487 (1999)

Costamagna, G., Mutignani, M., Rotondano, G., Cipolletta, L., Ghezzo, L., Foco, A., Zambelli, A.: Hydrophilic hydromer-coated polyurethane stents versus uncoated stents in malignant biliary obstruction: a randomized trial. Gastrointest Endosc **51**, 8–11 (2000)

Davids, P.H., Groen, A.K., Rauws, E.A., Tytgat, G.N., Huibregtse, K.: Randomised trial of self-expanding metal stents versus polyethylene stents for distal malignant biliary obstruction. Lancet **340**, 1488–1492 (1992)

Dormann, A., Meisner, S., Verin, N., Wenk, L.A.: Self-expanding metal stents for gastroduodenal malignancies: systematic review of their clinical effectiveness. Endoscopy **36**, 543–550 (2004)

Dowidar, N., Moesgaard, F., Matzen, P.: Clogging and other complications of endoscopic biliary endoprostheses. Scand J Gastroenterol **26**, 1132–1136 (1991)

Familiari, P., Bulajic, M., Mutignani, M., Lee, L.S., Spera, G., Spada, C., Tringali, A., Costamagna, G.: Endoscopic removal of malfunctioning biliary self-expandable metallic stents. Gastrointest Endosc **62**, 903–910 (2005)

Ferlitsch, A., Oesterreicher, C., Dumonceau, J.M., Deviere, J., Leban, T., Born, P., Rosch, T., Suter, W., Binek, J., Meyenberger, C., Mullner, M., Schneider, B., Schofl, R.: Diamond stents for palliation of malignant bile duct obstruction: A prospective multicenter evaluation. Endoscopy **33**, 645–650 (2001)

Freeman, M.L.: Adverse outcomes of ERCP. Gastrointest Endosc **56**, S273–S282 (2002)

Fritz, P., Brambs, H.J., Schraube, P., Freund, U., Berns, C., Wannenmacher, M.: Combined external beam radiotherapy and intraluminal high dose rate brachytherapy on bile duct carcinomas. Int J Radiat Oncol Biol Phys **29**, 855–861 (1994)

Fumex, F., Coumaros, D., Napoleon, B., Barthet, M., Laugier, R., Yzet, T., Le, S.A., Desurmont, P., Lamouliatte, H., Letard, J.C., Canard, J.M., Prat, F., Rey, J.F., Ponchon, T.: Similar performance but higher cholecystitis rate with covered biliary stents: results from a prospective multicenter evaluation. Endoscopy **38**, 787–792 (2006)

Gress, F., Schmitt, C., Sherman, S., Ciaccia, D., Ikenberry, S., Lehman, G.: Endoscopic ultrasound-guided celiac plexus block for managing abdominal pain associated with chronic pancreatitis: a prospective single center experience. Am J Gastroenterol **96**, 409–416 (2001)

Gunaratnam, N.T., Sarma, A.V., Norton, I.D., Wiersema, M.J.: A prospective study of EUS-guided celiac plexus neurolysis for pancreatic cancer pain. Gastrointest Endosc **54**, 316–324 (2001)

Herzog, T., Belyaev, O., Muller, C.A., Mittelkotter, U., Seelig, M.H., Weyhe, D., Felderbauer, P., Schlottmann, R., Schrader, H., Schmidt, W.E., Uhl, W.: Bacteribilia after preoperative bile duct stenting: a prospective study. J Clin Gastroenterol **43**, 457–462 (2009)

Ho, H., Mahajan, A., Gosain, S., Jain, A., Brock, A., Rehan, M.E., Ellen, K., Shami, V.M., Kahaleh, M.: Management of complications associated with partially covered biliary metal stents. Dig Dis Sci **55**, 516–522 (2010)

Holt, A.P., Patel, M., Ahmed, M.M.: Palliation of patients with malignant gastroduodenal obstruction with self-expanding metallic stents: the treatment of choice? Gastrointest Endosc **60**, 1010–1017 (2004)

Hosono, S., Ohtani, H., Arimoto, Y., Kanamiya, Y.: Endoscopic stenting versus surgical gastroenterostomy for palliation of malignant gastroduodenal obstruction: a meta-analysis. J Gastroenterol **42**, 283–290 (2007)

Huibregtse, K.: Plastic or expandable biliary endoprostheses? Scand J Gastroenterol Suppl **200**, 3–7 (1993)

Ikeda, H., Kuroda, C., Uchida, H., Miyata, Y., Masaki, N., Shigematsu, Y., Monden, M., Okamura, J.: Intraluminal irradiation with iridium-192 wires for extrahepatic bile duct carcinoma–a preliminary report (author's transl). Nippon Igaku Hoshasen Gakkai Zasshi **39**, 1356–1358 (1979)

Isayama, H., Komatsu, Y., Tsujino, T., Sasahira, N., Hirano, K., Toda, N., Nakai, Y., Yamamoto, N., Tada, M., Yoshida, H., Shiratori, Y., Kawabe, T., Omata, M.: A prospective randomised study of "covered" versus "uncovered" diamond stents for the management of distal malignant biliary obstruction. Gut **53**, 729–734 (2004)

Isayama, H., Kawabe, T., Nakai, Y., Tsujino, T., Sasahira, N., Yamamoto, N., Arizumi, T., Togawa, O., Matsubara, S., Ito, Y., Sasaki, T., Hirano, K., Toda, N., Komatsu, Y., Tada, M., Yoshida, H., Omata, M.: Cholecystitis after metallic stent placement in patients with malignant distal biliary obstruction. Clin Gastroenterol Hepatol **4**, 1148–1153 (2006)

Isayama, H., Nakai, Y., Toyokawa, Y., Togawa, O., Gon, C., Ito, Y., Yashima, Y., Yagioka, H., Kogure, H., Sasaki, T., Arizumi, T., Matsubara, S., Yamamoto, N., Sasahira, N., Hirano, K., Tsujino, T., Toda, N., Tada, M., Kawabe, T., Omata, M.: Measurement of radial and axial forces of biliary self-expandable metallic stents. Gastrointest Endosc **70**, 37–44 (2009)

Jeurnink, S.M., van Eijck, C.H., Steyerberg, E.W., Kuipers, E.J., Siersema, P.D.: Stent versus gastrojejunostomy for the palliation of gastric outlet obstruction: a systematic review. BMC Gastroenterol **7**, 18 (2007a)

Jeurnink, S.M., Steyerberg, E.W., Hof, G., van Eijck, C.H., Kuipers, E.J., Siersema, P.D.: Gastrojejunostomy versus stent placement in patients with malignant gastric outlet obstruction: a comparison in 95 patients. J Surg Oncol **96**, 389–396 (2007b)

Johanson, J.F., Schmalz, M.J., Geenen, J.E.: Incidence and risk factors for biliary and pancreatic stent migration. Gastrointest Endosc **38**, 341–346 (1992)

Jung, G.S., Song, H.Y., Kang, S.G., Huh, J.D., Park, S.J., Koo, J.Y., Cho, Y.D.: Malignant gastroduodenal obstructions: Treatment by means of a covered expandable metallic stent-initial experience. Radiology **216**, 758–763 (2000)

Kaassis, M., Boyer, J., Dumas, R., Ponchon, T., Coumaros, D., Delcenserie, R., Canard, J.M., Fritsch, J., Rey, J.F., Burtin, P.: Plastic or metal stents for malignant stricture of the common bile duct? Results of a randomized prospective study. Gastrointest Endosc **57**, 178–182 (2003)

Kahaleh, M., Tokar, J., Conaway, M.R., Brock, A., Le, T., Adams, R.B., Yeaton, P.: Efficacy and complications of covered Wallstents in malignant distal biliary obstruction. Gastrointest Endosc **61**, 528–533 (2005)

Katsinelos, P., Kountouras, J., Paroutoglou, G., Paikos, D., Moschos, J., Chatzimavroudis, G., Zavos, C., Makrigiannis, E.: Uncovered Hanaro versus Luminex metal stents for palliation of malignant biliary strictures. J Clin Gastroenterol **42**, 539–545 (2008)

Kaufman, M., Singh, G., Das, S., Concha-Parra, R., Erber, J., Micames, C., Gress, F.: Efficacy of endoscopic ultrasound-guided celiac plexus block and celiac plexus neurolysis for managing abdominal pain associated with chronic pancreatitis and pancreatic cancer. J Clin Gastroenterol **44**, 127–134 (2010)

Kaw, M., Singh, S., Gagneja, H.: Clinical outcome of simultaneous self-expandable metal stents for palliation of malignant biliary and duodenal obstruction. Surg Endosc **17**, 457–461 (2003)

Kim, H.S., Lee, D.K., Kim, H.G., Park, J.J., Park, S.H., Kim, J.H., Yoo, B.M., Roe, I.H., Moon, Y.S., Myung, S.J.: Features of malignant biliary obstruction affecting the patency of metallic stents: a multicenter study. Gastrointest Endosc **55**, 359–365 (2002)

Kim, J.H., Song, H.Y., Shin, J.H., Choi, E., Kim, T.W., Jung, H.Y., Lee, G.H., Lee, S.K., Kim, M.H., Ryu, M.H., Kang, Y.K., Kim, B.S., Yook, J.H.: Metallic stent placement in the palliative treatment of malignant gastroduodenal obstructions: prospective evaluation of results and factors influencing outcome in 213 patients. Gastrointest Endosc **66**, 256–264 (2007)

Kocak, Z., Ozkan, H., Adli, M., Garipagaoglu, M., Kurtman, C., Cakmak, S.: Intraluminal brachytherapy with metallic stenting in the palliative treatment of malignant obstruction of the bile duct. Radiat Med **23**, 200–207 (2005)

Laasch, H.U., Martin, D.F., Maetani, I.: Enteral stents in the gastric outlet and duodenum. Endoscopy **37**, 74–81 (2005)

Landoni, N., Wengrower, D., Chopita, N., Goldin, E.: Randomized prospective study to compare the efficiency between standard plastic and polyurethane stents in biliary tract malignant obstruction. Acta Gastroenterol Latinoam **30**, 501–504 (2000)

Lee, D.K., Kim, H.S., Kim, K.S., Lee, W.J., Kim, H.K., Won, Y.H., Byun, Y.R., Kim, M.Y., Baik, S.K., Kwon, S.O.: The effect on porcine bile duct of a metallic stent covered with a paclitaxel-incorporated membrane. Gastrointest Endosc **61**, 296–301 (2005)

Lee, S.M., Kang, D.H., Kim, G.H., Park, W.I., Kim, H.W., Park, J.H.: Self-expanding metallic stents for gastric outlet obstruction resulting from stomach cancer: a preliminary study with a newly designed double-layered pyloric stent. Gastrointest Endosc **66**, 1206–1210 (2007)

Lermite, E., Pessaux, P., Teyssedou, C., Etienne, S., Brehant, O., Arnaud, J.P.: Effect of preoperative endoscopic biliary drainage on infectious morbidity after pancreatoduodenectomy: a case-control study. Am J Surg **195**, 442–446 (2008)

Leung, J., Rahim, N.: The role of covered self-expandable metallic stents in malignant biliary strictures. Gastrointest Endosc **63**, 1001–1003 (2006)

Leung, J.W., Lau, G.T., Sung, J.J., Costerton, J.W.: Decreased bacterial adherence to silver-coated stent material: an in vitro study. Gastrointest Endosc **38**, 338–340 (1992)

Levy, M., Rajan, E., Keeney, G., Fletcher, J.G., Topazian, M.: Neural ganglia visualized by endoscopic ultrasound. Am J Gastroenterol **101**, 1787–1791 (2006)

Lillemoe, K.D., Pitt, H.A.: Palliation. Surgical and otherwise. Cancer **78**, 605–614 (1996)

Lo, C.H., Chung, S., Bohmer, R.D.: A devastating complication: duodenal perforation due to biliary stent migration. Surg Laparosc Endosc Percutan Tech **18**, 608–610 (2008)

Lowe, A.S., Beckett, C.G., Jowett, S., May, J., Stephenson, S., Scally, A., Tam, E., Kay, C.L.: Self-expandable metal stent placement for the palliation of malignant gastroduodenal obstruction: experience in a large, single, UK centre. Clin Radiol **62**, 738–744 (2007)

Luman, W., Cull, A., Palmer, K.R.: Quality of life in patients stented for malignant biliary obstructions. Eur J Gastroenterol Hepatol **9**, 481–484 (1997)

Machan, L.: Clinical experience and applications of drug-eluting stents in the noncoronary vasculature, bile duct and esophagus. Adv Drug Deliv Rev **58**, 447–462 (2006)

Maetani, I., Ukita, T., Inone, H., Yoshida, M., Igarashi, Y., Sakai, Y.: Knitted nitinol stent insertion for various intestinal stenoses with a modified delivery system. Gastrointest Endosc **54**, 364–367 (2001)

Maetani, I., Tada, T., Shimura, J., Ukita, T., Inoue, H., Igarashi, Y., Hoshi, H., Sakai, Y.: Technical modifications and strategies for stenting gastric outlet strictures using esophageal endoprostheses. Endoscopy **34**, 402–406 (2002)

Maetani, I., Tada, T., Ukita, T., Inoue, H., Sakai, Y., Nagao, J.: Comparison of duodenal stent placement with surgical gastrojejunostomy for palliation in patients with duodenal obstructions caused by pancreaticobiliary malignancies. Endoscopy **36**, 73–78 (2004)

Maetani, I., Akatsuka, S., Ikeda, M., Tada, T., Ukita, T., Nakamura, Y., Nagao, J., Sakai, Y.: Self-expandable metallic stent placement for palliation in gastric outlet obstructions caused by gastric cancer: a comparison with surgical gastrojejunostomy. J Gastroenterol **40**, 932–937 (2005)

Maetani, I., Isayama, H., Mizumoto, Y.: Palliation in patients with malignant gastric outlet obstruction with a newly designed enteral stent: A multicenter study. Gastrointest Endosc **66**, 355–360 (2007)

Matsuda, Y., Shimakura, K., Akamatsu, T.: Factors affecting the patency of stents in malignant biliary obstructive disease: univariate and multivariate analysis. Am J Gastroenterol **86**, 843–849 (1991)

Menon, K., Barkun, A.: Management of occluded biliary Wallstents. Gastrointest Endosc **49**, 403–405 (1999)

Mezhir, J.J., Brennan, M.F., Baser, R.E., D'Angelica, M.I., Fong, Y., Dematteo, R.P., Jarnagin, W.R., Allen, P.J.: A matched case-control study of preoperative biliary drainage in patients with pancreatic adenocarcinoma: Routine drainage is not justified. J Gastrointest Surg **13**(12), 2163–2169 (2009)

Mishra, G., Liu, T.F., Frankel, A.E.: Recombinant toxin DAB389EGF is cytotoxic to human pancreatic cancer cells. Expert Opin Biol Ther **3**, 1173–1180 (2003)

Mittal, A., Windsor, J., Woodfield, J., Casey, P., Lane, M.: Matched study of three methods for palliation of malignant pyloroduodenal obstruction. Br J Surg **91**, 205–209 (2004)

Moss, A.C., Morris, E., Mac, M.P.: Palliative biliary stents for obstructing pancreatic carcinoma. Cochrane Database Syst Rev 2006;CD004200.

Moss, A.C., Morris, E., Leyden, J., MacMathuna, P.: Do the benefits of metal stents justify the costs? A systematic review and meta-analysis of trials comparing endoscopic stents for malignant biliary obstruction. Eur J Gastroenterol Hepatol **19**, 1119–1124 (2007)

Mutignani, M., Shah, S.K., Morganti, A.G., Perri, V., Macchia, G., Costamagna, G.: Treatment of unresectable pancreatic carcinoma by intraluminal brachytherapy in the duct of Wirsung. Endoscopy **34**, 555–559 (2002)

Mutignani, M., Tringali, A., Shah, S.G., Perri, V., Familiari, P., Iacopini, F., Spada, C., Costamagna, G.: Combined endoscopic stent insertion in malignant biliary and duodenal obstruction. Endoscopy **39**, 440–447 (2007)

Mutignani, M., Iacopini, F., Perri, V., Familiari, P., Tringali, A., Spada, C., Ingrosso, M., Costamagna, G.: Endoscopic gallbladder drainage for acute cholecystitis: technical and clinical results. Endoscopy **41**, 539–546 (2009)

Nakai, Y., Isayama, H., Komatsu, Y., Tsujino, T., Toda, N., Sasahira, N., Yamamoto, N., Hirano, K., Tada, M., Yoshida, H., Kawabe, T., Omata, M.: Efficacy and safety of the covered Wallstent in patients with distal malignant biliary obstruction. Gastrointest Endosc **62**, 742–748 (2005)

Ornellas, L.C., Stefanidis, G., Chuttani, R., Gelrud, A., Kelleher, T.B., Pleskow, D.K.: Covered Wallstents for palliation of malignant biliary obstruction: Primary stent placement versus reintervention. Gastrointest Endosc **70**, 676–683 (2009)

Park, D.H., Kim, M.H., Choi, J.S., Lee, S.S., Seo, D.W., Kim, J.H., Han, J., Kim, J.C., Choi, E.K., Lee, S.K.: Covered versus uncovered wallstent for malignant extrahepatic biliary obstruction: a cohort comparative analysis. Clin Gastroenterol Hepatol **4**, 790–796 (2006)

Pausawasdi, N., Scheiman, J.: Endoscopic evaluation and palliation of pancreatic adenocarcinoma: current and future options. Curr Opin Gastroenterol **23**, 515–521 (2007)

Pedersen, F.M.: Endoscopic management of malignant biliary obstruction. Is stent size of 10 French gauge better than 7 French gauge? Scand J Gastroenterol **28**, 185–189 (1993)

Perdue, D.G., Freeman, M.L., DiSario, J.A., Nelson, D.B., Fennerty, M.B., Lee, J.G., Overby, C.S., Ryan, M.E., Bochna, G.S., Snady, H.W., Moore, J.P.: Plastic versus self-expanding metallic stents for malignant hilar biliary obstruction: A prospective multicenter observational cohort study. J Clin Gastroenterol **42**, 1040–1046 (2008)

Piesman, M., Kozarek, R.A., Brandabur, J.J., Pleskow, D.K., Chuttani, R., Eysselein, V.E., Silverman, W.B., Vargo, J.J., Waxman, I., Catalano, M.F., Baron, T.H., Parsons III, W.G., Slivka, A., Carr-Locke, D.L.: Improved oral intake after palliative duodenal stenting for malignant obstruction: a prospective multicenter clinical trial. Am J Gastroenterol **104**, 2404–2411 (2009)

Raijman, I.: Biliary and pancreatic stents. Gastrointest Endosc Clin North Am **13**, 561–592 (2003)

Rogart, J.N., Boghos, A., Rossi, F., Al-Hashem, H., Siddiqui, U.D., Jamidar, P., Aslanian, H.: Analysis of endoscopic management of occluded metal biliary stents at a single tertiary care center. Gastrointest Endosc **68**, 676–682 (2008)

Sarr, M.G., Cameron, J.L.: Surgical management of unresectable carcinoma of the pancreas. Surgery **91**, 123–133 (1982)

Schiefke, I., Zabel-Langhennig, A., Wiedmann, M., Huster, D., Witzigmann, H., Mossner, J., Berr, F., Caca, K.: Self-expandable metallic stents for malignant duodenal obstruction caused by biliary tract cancer. Gastrointest Endosc **58**, 213–219 (2003)

Schilling, D., Rink, G., Arnold, J.C., Benz, C., Adamek, H.E., Jakobs, R., Riemann, J.F.: Prospective, randomized, single-center trial comparing 3 different 10F plastic stents in malignant mid and distal bile duct strictures. Gastrointest Endosc **58**, 54–58 (2003)

Schmassmann, A., von Gunten, E., Knuchel, J., Scheurer, U., Fehr, H.F., Halter, F.: Wallstents versus plastic stents in malignant biliary obstruction: effects of stent patency of the first and second stent on patient compliance and survival. Am J Gastroenterol **91**, 654–659 (1996)

Shah, R.J., Howell, D.A., Desilets, D.J., Sheth, S.G., Parsons, W.G., Okolo III, P., Lehman, G.A., Sherman, S., Baillie, J., Branch, M.S., Pleskow, D., Chuttani, R., Bosco, J.J.: Multicenter randomized trial of the spiral Z-stent compared with the Wallstent for malignant biliary obstruction. Gastrointest Endosc **57**, 830–836 (2003)

Shepherd, H.A., Royle, G., Ross, A.P., Diba, A., Arthur, M., Colin-Jones, D.: Endoscopic biliary endoprosthesis in the palliation of malignant obstruction of the distal common bile duct: a randomized trial. Br J Surg **75**, 1166–1168 (1988)

Shin, H.S., Seong, J., Kim, W.C., Lee, H.S., Moon, S.R., Lee, I.J., Lee, K.K., Park, K.R., Suh, C.O., Kim, G.E.: Combination of external beam irradiation and high-dose-rate intraluminal brachytherapy for inoperable carcinoma of the extrahepatic bile ducts. Int J Radiat Oncol Biol Phys **57**, 105–112 (2003)

Siddiqui, A., Spechler, S.J., Huerta, S.: Surgical bypass versus endoscopic stenting for malignant gastroduodenal obstruction: a decision analysis. Dig Dis Sci **52**, 276–281 (2007)

Simmons, D.T., Petersen, B.T., Gostout, C.J., Levy, M.J., Topazian, M.D., Baron, T.H.: Risk of pancreatitis following endoscopically placed large-bore plastic biliary stents with and without biliary sphincterotomy for management of postoperative bile leaks. Surg Endosc **22**, 1459–1463 (2008)

Smith, A.C., Dowsett, J.F., Russell, R.C., Hatfield, A.R., Cotton, P.B.: Randomised trial of endoscopic stenting versus surgical bypass in malignant low bileduct obstruction. Lancet **344**, 1655–1660 (1994)

Soderlund, C., Linder, S.: Covered metal versus plastic stents for malignant common bile duct stenosis: a prospective, randomized, controlled trial. Gastrointest Endosc **63**, 986–995 (2006)

Soehendra, N., Maydeo, A., Eckmann, B., Bruckner, M., Nam, V.C., Grimm, H.: A new technique for replacing an obstructed biliary endoprosthesis. Endoscopy **22**, 271–272 (1990)

Song, H.Y., Yang, D.H., Kuh, J.H., Choi, K.C.: Obstructing cancer of the gastric antrum: Palliative treatment with covered metallic stents. Radiology **187**, 357–358 (1993)

Speer, A.G., Cotton, P.B., Russell, R.C., Mason, R.R., Hatfield, A.R., Leung, J.W., MacRae, K.D., Houghton, J., Lennon, C.A.: Randomised trial of endoscopic versus percutaneous stent insertion in malignant obstructive jaundice. Lancet **2**, 57–62 (1987)

Stawowy, M., Kruse, A., Mortensen, F.V., Funch-Jensen, P.: Endoscopic stenting for malignant gastric outlet obstruction. Surg Laparosc Endosc Percutan Tech **17**, 5–9 (2007)

Stoeckel, D., Pelton, A., Duerig, T.: Self-expanding nitinol stents: material and design considerations. Eur Radiol **14**, 292–301 (2004)

Storkson, R.H., Edwin, B., Reiertsen, O., Faerden, A.E., Sortland, O., Rosseland, A.R.: Gut perforation caused by biliary endoprosthesis. Endoscopy **32**, 87–89 (2000)

Suk, K.T., Kim, J.W., Kim, H.S., Baik, S.K., Oh, S.J., Lee, S.J., Kim, H.G., Lee, D.H., Won, Y.H., Lee, D.K.: Human application of a metallic stent covered with a paclitaxel-incorporated membrane for malignant biliary obstruction: multicenter pilot study. Gastrointest Endosc **66**, 798–803 (2007)

Sunpaweravong, S., Ovartlarnporn, B., Khow-ean, U., Soontrapornchai, P., Charoonratana, V.: Endoscopic stenting versus surgical bypass in advanced malignant distal bile duct

obstruction: cost-effectiveness analysis. Asian J Surg **28**, 262–265 (2005)

Telford, J.J., Carr-Locke, D.L., Baron, T.H., Tringali, A., Parsons, W.G., Gabbrielli, A., Costamagna, G.: Palliation of patients with malignant gastric outlet obstruction with the enteral Wallstent: outcomes from a multicenter study. Gastrointest Endosc **60**, 916–920 (2004)

Tham, T.C., Carr-Locke, D.L., Vandervoort, J., Wong, R.C., Lichtenstein, D.R., Van, D.J., Ruymann, F., Chow, S., Bosco, J.J., Qaseem, T., Howell, D., Pleskow, D., Vannerman, W., Libby, E.D.: Management of occluded biliary Wallstents. Gut **42**, 703–707 (1998)

Tham, T.C., Lichtenstein, D.R., Vandervoort, J., Wong, R.C., Slivka, A., Banks, P.A., Yim, H.B., Carr-Locke, D.L.: Pancreatic duct stents for "obstructive type" pain in pancreatic malignancy. Am J Gastroenterol **95**, 956–960 (2000)

Topazian, M., Baron, T.H.: Endoscopic fenestration of duodenal stents using argon plasma to facilitate ERCP. Gastrointest Endosc **69**, 166–169 (2009)

Tringali, A., Mutignani, M., Perri, V., Zuccala, G., Cipolletta, L., Bianco, M.A., Rotondano, G., Philipper, M., Schumacher, B., Neuhaus, H., Schmit, A., Deviere, J., Costamagna, G.: A prospective, randomized multicenter trial comparing double layer and polyethylene stents for malignant distal common bile duct strictures. Endoscopy **35**, 992–997 (2003)

Truong, S., Bohndorf, V., Geller, H., Schumpelick, V., Gunther, R.W.: Self-expanding metal stents for palliation of malignant gastric outlet obstruction. Endoscopy **24**, 433–435 (1992)

van Berkel, A.M., Boland, C., Redekop, W.K., Bergman, J.J., Groen, A.K., Tytgat, G.N., Huibregtse, K.: A prospective randomized trial of Teflon versus polyethylene stents for distal malignant biliary obstruction. Endoscopy **30**, 681–686 (1998)

van Berkel, A.M., van Marle, J., Groen, A.K., Bruno, M.J.: Mechanisms of biliary stent clogging: confocal laser scanning and scanning electron microscopy. Endoscopy **37**, 729–734 (2005)

van Hooft, J., Mutignani, M., Repici, A., Messmann, H., Neuhaus, H., Fockens, P.: First data on the palliative treatment of patients with malignant gastric outlet obstruction using the WallFlex enteral stent: a retrospective multicenter study. Endoscopy **39**, 434–439 (2007)

van Steenbergen, W., van Aken, L., Ponette, E.: Acute pancreatitis complicating the insertion of a self-expandable biliary metal stent. Endoscopy **24**, 440–442 (1992)

Wang, Q., Gurusamy, K.S., Lin, H., Xie, X., Wang, C.: Preoperative biliary drainage for obstructive jaundice. Cochrane Database Syst Rev 2008;CD005444.

Warshaw, A.L., Fernandez-del, C.C.: Pancreatic carcinoma. N Engl J Med **326**, 455–465 (1992)

Watanapa, P., Williamson, R.C.: Surgical palliation for pancreatic cancer: developments during the past two decades. Br J Surg **79**, 8–20 (1992)

Weber, A., Mittermeyer, T., Wagenpfeil, S., Schmid, R.M., Prinz, C.: Self-expanding metal stents versus polyethylene stents for palliative treatment in patients with advanced pancreatic cancer. Pancreas **38**, e7–e12 (2009)

Weickert, U., Zimmerling, S., Eickhoff, A., Riemann, J.F., Reiss, G.: A comparative scanning electron microscopic study of biliary and pancreatic stents. Z Gastroenterol **47**, 347–350 (2009)

Wiersema, M.J., Wiersema, L.M.: Endosonography-guided celiac plexus neurolysis. Gastrointest Endosc **44**, 656–662 (1996)

Wong, Y.T., Brams, D.M., Munson, L., Sanders, L., Heiss, F., Chase, M., Birkett, D.H.: Gastric outlet obstruction secondary to pancreatic cancer: Surgical vs endoscopic palliation. Surg Endosc **16**, 310–312 (2002)

Yan, B.M., Myers, R.P.: Neurolytic celiac plexus block for pain control in unresectable pancreatic cancer. Am J Gastroenterol **102**, 430–438 (2007)

Yang, K.Y., Ryu, J.K., Seo, J.K., Woo, S.M., Park, J.K., Kim, Y.T., Yoon, Y.B.: A comparison of the Niti-D biliary uncovered stent and the uncovered Wallstent in malignant biliary obstruction. Gastrointest Endosc **70**, 45–51 (2009)

Yeoh, K.G., Zimmerman, M.J., Cunningham, J.T., Cotton, P.B.: Comparative costs of metal versus plastic biliary stent strategies for malignant obstructive jaundice by decision analysis. Gastrointest Endosc **49**, 466–471 (1999)

Yim, H.B., Jacobson, B.C., Saltzman, J.R., Johannes, R.S., Bounds, B.C., Lee, J.H., Shields, S.J., Ruymann, F.W., Van, D.J., Carr-Locke, D.L.: Clinical outcome of the use of enteral stents for palliation of patients with malignant upper GI obstruction. Gastrointest Endosc **53**, 329–332 (2001)

Yoon, W.J., Lee, J.K., Lee, K.H., Lee, W.J., Ryu, J.K., Kim, Y.T., Yoon, Y.B.: A comparison of covered and uncovered Wallstents for the management of distal malignant biliary obstruction. Gastrointest Endosc **63**, 996–1000 (2006)

Yoon, W.J., Ryu, J.K., Yang, K.Y., Paik, W.H., Lee, J.K., Woo, S.M., Park, J.K., Kim, Y.T., Yoon, Y.B.: A comparison of metal and plastic stents for the relief of jaundice in unresectable malignant biliary obstruction in Korea: an emphasis on cost-effectiveness in a country with a low ERCP cost. Gastrointest Endosc **70**, 284–289 (2009)

Local Ablative Techniques in the Treatment of Locally Advanced Pancreatic Cancer

Franco Orsi, Mario Bezzi, and Gianluigi Orgera

Contents

Abstract

› Pancreatic cancer has an extremely poor prognosis and prolonged survival is achieved only by resection with macroscopic tumor clearance. In recent years there has been a growing interest in ablative therapies for the treatment of unresectable tumors in various organs. Local ablative techniques have been developed to enable local control of tumors and cytoreduction, above all for primitive liver tumors, without damage of the healthy parenchyma.

› Tumor ablation is defined as the direct application of chemical or thermal energy to a tumor to obtain cellular necrosis. Ablation has been performed with several modalities including ethanol ablation, laser ablation, cryoablation, and radiofrequency ablation. Numerous preclinical studies have testified the tecnical feasibility, safety, and efficacy of different techniques in ablating the pancreatic parenchyma, but there are very few clinical studies. The purpose of this chapter is to evaluate current status of local ablative therapies in the treatment of pancreatic cancer and future trends.

1 Introduction

Treatment of locally advanced Pancreatic Cancer (PC) is challenging and no clinically meaningful gains have been made in the outcome of these patients in the past 40 years. Despite continuing advances in diagnostic imaging and staging, improvements in radiation therapy techniques and availability of new systemic

F. Orsi (✉) and G. Orgera
Interventional Radiology Unit, European Institute of Oncology,
Via Ripamonti 435, 20141 Milan, Italy
e-mail: franco.orsi@ieo.it

M. Bezzi
Department of Radiology, Sapienza – University of Rome,
Viale Regina Elena 324, 00161 Rome, Italy

A. Laghi (ed.), *New Concepts in Diagnosis and Therapy of Pancreatic Adenocarcinoma*,
Medical Radiology, DOI: 10.1007/174_2010_47, © Springer-Verlag Berlin Heidelberg 2011

therapies, the survival and mortality from PC have remained relatively constant. For all stages combined, the 1-year survival rate is around 20%, and the overall 5-year survival rate has remained dismally poor at <5% (Jemal et al. 2002).

Complete surgical resection remains the only curative treatment for PC. Unfortunately, because of the typically late onset of symptoms, only about 15–20% of cases of PC are amenable to surgical resection at the time of diagnosis. Of the remaining 80–85% of patients, 40% present with advanced locoregional disease precluding complete resection, with a median survival time of 6–11 months, and the other 45% of patients present with metastatic disease, with a median survival time of 3–6 months (Ghaneh et al. 1999).

Chemoradiation therapy (CRT) plays an important role in locally advanced PC. Favorable positive effects have been obtained in respect of local pain control, local control of disease, and overall survival with different radiotherapy techniques such as intraoperative radiation therapy with or without external chemo-/radiation therapy or with CRT alone. By administering up-to-date primary CRT, especially with gemcitabine-associated CRT, local remission in up to 50% of patients can be observed. By applying neoadjuvant CRT, better resectability and the reduction of the number of postoperative positive lymph node metastasis has been seen in patients with resectable or possibly resectable PC. With primary CRT, resectability can also be achieved in patients with primary unresectable PC (Cardenes et al. 2006).

The management of patients with locally advanced PC involves a multidisciplinary approach among the pancreatic surgeon, gastroenterologist, and medical and radiation oncologists. The main consideration is whether a patient is ultimately a candidate for combined chemoradiotherapy (chemo-RT) or chemotherapy alone, and this decision is reflected by the patient's performance status, extent and intensity of symptoms, nutritional status, and potential toxicity of the proposed therapy as to its impact on quality of life.

Unfortunately, until now no effective modality has been identified for the treatment of patients with locally advanced pancreatic tumors, although during the past decade, minimally invasive therapies have been used in patients with unresectable tumors. Local ablative methods such as radiofrequency (RF) ablation, local hyperthermia, cryoablation, intratumoral instillation of chemotherapy, or ethanol and photodynamic therapy have been anecdotally used in some patients, but little information can be obtained from literature (Date 2006).

Recently, microwave therapy (Carrafiello et al. 2008) and high-intensity focused ultrasound (HIFU) (Wu et al. 2005) have been proposed as new techniques in the treatment of locally advanced pancreatic tumors. All of these minimally invasive image-guided therapies deliver various kinds of energy to induce coagulative necrosis of a target tumor and their clinical applications may play an important role in some patients who are not candidates for surgical resection.

2 Local Ablative Therapies

The term "ablation" refers to the direct application of chemical or thermal therapies to a specific organ or tissue in an attempt to achieve eradication or substantial tissue destruction. The methods of tumor ablation most commonly used in current practice are divided into two main categories, namely, chemical ablation and thermal ablation.

Chemical ablation includes therapies that are classified on the basis of universally accepted chemical nomenclature, such as ethanol and acetic acid that induce coagulation necrosis and cause tumor death. Thermal ablation includes several different techniques that employ various sources of energy to destroy tumors, by using either heat produced by RF, microwaves, and ultrasound, or cold (cryoablation). The main aim of heat-induced thermal ablation is to destroy an entire tumor by using a source of heat to kill the malignant cells in a minimally invasive fashion without damaging adjacent vital structures. Heat from various sources can be used with equal effectiveness to destroy tumor cells. As long as adequate heat can be generated throughout the tumor volume, it is possible to eradicate the tumor.

Multiple energy sources can be used to provide the heat necessary to induce coagulation of malignant tissue by causing direct cell destruction. In general, "low-level" thermal therapy with temperatures ranging from 45 to 55°C results in limited tissue ablation. On the other hand, thermal therapy with temperatures greater than 55°C (particularly temperatures ranging from 60 to 100°C or more) results in significant tissue ablation and a successful outcome. Cell death results from coagulative necrosis, which occurs after a 2 min exposure to temperatures above 50°C.

Improvements in imaging technologies have enabled the development of minimally invasive tumor therapies, which rely on imaging guidance for the accurate percutaneous placement of needle-like applicators (Habash et al. 2007). The goal is to ablate the tumor and a margin of approximately 1 cm of surrounding normal tissue.

The potential benefits of minimally invasive, image-guided ablation of focal pancreatic neoplasms, as compared with conventional surgical options, include the ability to ablate and/or palliate tumors in nonsurgical candidates, thus obtaining a reduction in morbidity and an improvement in quality of life.

The typical PC has a volume doubling time of 50 days and, at the time of the patient's death, it consists of approximately 80–100 g of tumor tissue. Even small PCs are often inoperable, and, in theory, efficient cytoreduction (greater than 90%) could lead to prolongation of survival because death is rarely caused by systemic progression, but mainly due to the local and biochemical effects of the primary tumor. For this reasons, local ablative techniques would be particularly useful in the management of inoperable PC.

The delicate nature of the pancreatic parenchyma, predisposing to pancreatitis, along with the risk of injury to important structures, such as duodenum, common bile duct, or major arteries and veins, have been the main limiting factors in the application of ablative techniques to the pancreas. Numerous preclinical studies, however, have documented the technical feasibility, safety, and efficacy of different techniques in ablating the pancreatic parenchyma, but to date there are very few clinical studies.

A literature search on local ablative therapies used for the treatment of PC in humans shows radiofrequency ablation (RFA) to be the most frequently used ablative technique worldwide (Date 2006). Some animal studies on RFA of the pancreas have shown that RFA is relatively safe and could be applied to human subjects. Goldberg et al. (1999) studied the safety and efficacy of RFA in experimental models and concluded that RFA can be used in small neuroendocrine tumors and possibly in palliation of unresectable PC. Date et al. (2005) demonstrated the safety and efficacy of RFA in the normal pancreas of a porcine model. One report of 20 patients who had unresectable PC and were treated with RF hyperthermia confirmed the results in animal studies. This study reported two major complications – one septic shock and one major gastrointestinal bleeding (Matsui et al. 2000). Elias et al. (2004) reported two cases of multiple pancreatic metastases from renal tumors treated with RFA; unfortunately, both patients developed severe necrotizing pancreatitis, probably due

to multiple thermal injuries of the gland and died. Spiliotis et al. (2007) recently reported good results using RFA in 12 patients with inoperable PC. Varshney et al. (2006) demonstrated, on a small sample of patients, that RFA of unresectable pancreatic tumors is feasible and safe with minimum morbidity and mortality. The ablated area should be restricted within the tumor to avoid chances of acute pancreatitis or a pancreatic fistula. These reports confirm that RFA of pancreatic tumors may induce various complications such as acute pancreatitis, pancreatic fistula, pancreatic ascites and gastrointestinal hemorrhage, etc. Tumors located in the head of the pancreas seem to be more prone to complications than tumors located in the body/tail (Date et al. 2005). In addition, one of the most frequently encountered problems in RFA is pain, which may be related to the size and location of the ablated lesion (Friedman et al. 2004).

As regards imaging guidance, computed tomography (CT) is extremely accurate and probably the most commonly used guidance technique. However, endoscopic ultrasound may prove the most effective method of electrode placement after appropriate electrode design. Goldberg et al. demonstrated endoscopic ultrasound-guided ablation in a porcine model by using 1- and 1.5-cm electrodes that produced 10- to 12-mm diameters of necrosis around each electrode. Larger volumes of necrosis would require multiple electrodes or water cooling (Goldberg et al.1999).

Microwave ablation is a relatively new technology under development and testing that can be used to treat the same types of cancer that can be treated with RF ablation. Microwave technology provides all the benefits of RF and preliminary works show that it may be used as a viable alternative to other ablation techniques in selected patients. Microwave radiation lies between infrared radiation and radiowaves with frequencies from 900 to 2,450 MHz. Heating of the tissue is based on agitation of water molecules inducing cellular death via coagulation necrosis; electrical charge on the water molecule flips back and forth 2–5 billion times a second depending on the frequency of the microwave energy (Simon et al. 2005). Microwave ablation offers many of the benefits of others ablation techniques, in particular RF, and has several advantages, including higher intratumoral temperatures, larger tumor ablation volumes, faster ablation times, ability to use simultaneously multiple applicators (Wright et al. 2003), optimal heating of cystic masses and tumors close to the vessels, and less procedural pain (Simon et al. 2005; Shock et al. 2004). Due to this last advantage, microwave ablation can be proposed also as a treatment in outpatients.

The basic microwave ablation system contains many of the same components of a RF ablation system: a generator, a power distribution system, and an interstitial applicator (usually a needle). Treatment with microwave ablation is feasible and safe, with acceptable minor complications, in locally advanced PC and can be used as part of a palliative or multimodality treatment. Lygidakis et al. (2007) evaluated the safety, efficacy, feasibility, and complications of microwave ablation in unresectable locally advanced pancreatic carcinoma achieving partial necrosis in all cases without major procedure-related morbidity or mortality. In this study, location of tumor was predominantly in the head and/or uncinate portion of the pancreas with an average size of 6 cm. The authors did not have any major procedure-related morbidity or mortality. Minor complications were represented by mild pancreatitis, asymptomatic hyperamylasemia, pancreatic ascites, and minor bleeding. All patients had close follow-up and the longest surviving patient had a follow-up of 22 months (Lygidakis et al. 2007).

The most innovative and revolutionary technique is represented by HIFU ablation that is a noninvasive modality for the treatment of localized tumors. An ultrasound beam can be focused as it passes through soft tissues. During treatment, ultrasound waves are emitted from a transducer and focused to a small ellipsoid-shaped spot known as a sonication. HIFU transducers deliver ultrasound with intensities in the range of $100–10,000$ W/cm^2 to the focal region, with peak compression pressures of up to 30 MPa and peak rarefaction pressures up to 10 MPa. The major effect is heat generation due to absorption of the acoustic energy. The focused ultrasound energy delivered to the lesion during each sonication raise the tissue temperature to a degree that exceeds the thermal dose threshold required to obtain a coagulative necrosis. The heat raises the temperature rapidly to 60°C or higher in the tissue, causing coagulation necrosis within a few seconds. Focusing of the ultrasound beam results in high intensities at a specific location and over only a small volume (e.g., 1-mm diameter and 9-mm length). This focusing minimizes the potential for thermal damage to tissue located between the transducer and the focal point because the intensities are much lower outside the focal region. In addition to thermal effects, other mechanical

phenomena are caused by HIFU and include cavitation, microstreaming, and radiation forces, although HIFU-induced biologic effects are primarily caused by thermal and cavitation mechanisms.

The main advantages of HIFU are that it is noninvasive, conformal, and enables ablation of large-volume tumors. Guidance and monitoring of acoustic therapy is most important to ensure that the desired region is treated and to minimize damage to adjacent structures. The focused energy can be delivered under real-time ultrasonographic (US) imaging or under Magnetic Resonance (MR) guidance; both guidance techniques can obtain ablation of a three-dimensional target. Both methods have their advantages and disadvantages. MR has the advantage of providing temperature data within seconds after HIFU exposure. However, MRI guidance is expensive, labor-intensive, and of lower spatial resolution in some cases, although it is superior to sonography in obese patients. Sonographic guidance provides the benefit of imaging using the same form of energy that is being used for therapy. The significance of this is that the acoustic window can be verified with sonography (Fig. 1). Therefore, if the target cannot be well-visualized with sonography, it is unlikely that HIFU therapy will be effective in the target region, and it may potentially cause thermal injury to unintended tissue (Dubinsky et al. 2008). In the past decade, HIFU ablation has been used to treat disease in several organs. One of the most common applications is the

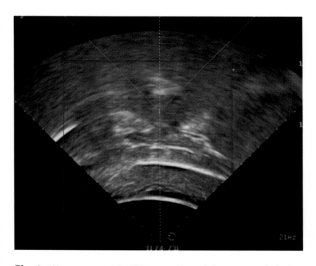

Fig. 1 Ultrasonographic (US) targeting of the pancreatic lesion during high-intensity focused ultrasound (HIFU) procedure. Consistent ecogenicity change was observed in the lesion after first cluster of sonications

management of patients with benign prostatic hyperplasia (Mulligan et al. 1997; Uchida et al. 1998) and localized prostate cancer (Beerlage et al. 1999; Gelet et al. 2000) by using transrectal US devices.

With most of the techniques described above (e.g., RFA, microwaves), the energy is applied percutaneously through needle applicators. The energy is, therefore, concentrated around the applicator, and there is heterogeneous distribution of heat throughout a target lesion. The result is that a maximum tumor diameter of 5 cm can be generally treated. HIFU is not restricted by these limitations. It does not require the insertion of an applicator into a target tissue, and an extracorporeal source can be used to treat large-volume tumors with imaging guidance.

Results from an open-label study in China in 251 patients with advanced PC (TNM stages II–IV) suggested that HIFU treatment can reduce the size of pancreatic tumors without causing pancreatitis and thus prolong survival (He and Wang 2002). An interesting finding was that 84% of patients with pain due to PC obtained significant pain relief after treatment with HIFU. Initial nonrandomized open-label human studies in China have provided additional evidence to suggest that HIFU treatment of pancreatic tumors indeed relieves PC-related pain and focally ablates malignant tissue (Wu et al. 2001; Yuan et al. 2003). Although HIFU is a noninvasive, nonsurgical treatment that has the potential to eliminate or significantly reduce pain associated with PC, no rigorously designed prospective randomized controlled trials have been conducted to determine whether treatment of pancreatic tumors with HIFU will result in local tumor response or in a clear clinical benefit by improving pain, functional status, quality of life, or survival.

At the European Institute of Oncology in Milan (Italy), a comprehensive cancer center, 11 patients with 11 pancreatic lesions underwent US-guided HIFU treatment within a feasibility study. Patients had histologically confirmed pancreatic adenocarcinoma in nine and neuroendocrine tumors in two cases. All were pretreated with chemotherapy, biological therapy, and/or radiotherapy, with no response. Patients were judged to be unsuitable for surgical resection and referred to HIFU. The procedure was performed by the JC HIFU system (Chongqing Haifu, Chongqing-China), under general anesthesia. All patients were evaluated clinically and by PET–CT, MRI, and CT (Fig. 2 and 3a). Nine patients presented a cephalo-pancreatic lesion, in

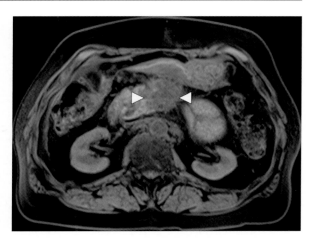

Fig. 2 Sixty-year-old patient with pancreatic cancer (PC). MRI after administration of contrast medium, performed before HIFU ablation, shows a 3.9 cm lesion in the body of the pancreas (*arrowheads*)

two cases tumor was located respectively to the isthmus and pancreatic tail. Mean age was 63.3 years (range 43–77 years). Tumors' average diameter was 5.2 cm (range 2.4–7.6 cm). CT and PET–CT showed a tissue volume control in 10/11 patients (Fig. 3b); one stable disease was observed. Eleven out of ten patients were rapidly palliated in symptoms with long-lasting pain control after a mean follow-up of 8 months. Five patients are still under treatment. One complication occurred after HIFU, with complete occlusion of the portal vein which was already involved by the tumor. All the patients but one returned home within 3 days after treatment. This study concluded that US-guided HIFU ablation is a safe and feasible treatment modality with a good efficacy in controlling pain in patients with solid pancreatic tumors (Orgera et al. 2010).

Inasmuch as the ablative techniques used in these studies were different, the results of these clinical experiences cannot be compared or added. To summarize, we can state that RF, Microwave, and HIFU may have role in ablation of pancreatic tumors in next future. RFA and high-intensity ultrasound ablation can ablate large volumes of tumor with high precision. Microwave is promising, but is still under development and testing on pancreatic tumors. Many specialist units are using RFA for the ablation of liver tumors, and the same set up can be used for ablation of pancreatic tumors as well. Eventually the choice of ablative therapy will be dictated by the local expertise, availability of equipment, and the cost involved.

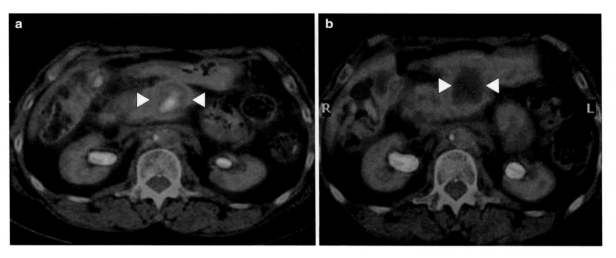

Fig. 3 (**a**) PET–CT images. Pretreatment PET–CT image showing positive uptake of the tumor (*arrowheads*). (**b**) Three months after treatment, PET–CT image showing complete disappearance of the positive uptake of the tumor (*arrowheads*)

3 Future Trends and Ongoing Research

In the future, the relative risks and benefits of local ablation techniques must be rigorously measured to better define their role in the treatment of locally advanced pancreatic tumors. The safety of each type of treatment will have to be assessed. In addition, the role of these cytoreductive measures in an adjuvant setting must also be explored. As a matter of fact, further studies on ablative therapy with or without chemotherapy and chemoradiation are warranted to study the impact of all available techniques on survival and quality of life in unresectable PC.

Once these issues are clarified, ablative techniques may, in the next future, have a role in:

1. Palliation of symptoms, in particular pain
2. Local tumor control in unresectable locally advanced disease
3. Treatment of small endocrine pancreatic tumors in patients who cannot undergo surgery

In addition, over the next several years, we expect substantial technological advances. Technology improvements will allow better image guidance for targeting the tumors to be ablated, more efficient detection of residual disease, easier therapy application by reducing device complexity, and the overall time required to ablate a given tumor.

References

Beerlage HP, Thueroff S, Debruyne FM, Chaussy C, de la Rosette JJ (1999) Transrectal high-intensity focused ultrasound using the Ablatherm device in the treatment of localised prostate carcinoma. Urology 54:273–277

Cardenes HR, Chiorean EG, Dewitt J, Schmidt M, Loehrer P (2006) Locally advanced pancreatic cancer: current therapeutic approach. Oncologist 11:612–623

Carrafiello G, Laganà D, Mangini M, Fontana F, Dionigi G, Boni L, Rovera F, Cuffari S, Fugazzola C (2008) Microwave tumors ablation: principles, clinical applications and review of preliminary experiences. Int J Surg 6(suppl 1):S65–S69

Date RS (2006) Current status of local ablative techniques in the treatment of pancreatic cancer. Pancreas 33:198–199

Date RS, Biggins J, Paterson I, Denton J, McMahon RF, Siriwardena AK (2005) Development and validation of an experimental model for the assessment of radiofrequency ablation of pancreatic parenchyma. Pancreas 30:266–271

Dubinsky TJ, Cuevas C, Dighe MK, Kolokythas O, Hwang JH (2008) High-intensity focused ultrasound: current potential and oncologic applications. AJR Am J Roentgenol 190: 191–199

Elias D, Baton O, Sideris L, Lasser P, Pocard M (2004) Necrotizing pancreatitis after radiofrequency destruction of pancreatic tumours. Eur J Surg Oncol 30:85–87

Friedman M, Mikityansky I, Kam A, Libutti SK, Walther MM, Neeman Z, Locklin JK, Wood BJ (2004) Radiofrequency ablation of cancer. Cardiovasc Intervent Radiol 27:427–434

Gelet A, Chapelon JY, Bouvier R, Rouvière O, Lasne Y, Lyonnet D, Dubernard JM (2000) Transrectal high-intensity focused ultrasound: minimally invasive therapy of localised prostate cancer. J Endourol 14:519–528

Ghaneh P, Kawesha A, Howes N, Jones L, Neoptolemos JP (1999) Adjuvant therapy for pancreatic cancer. World J Surg 23:937–945

Goldberg SN, Mallery S, Gazelle GS, Brugge WR (1999) EUS-guided radiofrequency ablation in the pancreas: results in a porcine model. Gastrointest Endosc 50:392–401

Habash RW, Bansal R, Krewski D, Alhafid HT (2007) Thermal therapy, Part III: ablation techniques. Crit Rev Biomed Eng 35:37–121

He SX, Wang GM (2002) The non invasive treatment of 251 cases of advanced pancreatic cancer with focused ultrasound surgery. In: Andrew MA, Crum LA, Vaezy S (eds) Proceedings from the 2nd international symposium on therapeutic ultrasound. University of Washington, Seattle, WA, pp 51–56

Jemal A, Thomas A, Murray T, Thun M (2002) Cancer statistics 2002. CA Cancer J Clin 52:23–47

Lygidakis NJ, Sharma SK, Papastratis P, Zivanovic V, Kefalourous H, Koshariya M, Lintzeris I, Porfiris T, Koutsiouroumba D (2007) Microwave ablation in locally advanced pancreatic carcinoma – a new look. Hepatogastroenterology 54:1305–1310

Matsui Y, Nakagawa A, Kamiyama Y, Yamamoto K, Kubo N, Nakase Y (2000) Selective thermocoagulation of unresectable pancreatic cancers by using radiofrequency capacitive heating. Pancreas 20:14–20

Mulligan ED, Lynch TH, Mulvin D, Greene D, Smith JM, Fitzpatrick JM (1997) High-intensity focused ultrasound in the treatment of benign prostatic hyperplasia. Br J Urol 79:177–180

Orgera G, Della Vigna P, Bonomo G, Monfardini L, Curigliano G, Orsi F; European Institute of Oncology, Milan, Italy (2010) High-Intensity Focused Ultrasound Treatment in patients with Advanced Pancreatic Cancer: assessment of local tumor response and clinical results. Original Scientific Research (Abstract No: 303). In: SIR 35th annual scientific meeting, 2010, Tampa, FL, USA

Shock SA, Meredith K, Warner TF, Sampson LA, Wright AS, Winter TC III, Mahvi DM, Fine JP, Lee FT Jr (2004) Microwave ablation with loop antenna: in vivo porcine liver model. Radiology 231:143–149

Simon CJ, Dupuy DE, Mayo-Smith WW (2005) Microwave ablation: principles and applications. Radiographics 25(suppl 1):S69–S83

Spiliotis JD, Datsis AC, Michalopoulos NV, Kekelos SP, Vaxevanidou A, Rogdakis AG, Christopoulou AN (2007) Radiofrequency ablation combined with palliative surgery may prolong survival of patients with advanced cancer of the pancreas. Langenbecks Arch Surg 392:55–60

Uchida T, Muramoto M, Kyunou H, Iwamura M, Egawa S, Koshiba K (1998) Clinical outcome of high-intensity focused ultrasound for treating benign prostatic hyperplasia: preliminary report. Urology 52:66–71

Varshney S, Sewkani A, Sharma S, Kapoor S, Naik S, Sharma A, Patel K (2006) Radiofrequency ablation of unresectable pancreatic carcinoma: feasibility, efficacy and safety. JOP 11:74–78

Wright SA, Lee FT, Mahvi DM (2003) Hepatic microwave ablation with multiple antennae results in synergistically larger zones of coagulation necrosis. Ann Surg Oncol 10:275–283

Wu F, Chen WZ, Bai J, Zou JZ, Wang ZL, Zhu H, Wang ZB (2001) Pathological changes in human malignant carcinoma treated with high-intensity focused ultrasound. Ultrasound Med Biol 27:1099–1106

Wu F, Wang ZB, Zhu H, Chen WZ, Zou JZ, Bai J, Li KQ, Jin CB, Xie FL, Su HB (2005) Feasibility of US-guided high-intensity focused ultrasound treatment in patients with advanced pancreatic cancer: initial experience. Radiology 236:1034–1040

Yuan C, Yang L, Yao C (2003) Observation of high intensity focused ultrasound treating 40 cases of pancreatic cancer (in Chinese). Chin J Clin Hepatol 19:145–146

Index

Printing and Binding: Stürtz GmbH, Würzburg